BOOKS BY JACK OLSEN

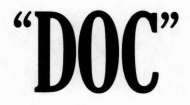

"DOC"

The Rape of the Town of Lovell

JACK OLSEN

New York **ATHENEUM** 1989

Atheneum
Macmillan Publishing Company
866 Third Avenue, New York, NY 10022
Collier Macmillan Canada, Inc.

Library of Congress Cataloging-in-Publication Data
Olsen, Jack.
"Doc" : the rape of the town of Lovell.
1. Rape—Wyoming—Lovell—Case studies. 2. Story,
John. 3. Physicians—Wyoming—Lovell—Case studies.
4. Women, Mormon—Wyoming—Lovell—Case studies.
5. Secrecy—Case studies. I. Title.
HV6568.L68047   1989   364.1'532'0978733   89-6545
ISBN 0-689-11959-3

Macmillan books are available at special discounts for bulk purchases
for sales promotions, premiums, fund-raising, or educational use.
For details contact:

Special Sales Director
Macmillan Publishing Company
866 Third Avenue
New York, NY 10022

10 9 8 7 6 5 4 3 2 1

Designed by Jack Meserole

PRINTED IN THE UNITED STATES OF AMERICA

For Su forever

Lovell, Cowley and Byron—we call it the devil's triangle. A few years ago a psychologist came here to practice. I met him and said, "Welcome to the twilight zone." He laughed and said that was a negative statement. Six months later he was gone.

—Cheryl Nebel

Sex is a topic so fraught with anxiety in the Mormon church that it is no surprise that countless distortions have arisen around it.

—Sonia Johnson,
From Housewife to Heretic

"There are very few acts of volition. I don't believe in individual guilt. . . . And yet I do believe that the intelligent person, the moral individual, must avoid evil and cruelty and dishonesties. I once wrote that the only crime is deliberate cruelty. I still believe that."

—Tennessee Williams,
quoted by Dotson Rader in
Tennessee: Cry of the Heart

Contents

"DOC"

Prologue

i.

DRIVING into town on State Highway 310, the motorist sees:

A railroad spur leading to a bulky brick building. A four-pack of thick white silos next to a towering smokestack. An aging maroon and gray boxcar, BRACH'S CANDY faintly lettered on its side. Mottled brown sugar beets in mounds higher than houses. An oblong little park, accented by rosebushes. Block after block of one-story frame homes in need of paint. Heavy-limbed honey locusts, cottonwoods, maples; weeping birches drooping to the ground; tall stiff firs. Street-corner flower boxes, most of them displaying weeds. Broad avenues with deep gutters. One traffic light. Signs:

THE ROSE CITY
POP 2447 ELEV 3814
Minnows-crawlers
Murphey Ford is still open!
Hunter's welcome

And a low-slung red-brick edifice set back from the street on a manicured lawn a block long: "Church of Jesus Christ of Latter-Day Saints." A deserted bank building, spiders spinning in cracked windows. The

Hyart Theater, "open two nights a week, one show only, shorts repeated after feature." Empty storefronts with old signs—Montgomery Ward, Kids Are Special Clothes, Busy Corner Pharmacy, Williams Family Restaurant, John's Auto Clinic, Ponderosa Floral. Abandoned gas stations and souvenir shops and cafés. A ruined carwash, windows out, the smashed clock on the facade stopped at 2:14.

And a brace of mallards in a taxidermist's window. A Rexall Drug with soda fountain. Three bars, two restaurants, an IGA market, a few small shops, a secondhand store, vacant lots littered with rubble, earth-moving equipment with rusted gears, disused balers and tractors.

And older model Darts, Blazers, Dusters, Broncos, some with flapping fenders. Pickups bearing dogs. Tired drivers in faded cowboy clothes. Teenagers lounging in front of Pizza on the Run. Patriarchs under a tree.

Lovell, Wyoming. Dry, dusty, demoralized, dying. Even on sunstruck days when heat blisters the asphalt, the town seems to lie in shadow. Most drivers pass on through.

ii.

LESS THAN A BLOCK from the thin gray-and-white steeple of the Mormon church, a Harvard alumnus named William Watts Horsley once practiced medicine on Park Avenue. The white frame sides of his two-story house seemed to blush from the glow of fifteen hundred rosebushes. For years he served as a director of the American Rose Society, and he was renowned for his studies of the life cycle of the rose midge. Garden companies sent him their latest specimens to critique. He was known as the Rose Doctor.

A public-spirited man, Dr. Horsley made it a practice to present a selection of rosebushes to every home buyer. New mothers received offerings in their babies' honor. The gifts often included the lovely pink-and-yellow Peace Rose, which Dr. Horsley and Jinx Falkenburg had officially named at a Rose Society ceremony in San Diego. As Lovell's volunteer parks director, he established public gardens that were dense with red, white, pink and yellow roses. He and his devoted sons planted bushes around the hospital, in front of stores, even in vacant lots. Because of Dr. Horsley, the community became known, first informally and then by edict of its leaders, as the Rose Town of Wyoming.

W.W. Horsley was a skilled surgeon, a balding near-genius with odd but formidable talents. He could shoot the eye out of a mudhen with a .22. With his slingshot of surgical tubing, he killed sage grouse at fifty yards. He was a mnemonics expert who could make twenty-five new friends at a convention and, a year or two later, recite the name and favorite rose of each.

He also had a dark side. In the final years of his practice, he was forced off the staff of the local hospital. The management leaked a cover story to the effect that he'd breached drug rules, but the truth was that he'd been caught flagrante delicto with another doctor's male patient.

Only a few insiders knew that the brilliant Horsley had indulged himself with boys and young men for years. After his resignation, he resumed his sexual practices in the privacy of his office. Thus the doctor who'd expected to be remembered for his love of roses left a different kind of legacy when he died in 1971. His home at 127 Park Avenue slipped into other hands and soon was barren of the bushes that he'd tended branch by branch and flower by flower.

Not everyone mourned. Some said that in his own way, the Rose Doctor was responsible for the disgrace that befell the town in the 1980s. But by then he'd been dead for years and didn't have to share the blame.

BOOK ONE

Love Among the Mormons

1

Arden McArthur

SHE LIKED to tell her friends that the first time she laid eyes on Dr. John Story he seemed like a pluperfect geek. That was back in 1958, shortly after he arrived in the small Wyoming town east of Yellowstone Park. At the time, Arden's regular physician was away, and the new man had set up his practice in a squat little building across the street from the town hall. Arden hated to leave her beet field—it was June, time for the first hoeing—but baby Minda was running a fever.

Right from the start (as she explained later) she was put off by the tight-lipped way this Dr. Story treated the three-month-old girl. Lovellites were used to folksy, friendly doctors, but the new man didn't have a shred of personality. He was just . . . blah. He reminded her of Mr. Peepers.

She warned herself to stop being judgmental. She disliked that particular fault and constantly fought against it. Like almost everyone else in this isolated outpost, she was deeply religious. She believed that judgment was for Father in Heaven, not for his children, even if the children were "LDS," members of the Church of Jesus Christ of Latter-day Saints and candidates for godhood themselves.

When she left the new doctor's office, she asked for the bill. The geek said he would send it.

7

Three years later a bill for $8 arrived. She paid it and wondered what kind of an operation he was running. Luckily it didn't matter. Good old Dr. Tom Croft, brother-in-law and former medical partner of the disgraced Dr. Horsley, continued to treat the McArthur clan as he had for years. He knew his medicine, and he didn't natter around as though he'd just got out of medical school.

When Dr. Tom announced that he was leaving Lovell for good, Arden rushed to his office. She knew too much about the Rose Doctor to consider switching to him, and she didn't want to return to the geek. "If you leave, then I can't have any more babies," she complained to Dr. Tom in her slight lisp. He'd delivered six of hers, but she wanted more. The Bible said, "Be fruitful, and multiply, and replenish the earth"— not that the McArthurs needed the advice. In addition to their own brood, there was always an orphan or two underfoot in their two-story farmhouse, or a neighbor child whose parents were having problems, or a derelict teener. The Mormon prophet Mosiah had instructed: "Ye yourselves will succor those that stand in need of your succor." Arden and Dean were known throughout the Lovell stake for succoring those in need, especially children. Once they'd found themselves caring for three sets of twins, none their own.

"I'm leaving for good, Ard," Tom Croft said in his soothing voice, "but you needn't worry. Dr. Story's here now."

Arden said, "But I need a *good* doctor."

"Well, let me tell you something," the old Mormon said (and years later she remembered it word for word). "Whenever I've gone out of town and turned a patient over to Dr. Story, she's never come back to me."

Dr. Tom seemed to mean it as a compliment.

When she became pregnant and returned to the little clinic off Main Street, she found Dr. Story unchanged. He still mumbled, still talked in circles, still seemed . . . different. Along with other patients, Arden sat in his waiting room for hours. She would say to herself, Five more minutes and I'm walking out. But she never did. She had a reputation for forcefulness, but underneath she was still a subservient little Mormon girl, raised in a time warp, untouched by the sexual revolution or the women's movement or any of the other main currents of American life. Lovell women knew their place and stayed in it. This Story person wasn't a very impressive specimen, with his dark-rimmed glasses and wispy build and conservatively combed black hair, but in an LDS community he enjoyed an exalted station. He was a doctor, and a male.

It took Arden several visits to change her mind about the new man. When she was asked later why she hadn't quit him at the beginning, she wasn't exactly sure. There'd never been more than two or three doctors in Lovell; it seemed they were always coming or going, and at least the geek from Nebraska seemed permanent.

At that stage of her life, in the early 1960s, long before things started to go bad, Arden Loraine Tanner McArthur was considered a success by nearly everyone in town, but not for reasons that mattered to her. She and her husband Dean, who was descended from an old Lovell family, owned 160 irrigated acres at the eastern edge of town and leased 600 more. Dean was the quiet master of his domain. On the rare occasions when he raised his voice, everyone jumped.

With help from his aging parents across the road, Dean and Arden reared a brood of singing children in a two-story brick house a quarter mile off the Globe Canal. In their yard and along the ditch, billowing cottonwood trees threw up shade against the desert sun and turned into big golden globes in the fall. The lady of the house, despite the finely articulated features and wide-set blue eyes of a fashion model, was renowned for her typically Mormon zest for work. In her four decades of life, she'd known little else. Mosiah had spoken on that subject, too: "And I did cause that the women should spin, and toil, and work . . ."

Arden enjoyed the feel of rich, moist earth and the view from the undersides of cows, but she tried not to look the part. Neither Mosiah nor any other prophet had ordered farm wives to walk with their shoulders slumped or let their backsides expand like prize pumpkins. ("Chunk City," a newswoman nicknamed Lovell when the trouble erupted years later.) Arden always kept a close watch on her posture and her diet, and made her children do the same.

As a depression child on a forty-acre truck farm west of Lovell, Arden Tanner had helped her family raise the potatoes, corn, peas, string beans and asparagus that brought in a few cents a pound. She milked, slaughtered chickens, slopped hogs, mucked out stalls and rode the sprung seat of the old family tractor to plow and cultivate. By such diligent effort, the Tanners of Big Horn County, descended from five Mormon brothers who emigrated from England, managed to eat well, pay full tithe and keep their bills current. From grammar school on, Arden held a paid job ("there was no other money") as the janitor's helper. She and her nine siblings owned one pair of shoes each and went barefooted when the ground wasn't frozen. When she was asked how the Tanners weathered the depression, she joked, "What depression?"

Like all Latter-day Saints, Dean and Arden McArthur regarded their time on earth as preparation for the Celestial Kingdom. Arden accepted the literal truth of every pronouncement by the high priests, every dictum in the Book of Mormon and other holy texts, every crackling revelation sent from the Heavenly Father to the current LDS prophet in Salt Lake City. If the church counseled against enlightening teenagers about sex, Arden complied. When the revealed truth held that blacks were ineligible for the priesthood, she believed, and when the latest prophet proclaimed that God now held otherwise, she accommodated to the change. A century earlier, she might have accepted polygamy, subsequently outlawed by church and state. She firmly believed in the priesthood—the power to act for God bestowed on males from the age of twelve—and often asked her husband or one of her older sons to anoint her head with holy oil from the refrigerator. And she believed in what the prophets called "the burning in the bosom." Such rushes of feeling transcended reason and were understood to come straight from the Lord.

Early in her marriage, Arden had seen to it that she and Dean had been sealed "for time and all eternity" in a ceremony inside the cavernous temple in Salt Lake City, a ritual that made them eligible for the Celestial Kingdom. Sometimes she traveled 350 miles to the regional temple in Idaho Falls to perform the ordinance known as "baptism for the dead," retroactively saving not only every relative she could unearth from the family genealogies but a long list of other lost souls—LDS, Christian, Jew and atheist alike. It was one of her church's deepest obligations.

She held a "Temple Recommend," which required total obedience to church discipline, the most worthy thoughts and deeds, and the purest of ideals and practices, including "compassionate services" for others, needy or not, Mormons or not. From time to time she held office in the Relief Society, the women's auxiliary. Members fed the hungry and comforted the sick and bereaved, according to the words of the prophet Moroni: "And except ye have charity ye can in nowise be saved in the kingdom of God."

The Relief Society met every Sunday under another Moroni rubric: "Charity Never Faileth." Arden visited with suffering parishioners and sometimes counseled them for hours. Through the years she baked bread and cinnamon rolls and gave most of it away. When the first aromatic wisps curled up from her big oven, Dean would yell, "Who's it going to *this* time?" Arden's generosity was a family joke.

Eventually a few of her hot cinnamon rolls began showing up at the home of the new doctor and his family. Arden would drive the sweet-smelling tray up the easy slope of Nevada Street and wait in the family Buick while her daughter Meg or Marie or Michele ran it inside. Mrs. Story always gave a friendly wave.

By the mid-sixties, after the new doctor had been in town five or six years, Arden realized that she'd been doubly unfair—first by judging him and then by misjudging him. The Storys turned out to be active Baptists, nondrinkers, nonsmokers, as straitlaced as the most pious Saint. Arden told her friends, "Why, they even live like LDS!" One of her talents was barbering, and she began cutting the hair of the two Story children, Susan and Linda. She wouldn't take payment, but sometimes a nice gift turned up on her doorstep.

As a general practitioner, Dr. Story seemed the equal of Dr. Croft. His workups were precise; his pelvic examinations sometimes lasted a half hour or forty-five minutes, and he would take fifteen minutes to do a Pap smear. Arden was having female problems at the time and often found herself in the stirrups. Like many women, she hated the procedure, so "I willed my mind to be somewhere else, and I never felt discomfort or pain. Of course, I wasn't crazy about his surprises. You'd go in for a sore throat and he'd look at your chart and say, 'You haven't had a pelvic for a long time,' and then you'd be flat on your back."

Somehow the busiest doctor in Big Horn County always had time for the McArthurs. It seemed as though every time one of the kids had an accident, it was on Dr. Story's day off, but when they reached the emergency room he'd be waiting. "Arden," he said one day, blinking his owlish brown eyes, "I've told my office, 'If the McArthurs call in, beep me right away.' " He made house calls without complaint.

It hadn't occurred to Arden to wonder how her family rated such special treatment, so she was surprised when a friend asked: "What is it about your family and Dr. Story? He's got you way up on a pedestal."

Arden winced. "He'd better not," she said.

"He said that if all the Mormons were like you and Dean and your family, he'd be LDS himself. But the others are all hypocritical."

Arden bridled at any criticism of her church, and heights made her dizzy. She marched into the clinic. "You get me off that pedestal!" she told Dr. Story. "We McArthurs are just human beings. I don't want to be put in a position where I fall so hard that I can't be picked back up. And I don't want my family in that position, either."

"Oh, Arden," he said consolingly, and passed a few shy compliments about her style and looks. Sometimes he seemed like a sawed-off Cary Grant. To Arden, it was almost as though he realized he had to develop a warmer bedside manner. She wasn't sure what to make of all the compliments. She knew she had reasonably good looks, but didn't care. She dressed up for personal pride, not to attract males. And anyway, what difference did looks make to a doctor?

For another year or so she saw him off and on at his office, and now and then bumped into him on Main Street. Once she invited him to a political luncheon at her home. "How would that look?" he said. "We have to remember the doctor-patient relationship." She found it an odd comment; she hadn't been inviting him to a motel. He showed up at her meeting but left early.

The Storys seemed to limit their social lives to fellow Baptist church members—not that it mattered to Arden. Her time was spoken for and then some. Nevertheless, she began to realize that somehow, against all odds and probabilities, she and John Story had become good friends.

She remained aware of the proprieties and continued to address him as Dr. Story. He bristled when anyone called him Doc or John—"Don't first-name me," she heard him tell a patient. He seemed to relax a little when he saw her. He would slide his chair over to his power-driven examining table and tell her how nice she looked. When the nurse tapped on the door to remind him that he was running late, he said, "Yes, yes," and kept right on talking.

Her visits sometimes stretched to an hour. "Don't leave," he would say when he'd finished treating her. "I'll be right back." He would disappear into another examining room and return a while later, blinking behind those somnolent brown eyes that seemed overwhelmed by his glasses.

He showed a wide range of knowledge, but his favorite themes seemed to be bureaucratic incompetence, the wastefulness of the Social Security program and health insurance and public welfare, and the dangers of centralized control, not only in government but in religion and business. He'd quit the American Medical Association because it was too liberal. He spoke highly of Phyllis Schlafly, Barry Goldwater, the late Senator Joseph R. McCarthy and various other right-wing icons, and seemed to despise Lyndon Johnson, every Kennedy including those unborn, and "Commie sympathizers" like Hubert Humphrey, Wayne Morse and Eugene McCarthy. None of these attitudes struck Arden as particularly outlandish. Big Horn County was so conservative that its handful of dedicated liberals routinely registered Republican to keep from wasting their vote.

One midsummer afternoon when the sweet white steam from the sugar factory curled over town, Arden donned a favorite lemon-yellow frock and strolled the quarter mile to the downtown shopping strip along Main Street. She had a thin waist, a substantial bust and a shapely backside, and once in a while she liked to change out of her stiff old overalls and look like someone who didn't spend all day in the company of cows. She knew how to apply makeup. She liked to rub on a touch of blusher, pile her ginger hair high atop her head, and slip into four-inch heels that made her look even taller than her five feet seven. As she walked along the highway, shoulders back, head high, she knew that she attracted disapproving stares from local women who believed that dressing up was for church. There were even a few Lovell women (nonacquaintances, to be sure) who considered her conceited or cocky. Arden wasn't bothered; she knew what she was. Her wardrobe was sparse, but she'd learned how to mix and match, and she kept her best outfits in such pristine condition that her daughter Minda continually complained, "Oh, Mom, do I have to go to that dang dry cleaners *again*?"

After running a few errands on this sweltering day, Arden dropped into the Rose Bowl drive-in. Another well-dressed woman was sitting there, and Arden recognized Marilyn Story. It was a surprise. For the most part, the doctor's wife kept to herself. She was a petite, pretty woman with thick dark hair and a slightly hawkish nose that was said to come from an Indian ancestor. To the lanky Arden, Mrs. Story seemed a perfect match for her small husband. Together, they looked as though they'd just walked off the top of a wedding cake.

The two women pulled up chairs at the same table, and the subject turned to religion, as it so often did in this small town where the three main topics of conversation were God, the price of oil at the well-head, and the status of the beet crop. After a while, Mrs. Story said pleasantly, "You know, Arden, you and I don't believe in the same God."

Arden was accustomed to such comments from Gentiles, but she was so certain of her own theology that she never felt defensive or belligerent. The various religions had coexisted happily in Lovell ever since a new Lutheran pastor had preached against the Saints and watched as half his congregation walked out. "Those are our friends you're talking about," he'd been told. "We know the LDS and they're not like that."

Now Arden responded, "But Mrs. Story, there's only one God."

The doctor's wife said she would be teaching a Bible class that night at the Baptist church. "Why don't you come," she said, "and I'll show you the difference."

After forty years in the Mormon church, Arden felt no need for a Baptist Bible lesson, but she didn't mind listening while she finished her lemonade. Marilyn described an omnipotent God so big that he covered the universe and so small he could be in your heart. Then she added, "But of course you Mormons don't believe in Jesus Christ."

"Why, of course we do," Arden said patiently. Why else, she asked, would we call ourselves the Church of Jesus Christ of Latter-day Saints? Jesus was a prophet and so was the current president of the Mormon church in Salt Lake City. The main difference was that the president was alive and capable of receiving and revealing divine truth; Jesus was dead and his words were preserved in the Bible.

Arden issued a polite invitation of her own. "Marilyn, you can come to our church anytime, Sunday school, sacrament meetings, I don't care, and you'll hear about the life of Christ."

"Well, you don't understand what I mean."

"Perhaps I don't." She decided to try simple logic. "Do you believe Christ was born and grew up and he was crucified and hung on the cross?"

"Yes."

Arden held up her palms in a gesture that said Marilyn had just proved her point. "Well, if you believe that God and Christ are the same individual, why would he put his self into the womb of a woman and come forth as a child and grow up in normality as a mortal being on this earth? He wouldn't have to do that, Marilyn, not if he's God. It wouldn't make sense to go to all that trouble."

They batted the subject back and forth till it was time to go home and irrigate. As Arden left, she handed the doctor's wife her personal copy of the book *Jesus the Christ*, which was the LDS priesthood manual at the time. "Read this," she said, "and you'll see that we do believe in Christ."

Marilyn thanked her and said she would.

The next time Arden ran into the doctor's wife, neither woman mentioned the textbook or the evening Bible classes. Arden didn't push. Mormons were energetic proselytizers, and she liked to remind her children, "We're a missionary church." But something told her that Marilyn Story's religious beliefs were no more susceptible to change than her own.

Sometimes the two women chatted at the office while Arden waited to see the doctor. She learned that Marilyn had been brought up on a cattle ranch and revered her cowboy father. "My dad was a wonderful Christian," she said. "He taught Scripture."

To Arden, that explained a lot. She herself had a good knowledge of Scripture, but both the Storys could out-Bible her every time. "That Dr. Story!" she told Dean one night. "He just loves to banter Scripture." Non-Mormons had an unfair advantage; they only had to learn the Bible, not the four "sticks" studied by every devout Saint. Why, the Book of Mormon ran almost 800 pages, and there were two other sacred books, *Doctrine and Covenants*, and *The Pearl of Great Price*, plus the Bible itself. That was a lot to remember.

Gradually Arden came to admire the doctor's wife. Beneath her cool exterior, she showed a survivor's sense of humor. "And she's never ignorant toward others," Arden told Dean. (In the Big Horn Basin, "ignorant" meant "rude.") But Marilyn seemed to have a low opinion of herself, and Arden couldn't imagine why. "I was such an airhead," Marilyn described herself as a young woman. She didn't seem to think she was living up to her role as the town doctor's wife. Arden wondered if the self-deprecation had something to do with her life at home, some deficiency in love or warmth. Marilyn admitted that she'd never been tactile. "I love to have affection shown me," she said in a moment of candor, "but I'm not the one that's gonna go up and hug my little girls and stuff like that. I almost have to make myself do that. Doctor is different. He shows affection. He's a very touching person."

Apparently Marilyn wanted a larger family, but there was a problem. "There's more women come into this office with tipped uteruses," she complained one day. "He's more concerned with them than he is with me. My uterus is tipped so bad that my chances of getting pregnant are nil."

A few months later, Arden heard that the doctor's wife was pregnant. She telephoned her congratulations. "Oh, wouldn't it be nice," she said, "if you had a boy."

Marilyn said in a curiously flat voice: "We don't want a boy."

"Well, my lands!" Arden said. "Why not?"

Marilyn explained that she was five three and a half and her husband was only a few inches taller and "he doesn't want to bring another short boy into the world."

In later years, Arden hated to think about the little girl's tragic life. Annette Story was born in 1967, curiously hairless except for a faint blond fuzz. Arden thought she was the saddest child she'd ever seen. The other two daughters favored the Story side, but this child had a long unsmiling face and big sad eyes. Marilyn said the baby favored her own family, the Taussigs of Colorado.

At twenty months of age, Annette was playing in her front yard when Marilyn stepped inside her house just long enough for the child to toddle into the blind spot of a woman who was backing her car down a neighbor's driveway.

For a while, Arden and her friends hadn't been sure that Marilyn would survive. She was too distraught to go out and have her lovely black hair done for the funeral. Arden went to the house and did it for her.

Everyone knew that the old Baptist church would be too small to hold all the townspeople who wanted to offer their sympathies to the bereft doctor and his wife. Arden and some of the high priests saw to it that the Saints offered their much larger building, but Dr. Story chose the Lutheran church. The overflow crowd spilled under the maples and cottonwoods. Arden had never seen such a public display of sympathy in Lovell.

Dr. Story seemed to snap back, but Marilyn remained in deep mourning. "Listen here," Arden told him on an unannounced visit, "you've got to do something about your wife. She needs to get out and see people."

Story seemed surprised that anyone had noticed a problem. "She's working in the back of the office," he said. "She does the billing."

"Yes, in that dang back," Arden said angrily. "Get her out in front where she won't be stuck all by herself."

The next time she came in, she saw that Marilyn's desk had been moved from behind a closed door. But the poor woman still looked as though she'd cried all night.

A few months after the tragedy, Arden learned that Story had resigned his position as Sunday School teacher and led a rebellion in the Baptist church. The word was that the local Baptists had become too liberal for him, trying to interpret Scripture instead of following it. The splinter group was meeting at the Oddfellows Hall and already raising a building fund.

The Lovell Bible Church opened a year later, up among the small frame houses on West Eighth. It was a plain wooden building with a simple wooden cross on the front, no stained glass or other ornamentation, a church as simple as its founding principle that the Bible held all truth.

Arden and her pretty daughter Meg attended the dedication and open house. They hadn't taken two steps inside the foyer, walking across a rug that Dean McArthur had helped install on his part-time job, when Arden stopped short. She thought, They're building an edifice to our Father in Heaven and these geeks are smoking. Why, it smells like a pool hall!

Dr. Story took her by the elbow. She jerked away and said, "I can't believe that you would allow tobacco to be smoked in your church."

He promised to order a ban. He took her aside and said, "If you have any questions about our church, ask me." His face was never easy to read—he spoke in the same soft monotone no matter what he was discussing, and he seldom showed emotion—but on this day he radiated deep pride and satisfaction.

It wasn't long before Arden heard that the local Baptist church was going broke; Dr. Story's rebellion had cut heavily into the membership and the diminished congregation couldn't pay its bills. He argued that it was their own fault. "They were taking too much direction from out of town," he explained on her next office visit. "A new preacher was coming in and he told everybody, 'We'll start using the northern Baptist literature.' That means humanizing the Scriptures, teaching that the Bible isn't the word of God. How could a Christian accept that?"

Arden realized it was his old bugaboo again. How he hated to be controlled! It wasn't necessarily a bad trait, but he seemed to carry it to extremes.

He changed the subject to the Mormon church. She knew that he had strong opinions about the Saints, even though he expressed them without rancor.

She teased him by quoting a hallowed precept: "As man is, God once was, and as God is, man may become."

"That's just plain impossible," he exclaimed. "What makes you Mormons think you can put yourselves on the same plane as God? Why, that's audacious."

Arden said, "Can you put yourself on the same plane as your father?"

"No."

"Why not?"

"Because he's older. He's had other experiences."

"Okay, what's the difference? You could still grow. While you're growing, your father's growing, and it's a continual circle."

He looked put off, so she took another tack. "I want to ask you about your dedicatory prayer the other day. You always say that we Mormons use Canaanite language in our prayers, thee and thou and thine, but when you gave the prayer you talked to the Lord just like I was sitting here talking to you. And you say we put ourselves on the same plane as God?"

He tried to respond, but she plowed ahead. "You're bringing him down to your language. We speak to him as a deity, with thee and thine, because that's the way he talked when he was on earth. But you—you don't go to his level. You bring him down to yours."

Dr. Story seemed bored with the subject. He said, "What other questions do you have?"

She felt a little impish. "Well," she said, "I heard them call you Elder Story. Why do you settle for being an elder in your church when you could be a high priest in ours?"

He smiled. They both knew she was being facetious.

They talked off and on for two hours. He didn't yield and neither did she. At the end, she told him half-jokingly that he was "stiff-necked and impudent."

He seemed bemused and said, "That's Ezekiel, isn't it?"

Trying to build up its membership, Dr. Story's new church brought in a traveling speaker, an excommunicated Saint who was making a career out of "exposing" Mormons. Arden's church had never lacked apostates. They wrote books against LDS, published newsletters, sold cassettes, bought time on the radio. Mormon-bashing was big business, even in the shadow of the Salt Lake City Temple. "Mom," her daughter Minda once asked. "how come so many people write against us? We don't write against anybody."

"I don't know what they're so het up about, honey," she'd answered. "We work hard and mind our own business. I guess that bothers some folks."

Lovell history had been written in the Saints' sweat and blood. Mormonism thrived in barren regions; it was a religion of abstinence and cooperation, simple joys, pleasures deferred till the worthy stood together in flowing white robes. There was a time, early in the century, when the whole Big Horn Basin, towns like Cowley, Deaver, Frannie, Powell, Lovell and Arden's childhood village of Byron, were peopled almost entirely by Mormon colonizers dispatched by the high priests of the St. George temple in Utah. They'd broken through the alkali crust with pickaxes and laid track for the railroad and dug canals to irrigate badlands where only cactus and greasewood had grown. Making something out of nothing had always been a Mormon specialty.

The handful of non-Mormon settlers, including cattleman Henry Clay Lovell, had watched the colonization and concluded that the Saints could make water run uphill. LDS planners, following principles laid down by Brigham Young, partitioned the bottomland into one-acre plots with a house at each corner and communal property in the middle. The first streets were wider than most big-city thoroughfares, including New York City's Broadway. (Arden held the accepted belief that President Young had insisted on wide streets because he looked into the future and saw cars and trucks, while others claimed that he simply measured out the width required to turn a horse and wagon.) Trees and shrubs had sprung to life as platoons of colonists brought cuttings up from St. George.

Arden knew well that without those early Saints, Lovell might still be a flyblown way station where steers paused to drink at the Shoshone River and trudged on to the railhead at Billings, seventy miles north. She wondered if Dr. John Story and the Reverend Terwilliger and the other elders of the Lovell Bible Church had known any of this history as they sat for three days listening to the visiting speaker's anti-Mormon poison.

When she put in a complaint during her next visit to the clinic, the doctor apologized and told her that the lecture series was the result of a misunderstanding. He swore he'd had no idea that the visitor would attack the Mormons and promised it would never happen again.

Arden was a long way from mollified. "If you're really interested in our church," she said, "why don't you bring in someone who knows about it, not some poor fool who's been excommunicated? He doesn't know anything or he wouldn't've been excommunicated in the first place! If you want to know about LDS, I'll be glad to get you some instruction."

Dr. Story didn't take the bait, but she made a mental note to try again. What a coup it would be to convert a man who didn't drink or smoke, who firmly believed in God, who was loving and gentle and concerned about mankind and bored with money and possessions, and on top of that was the town doctor! He seemed to follow LDS principles in everything he did. He'd even gone to Latin America with a Christian doctors' group and treated the natives. What was that but "compassionate service"?

One day he complained that he'd been trying to find a copy of the *Doctrine and Covenants*, a compilation of 150 years of messages from God to the LDS prophets. He said, "I know I'll never see it because it's secret."

"Sacred," Arden corrected him. "Not secret." It was a distinction that the Saints often had to make to their unbelieving friends.

Dr. Story said that as far as he could see, the two words were synonymous in LDS doctrine. "That's why I've never been able to get ahold of that book. I can get the Book of Mormon and *The Pearl of Great Price*, but that's all."

By now she was onto his eccentricities. If he couldn't put his hands on a book owned by every Saint in town, it showed a lack of control.

And control, she suspected, was important to undersized men like him. "You listen to me," he'd told Arden's mother. "I'll make the diagnosis, not you." Everyone agreed that his favorite expression was, "I'm the doctor here."

She brought him a well-thumbed *Doctrine and Covenants*, and he seemed surprised and pleased. "Here's the secret document you ordered," she couldn't resist saying. "I bought it in a bookstore. I didn't even have to give a password."

After he'd had a few months to peruse the book, she asked, "Why don't you let me send a missionary out to see you?"

"Not unless they'll come after midnight," he said. "That's when I do all my studying."

"Well," she said, "I'm sure they could work that out."

He said he didn't want his wife and daughters involved. She took that to be another example of his need for control—he didn't want his family doing any independent thinking. Certainly his docile wife seemed to take most of her ideas from him, at least as far as Arden could see. When Marilyn spoke, you could hear his voice behind her words. Arden couldn't imagine him married to any other kind of woman.

She talked to the stake missionaries about the hot prospect and they made several nocturnal visits to the Story home. But they finally realized that the doctor had never been a sincere prospect; what he'd really wanted to do was convert them. The earnest young men in the neat dark suits and gleaming white shirts decided they had better uses for their time.

A year or so later, in the early 1970s, Arden got a phone call from her LDS friend Dottie Parry, a nervous woman who liked to gossip. Lovell's main street extended one mile, from the white colonnades of the sugar factory past the line of small homes and shops and out to the green McArthur fields, and sometimes the latest news seemed to travel that mile faster than sound or light—Lovell's own version of jungle drums.

Sister Parry rambled on disjointedly, and Arden only half-listened till she caught Dr. Story's name: ". . . And he told me there was nothing wrong with me, it was all in my mind, and then he gave me a pelvic examination and did something that I—well, I'd rather not say. Ard, some strange things go on in that office."

Arden cut her off. "People can say anything they want about anybody," she said. "Dr. Story's been good to us. When we need him, he's there."

"But—"

"I'm sorry, Dottie," Arden said. "I don't want to discuss it." She seldom altered a position once she'd made up her mind. There were *facts* and *nonfacts*, and Dottie was talking nonfacts.

Besides, Arden had been uncomfortable with sexual palaver ever since a traumatic childhood experience. She'd stayed overnight with close family friends. Before bedtime, the "aunt" warned, "Now Arden, if you get frightened you can come into bed with me and 'uncle.' *But be sure to crawl in on my side.*" Six-year-old Arden crawled in on the wrong side and "uncle" spent half the night trying to penetrate her. She was afraid to cry out. She never told a soul till she married Dean because, as she explained, "Nobody tells things like that." Her husband said she'd been right to keep quiet.

It wasn't long after the unpleasant conversation with Sister Parry that another bolt of gossip flashed from one end of Main Street to the other. It was all about Dr. Story, and all insubstantial. Arden's daughters reported that the girls at Lovell High School were calling him Stud Story for his behavior during their Girls Athletic Association physicals. They said he made them undress, stared at their bodies, uttered ignorant comments about their "buds" and pubic hair, and administered intimate examinations that weren't even required.

Sure, Arden said to herself after she'd heard the bill of particulars, and I'll bet he rapes and beats them and puts out cigarettes on their skin. *Kids!* She advised Meg and Michele that whispering campaigns were the devil's work. It was right there in the Book of Mormon, Helaman, 16:22. "Satan spreads rumors and contentions."

Just the same, she stayed in the examining room the next time she took her oldest daughter Marie in for a pelvic exam. He'd barely begun when Marie screamed and said, "It hurts!"

He flushed. "Oh, for heaven's sakes," he said angrily. "What's the matter with you? All girls your age masturbate!"

Marie sat up so forcefully that her long leg slammed into his shoulder and buckled his knees. "I beg your pardon, Dr. Story!" she said. "This is one girl who has *never* masturbated."

He composed himself and said, "Well, Marie, you're going away to school. You'll be dating. If you want a good marriage, you'll come back. I'll put you under and dilate you so that you won't have any problems with your husband."

Arden thought, How concerned he is. He's always been that way about our family.

As they were climbing into the car, Marie said, "I can't believe a doctor would say that to anybody, even if it were true."

"Sis," Arden said, "he's a doctor. He knows more than we do. He's seen things we don't know anything about."

"What if he has, Mom? Why does he have to tell me what the other girls do? I'm not interested. *I don't care!*" The child complained all the way home.

The following Monday, Arden had an appointment for an arthritis treatment. "My daughter's very upset with you," she said when Dr. Story entered the examining room.

"Why?" he asked as furrows broke across his high forehead.

"Because of what happened when you gave Marie the pelvic."

"What happened?"

"You don't remember?"

"No, Arden. I'm sorry. I don't remember. I see a lot of patients, you know."

She was astounded. "You don't remember telling Marie that all high school girls masturbate?"

He swore that he didn't. She recited every detail. "Nope," he responded cheerfully. "Not me, Arden. Why, that doesn't even sound like me."

"But you did. I heard it!"

When he made a clumsy switch to another subject, she decided that he must be upset about something. She wasn't offended. The poor man juggled a long list of jobs—G.P., emergency room physician, obstetrician, public health officer, gynecologist, school doctor, church elder, lay preacher, father, husband. Sometimes he rode shotgun on the hearse that doubled as the town ambulance. Lately he'd set aside one of his examining rooms for counseling, leaning heavily on his knowledge of the Bible.

Arden didn't know what had caused the outburst at Marie or the lapse of memory, but there had to be a logical reason. Maybe he'd lost a patient. Or maybe there was trouble at home. She wondered what would have happened if she hadn't been in the examining room with her daughter. Probably nothing, she thought. Maybe I'm the problem. Maybe I've begun to irritate him.

2

Meg McArthur Anderson

A YEAR LATER, the McArthur family's second oldest daughter, Meg, went to the clinic for her own precollege physical. She didn't look forward to the exam, but she wasn't nervous. Her mother revered Dr. Story, and Meg's own experiences on the examining table hadn't been all that traumatic. He'd given her three GAA physicals, each time kneading her breasts and putting his hands in her underpants. "I was just a kid and he was my doctor," she said later in her mellifluous voice. "Who knew what a sports physical consisted of?"

For this fourth physical, Meg stripped at the nurse's request and climbed on the cold table. Dr. Story told her how healthy she looked and instructed her to put her feet in the stirrups. The taut sheet across her upraised knees screened off the lower half of her body; all she could see was his head and shoulders as he moved closer. A painful jolt snapped her eyes open. "Ow!" she yelped. "That hurts!"

He stepped backward and said with an edge to his voice, "I can't finish this exam. You're just gonna have to keep coming back till I can."

She refused to return to such pain. She wondered what had gone wrong. As an eighteen-year-old virgin, could she have . . . a female problem? She was afraid to ask her mother; they were close, but intimate matters weren't discussed at home. Nothing she'd learned at school or church shed any light. She wondered if she had a growth down there—cancer or something. But wouldn't he have told her? She thought, Oh, lands, I'm scared. Then she took a look at the form for the precollege physical and discovered that no pelvic examination was required.

As of that summer of 1973, Meg gave every appearance of being another McArthur success story. She had slender arms and finely sculpted hands which she used to make graceful gestures that enhanced her speech. She had the same disarming lisp as her mother, a minor defect that made her other qualities more affecting. She wore her whitish-blond hair shoulder length, parted in the middle, sometimes braided or checked by barrettes or bows. Her fair skin burned but didn't tan. She had a strong straight nose and the deep blue-green eyes that ran in the family. She wore a size nine dress, with tucks and adjustments for her small waist, flaring hips and prominent breasts.

"Meg stood in the right line," complained her younger sister Minda, who felt that she hadn't. Their mother liked to joke that she herself had been large in the bust herself, "but I gave it to you girls an inch at a time."

Meg's GPA always hovered near 4.0; she was senior class president and National Honor Society member and a church teacher and leader. As a star drummer, she joined her trumpeting sister Minda in giving the high school band its tempo and drive.

Like most Mormon women, Meg lived in the shadow of males: the bishop, the stake president and other high priests, the current prophet and his twelve counselors in the Salt Lake temple. In a way, she was also subservient to her father and brothers, holders of a priesthood permanently denied to women, no matter how great their spirituality or accomplishments.

Dean McArthur opened his family's day at 4 A.M.; lying abed till daylight was considered "sleeping in." There were five phones in the two-story farmhouse and their father dialed a ringback number that made them go off together. The children would hear ten awful *brrrring-brrrring*s. The noise would stop, then start again. Even in the daytime, Meg jumped when she heard a phone.

By the time she dressed, her mother had breakfast on the table, robust farm food and plenty of it, and then the McArthur clan trooped to the barn, led by their father singing his favorite Mormon hymn in a voice that woke up the cows:

Let no one shirk.
Put your shoulder to the wheel.
Push along, do your duty
With a heart full of song.
We all have work.
Let no one shirk.
Put your shoulder to the wheel.

All her life, Meg loved to sing and talk about it. "To a Mormon, singing is a sign of courage and joy. We teach our kids—if you're afraid, think of a great hymn. 'Come, Come Ye Saints.' 'I Am a Child of God.' There's nothing scarier than walking into a cold dark barn, so we'd walk in singing. Then we'd sing and milk together—me, Marie, my big brother Max, Dad, and *his* dad—we called him Papa—and a hired hand or two. We milked a hundred cows and then did it all over again at four in the afternoon. No vacations, no days off.

"After the first milking, we'd all pitch in and do the beets, singing away. I'd help shovel the green tops onto the truck and my dad would run 'em out to the animals for fodder. Some mornings it was so cold you could see every note in your breath."

An uncle and aunt went on a two-year mission to New Zealand, and every morning and evening Meg and her year-older sister, Marie, saddled their uncle's two crazy horses—"they were green-broke but they didn't know it"—and rode to the relatives' farm to milk their cows. There was no mention of pay. Meg was happy to help bring the truth to a far-off land.

From the time she was twelve, her favorite childhood experience had been the visit to the temple in Idaho Falls to be baptized for the dead. For weeks the children would pore through family histories and genealogies and write out lists of candidates. Usually Meg would be baptized for ten or fifteen people at a time, but once she'd gone in with a thousand names. It was exciting to think about saving so many souls and meeting them later in the Celestial Kingdom.

Except for her experiences with Bob Asay, Meg reckoned that her childhood would have been close to perfect. He was "Uncle Bob" to the McArthur children, although he was really their father's distant cousin. Asay (pronounced "Acey") was a common name in Lovell. The first Asays had come to the Big Horn Basin in a wagon train in the spring of 1900, and by the 1970s there were twenty in the thin Lovell phone book and more in the back country. Dean McArthur sometimes laid rugs for his cousin's business, Bob Asay Carpet and Furniture, and was paid in sorely needed cash. Asay, a bachelor who lived in an apartment in his store, had been welcome in the McArthur farmhouse for as long as Meg could remember. He brought candy and ice cream, let the children sit on his lap and steer his car, took them on church excursions, regaled them in a lovely voice with songs that he composed himself, and stripped them of their innocence.

They had no means of defense. Like most LDS children, they'd been kept in the dark about sex. Meg had never seen her parents naked. Her earliest sexual memory was of a hot summer day when she'd taken her shirt off and her mother had yelled, "Put a shirt on! You're a girl." The two-year-old child had burst into tears.

None of the McArthur children ever gave sex much thought. Meg witnessed barnyard couplings but didn't relate them to human activity— and certainly not to her parents or herself. At school she learned how amoebas and frogs and worms reproduced, but nothing about the sexual practices of humans. At the end of her junior year, she went to her bishop, lowest-ranking officer in the Mormon hierarchy, to renew her Temple Recommend.

"Do you masturbate?" he asked.

She said no. Later she asked another girl what masturbation was. "Oh, my word," Meg exclaimed. "Who would do *that*?"

At nine or ten, she'd become the first of the McArthurs to be bothered by "Uncle Bob." She couldn't imagine why a devout LDS businessman in his late thirties would want her to stroke his thing or why it grew so large in her hand, but Uncle Bob was always nice about it.* A year or two passed before she began to feel that she was doing something wrong.

She thought of complaining to her mother, but the subject was still taboo. Something told her to keep her secret from her friends at church and school. Instead, she smiled, kept up her good works, and held her shame inside.

She didn't know how to turn Uncle Bob away. He was pleasant about his persistence, teasing and cajoling but never brutal. If he wasn't

---

*Robert Asay has denied all allegations of child abuse or molestation. He has never been charged with a criminal offense.

pestering her, he was pestering her siblings, sometimes in front of one another. By the time the children united against him, Meg had developed a pronounced aversion to sex and a morbid fear of rape. For most of her years in high school, she refused to go out alone at night. She wasn't positive what a rapist did, but she knew it would be torture.

Confused about sex, she didn't read any sinister significance into her painful GAA physical. Dr. Story was as unassailable in his lofty position as the Lovell stake president. Nor did she make any retroactive connections in college when she visited a Utah doctor for a pelvic examination. Meg asked him, "Are there different instruments that you use? My doctor back home said that I was so small that he could never give me an exam."

The gynecologist shook his head and went to work. There was a twinge of pain, and in about two minutes the exam was over. Meg asked, "Any problems?"

He said, "Did you feel the instrument?"

"No."

"You don't have any problems."

Meg felt self-conscious as she raised herself off the table, "Well," she said, "I was just under the impression that I was too small, because my other doctor said he couldn't give me a pelvic."

The Utah doctor didn't comment. Apparently doctors never discussed doctors. It was no big deal to Meg.

3

Minda McArthur Brinkerhoff

"DO YOU KNOW the middle-child syndrome?" she asked, her words flying out at a disk jockey's speed. "I was fifth out of nine—the syndrome is you don't get enough attention." She talked right through a deep breath. "Gosh, I would never go back to being a kid again." She sounded as though she expected to be interrupted any second. Like most of the McArthurs, she had a rich full voice. At the evening meetings of the Mormons' Mutual Improvement Association, "the Mutual," she rippled the curtains with her vibrato:

> Genealogy, I am doing it.
> My gen-e-a-lo-gy!
> And the reason why I am doing it
> Is very very plain to see.
> I will write my book of re-mem-ber-ance.
> I'll write my his-to-reeeee. . . .

Minda was as tall as her mother, with slender legs that turned shapely in heels and a willowy figure that she bemoaned. Her curly dark-blond hair hung long in back. She had the widest eyes in the family, a firm chin, a straight nose that tilted up at the end—and a tendency to slouch. "All my life I heard, 'Stand up straight,' and Mom would push my shoulders back. She used to get *so* mad. I wore a shoulder brace in my freshman and sophomore years, but no one could see it. I didn't like to stand straight because it looked as though I was pushing out something I didn't have."

When Minda discussed her childhood, she made it sound like a painful sequence of hardships and tragedies, mostly involving livestock. "I was the best milker, but I forgot to milk one night and the next morning, Oh, shoot! Their udders were painful and swollen! . . . My sister Michele slept on our goose and killed it. . . . My dad stepped backward and broke his pet goose's neck. We didn't have too much luck with geese. . . . A heifer knocked me off the fence onto the cement 'cause I got too close to her calf. Gol, we had the *meanest* bulls. It was a challenge to get across the pasture to the canal."

She remembered the way the pigs squealed when she held them down for her dad's knife. "They ate each other's bags when Dad threw 'em," she said, giggling and turning red. "Honest Injun! They fought over 'em and gobbled 'em down. *Uggggh!* Double *uggggh!*"

When she was in junior high, a dog maimed the chickens, "so we had to have a big chicken kill. We'd run 'em to Dad and he'd step on their heads, hang 'em up on the fence and let 'em drain. Then we'd run 'em to Mom and she'd dip 'em in the boiling water and we'd pluck the feathers." She laughed hysterically. "It was a warped childhood." She rolled her blue-green eyes at her own exaggeration.

One day her Aunt Ramona had hurt her feelings by saying, "Minda doesn't take life seriously enough. Everything's a big joke to her."

It was true that Minda never used one word when ten would suffice. To some she came across as a scatterbrain, but her friends and family knew better. She was nervous, bright and quick. Her popcorn-popper speech and loud spasms of laughter helped dissipate nervous energy. Sister Meg had a tendency to do the same, and so did her mother, though neither with the middle child's intensity. In between laughs, Minda berated herself about every little thing: "Well, gol, girl, you've got to do those dishes!" "Come on, you silly! *Move it!*" She would say, "Shame, shame, double shame! Minda, what is the *matter* with you?"

In Lovell High School she'd been a tomboy who barely spoke to girls, played football and "Army" with the boys, and starred as first trumpeter in the band. She loved to blow her horn; she bragged that she could play anything up to (but not including) "The Flight of the Bumble Bee." In church she usually got stuck with the third part harmony "because nobody else would play it." The Lovell church was the only known LDS congregation with a trumpeter playing third part. At informal church functions, her luminous sister Meg pounded the drums on uplifting songs like "Genealogy" or the rousing Mormon marches.

Minda's childhood problem was low self-esteem. "Everybody thinks I'm the outspoken one. But gosh, I wasn't that way as a kid. I hated housework, so I'd go out and help my dad. I'd milk, feed the animals, grind the hay, run the tractor. I love my mother, but we weren't as close as me and my dad. I got along with the other kids, I guess. The household rule was, don't mess with Minda. My sister Michele and I used to wrestle, and I always won. My little brother Mike, I could just clean his plow. When it came to wrestling, I knew little tricks, like get 'em in a leg-lock and squish 'em hard."

Her voice lowered. "I spoke my mind and didn't take anything off anybody." Her family advised her to soften, but she couldn't. Who would stand up for the middle child if she didn't stand up for herself? "I served my time in the principal's office. In those days, my best friend was my journal. Some subjects were just too personal. I filled notebook after notebook."

She giggled as she pulled a yellowing Stenopad from a box crammed with papers. "I wrote this on my thirteenth birthday in 1971. 'Everybody forgets my birthday, even the kids at school.' Two days later, Michele and I were baby-sitting our baby brother Marc. We let him play on the lawn while we cleaned house, and our dog Champ chomped him on the face. Dr. Story wasn't around and another doctor had to take stitches. Michele and I were gonna run away. We knew that Dad was gonna *kill* us."

For blood offenses, church doctrine called for blood atonement (one reason that the Mormon theocracy known as Utah permitted execution by firing squad). Minda and her sister feared that their father might follow the stricture, and they composed a plea called "Watch My Tiny Baby." It opened:

> We have run away cuz
> Champ bit Marc this very
> day.

And ended:

> We hope you keep your cool,
> So we can go to school.
> So we
> Can go so nice and clear with
> out bruises on the rear.

The two sisters were so frightened that night that they made their grandmother sit between them as their parents walked in the door. Dean McArthur ignored the girls and exacted his blood atonement on the dog.

Minda thought she could put her finger on the exact moment when she began to think of herself as a lower form of life. "Uncle Bob began on me when I was seven," she said, and burst into tears. "Oh, gol," she wailed, "I'm so ashamed." She composed herself and told her story in fits and starts:

"He did it to me dozens of times. I kept it to myself till I found out that he was bothering my sisters and brothers. Nobody would've believed me anyway. Shoot, I was a little kid and he was a businessman with mooga-bucks.

"After the first year or so, he'd be with us in our living room . . . and he'd have one of us massaging it in front of the others. He used the same technique, the same words. 'Come sit on my lap.' He always had bags of candy, *tons*. He'd say, 'Don't you want to drive my car?' Or 'Come over here. I have something for you.' He'd put your hand on his penis and make it go up and down, and he'd be saying, 'We sure been having good weather lately, haven't we?' 'How're things at school?'

"I don't know if he had, uh, orgasms. I wouldn't have known what they were. Meg says she's always hated the smell of semen, and she thinks the aversion might have started with Bob Asay. But she's blocked all the details out and . . . she's not sure.

"At night I was always cold, 'cause Dad set our thermostat at fifty-five, and I would sneak down and sleep in front of the old gas fireplace in our living room. Uncle Bob caught on and started coming into the house after Mom and Dad went to bed. I would be the only one in the living room. Once I panicked—a little kid with this huge man on top of me. I pushed him off and ran upstairs to my room. After that, I started sleeping in my mom's closet where there were warm pipes and ducts. He never found me there.

"I used to hide from him in the daytime—we all did. Mom and Dad wouldn't be out the door five minutes when he'd be on the phone. 'Are Dean and Arden there? Well, when'll they be back, honey?'

"We caught on and wouldn't answer, so he just started dropping in. He'd say, 'I called and nobody was home.' We hid in the dirt room under the floor till he found us there. I hid on a shelf in a walk-in closet. I'd drag in a box and hide behind it and pull a blanket over me. Mom and Dad would come home and be all upset 'cause the work wasn't done around the house. Uncle Bob was so close to them, we didn't dare tell.

"I was supposed to be baptized when I was eight, and I told my mom I wasn't worthy. I couldn't say why, so she had me baptized anyway. I cried a lot. My mom picked up that I didn't like myself. She put a sign on my mirror: 'I like what I see.' Gol, you gotta give her credit. She was in there trying.

"Uncle Bob kept at me till I was ten or eleven. Then one night we all got together and told our parents. It was very hard. We'd never talked about sex in our house. There was a lot of talking and crying that night. And then Bob walked in and we all had root beer floats together! He wasn't kicked out! Nothing! Dad was working part time for him, laying carpets. Maybe that's why."

Minda brushed at a watery streak of mascara. "Do you know what that does to a kid?" she asked. "As far as we knew, nothing was ever done about Bob, except that Mom and Dad wouldn't leave us alone with him after that." She raised her voice. "*Nothing was ever done about him!* That's what hurts the most."

She turned away and blew her nose. For once, she spoke slowly. "Later a teenager came to Dad and complained about Uncle Bob. He said, 'Dean, I can't take it anymore. You have to help me.' Nothing came of that, either."

She sniffed again. "I had to go to the new ward bishop to be interviewed for a Temple Recommend. Shoot, I knew he'd turn me down." Applicants had to meet seventeen requirements, including abstention from coffee, tea, alcohol, tobacco and cola drinks; total adherence to "commandments of the gospel"; attendance at church functions; refusal to associate with backsliders; and, above all else, moral cleanliness. "I was unclean," Minda said. "I told the bishop about Uncle Bob, and I remember crying and saying I wasn't worthy. When I was finished, he asked me when it had happened last, and then he assured me I hadn't done anything wrong. I got the Recommend and went off to our temple in Idaho Falls to be baptized for the dead. I've always had blind faith, I'm a total believer. It makes me feel better about myself."

Sex and sexuality remained taboo subjects in the McArthur household. Arden and Dean were demonstrative with each other but not with their children. "At night, Dad would sit in his big old chair and Mom would plop down in his lap or sit on the arm, and they'd be there the whole evening," Minda said, smiling at the memory. "Or Mom would be standing in the kitchen and Dad would give her a big kiss. But they kept their distance from us kids—maybe a little kiss on the cheek at bedtime, but never all huggy-huggy. Well, gol, of *course* they loved us. They showed it all the time, like my dad saying, 'Have a good day today. Turn the world over. You know you can do anything!' He'd say, 'Don't you look pretty today. You sure are beautiful!' "

After the Bob Asay revelations, the McArthurs tightened enforcement of the Mormon strictures about modesty. "Mom made me wear skirts below the knee," Minda recalled. "I always had to wear T-shirts for underwear. Mom said, 'When you grow up, you won't have a problem changing from skimpy clothes to modest clothes that'll cover your garment.' "

It was the sacred obligation of every committed Mormon to protect against Satan by wearing "the garment," disparaged by detractors as "magic underwear" and "angel chaps." In the required ritual, the high priest intoned: "It represents the garment given to Adam when he was found naked in the Garden of Eden, and is called the Garment of the Holy Priesthood. Inasmuch as you do not defile it, but are true and faithful to your covenants, it will be a shield and a protection to you against the power of the destroyer until you have finished your work here on earth."

The garment was a cotton sack in the shape of old-fashioned B.V.D.s, with a trapdoor in the rear and arcane slits and markings over the private areas. It was supposed to be worn next to the skin for life; fundamentalist Mormons made love in the garment, gave birth, underwent surgery, swam and showered and took part in sports in it. Every Mormon could recite tales attesting to the garment's efficacy. Believers believed that neither steel-jacketed bullet nor chain saw could pierce the godly weave.

Both McArthur parents wore the garment. Dean, though openly less pious than his wife, had been a bishop. On hot days Minda used to see her mother standing in front of the stove wearing nothing but the garment—the kids called it LDS air-conditioning.

The high neck and knee length presented a style problem, and Mormon mothers prepared their daughters by first dressing them in T-shirts and long skirts. Minda, of course, rebelled, but Arden was not one to yield on sacred matters. When Minda was in the sixth grade, "a visiting cousin left her bikini at our house and I changed into it every day at the pool. My mom never found out. Then there was a phone call to send the bikini back." She sighed. "These are the things that break a kid's heart."

When Minda entered junior high, the Lovell schools were just beginning to consider sex education. "My mother was adamant against it," Minda recalled. "She said the teachers would be single, and what did they know about sex? My sisters and I were indifferent. Sex wasn't discussed at home or in church. Why should it be taught in the schools?"

The closest the church came to offering sexual guidance came in the form of occasional instructions from Salt Lake City. A typical memo was entitled "Steps in Overcoming Masturbation" and recommended breaking off relationships with other self-abusers, leaving the bathroom immediately after a bath and avoiding the mirror, wearing tight clothes in bed "so that it would be difficult and time consuming for you to remove those clothes," yelling "stop!" and reciting Scripture or imagining "having to bathe in a tub of worms" when the urge became overwhelming, reading *How to Win Friends and Influence People* or holding the Book of Mormon firmly in hand through the night. "In very severe cases," the bulletin went on, "it may be necessary to tie a hand to the bed frame." Such pronouncements were aimed mainly at missionaries and insiders; they were seldom seen by the children and most ordinary members of the church.

An eighth-grade teacher showed a film about menstruation, and Minda was so embarrassed she refused to look. The prepubescent schoolboys were always pulling tampons from the girls' purses and waving them about. Minda turned purple. She spoke against a teacher who showed a movie about Elisabeth Kübler-Ross's theories on dying. So did most of her friends, and the teacher was pressured to send the film back. Lovell was a tight little Mormon town, barely affected by trends and happenings in Billings and Casper, let alone the rest of the country, and its children reflected their parents more strongly than most.

At thirteen, Minda told her mother, "Gol, Mom, I think I started my period."

Arden looked startled and said, "You did?" When Minda realized that her mother would have no more to say on the subject, she moped off to her room.

A year later, she cut her hand while doing the dishes, and the family doctor took stitches at the hospital. At school the next day a senior boy asked, "Who sewed you up?"

"Dr. Story," Minda answered.

"Is *he* your doctor?"

"Yeah."

The senior asked, "Don't you know what he's like?"

"What do you mean?"

"Don't you know that he fools with girls in his office?"

"Oh, for crying out loud!" Minda said. "I've been going to him since I was three months old. Shoot, if he did things like that, don't you think I'd know?"

The boy said, "I just can't believe you'd keep going back to him."

Minda blew up. "You can't say things like that!" she yelled. "You weren't there! You don't know!"

Nor could she fathom her classmates' warnings about the GAA physicals. All Dr. Story ever did was check her heart and reflexes and sign the form. The other girls insisted that he took liberties. "No way," Minda said. She knew malicious gossip when she heard it. If Dr. Story were kinky, her mother would have been the first to know. And she was his number-one backer.

4

Meg Anderson

FOUR HUNDRED MILES AWAY, Meg was majoring in drama and speech at her father's alma mater, Utah State. She was interested in marriage but still too afraid of men to join in the mating game that preoccupied the other students. All her life, she'd felt like an insect looking up the pant legs of men. Her female teachers had been imitation males; she could hear their fathers speaking through them. Bob Asay had saddled her with an irrational fear of sexual mistreatment. At night she forced herself to walk down the long dark hill toward town, but she always wound up shaking and shuddering and running back to the dorm.

From the first, she'd liked Logan. It looked like Lovell, only bigger. Like every other town in Utah, it was strongly LDS. The college sat in groves of trees; there were flowers everywhere and a comforting Mormon expansiveness to the streets and buildings.

She did odd jobs all week, cleaned houses on weekends, and managed a full curriculum. After eighteen years of hoeing beets and milking cows, it almost seemed like a vacation. She acted in school plays, sang in the college chorus, pounded on a used set of traps in a basement practice room, dabbled in piano, and let a friendly cowboy teach her "Night Rider's Lament" and "The Streets of Laredo." She took out a loan from a Lovell bank to buy guitars for herself and her upperclass-man sister Marie so they could practice together, then strummed till her fingertips split.

Meg's first man turned up in the unexpected setting of Family Home Evening, the Mormons' traditional Monday night of prayer, play and song. In the campus setting, Meg was named Family Home Evening "mother," responsible for the moral and spiritual health of her group. The role fit; she'd been a church leader since junior high.

After a few meetings, a clean-cut young member named Greg Hagan asked for a date. She couldn't say no. She certainly wasn't going to tell him that she had a morbid fear of rape. When he returned her to her door, he slammed her against the wall and grabbed her breasts. She screamed and locked him out.

She reported the incident to her LDS branch president the next day. "Don't worry, Meg," he said grimly. "We'll take care of him."

A month later Greg Hagan was married in the temple. Meg was crushed. She told herself, Every day of my life I've been taught morality. It's our shining ideal, way up here, out of sight. Why, immorality is the greatest sin next to murder! *And yet the branch president signed Greg Hagan's Temple Recommend!* She pondered and prayed but received no enlightenment.

When she was twenty, she met the man she would always think of as "Mr. Expert." His area of expertise was sex, but he kept his talent concealed till she was hopelessly in love. She fought the sofa wars for two years and lost four or five times. When the relationship ended, she felt so degraded that she confessed every detail to her bishop. He brought her before a church court—the Mormons called them courts of love—and she was disfellowshipped by a jury consisting of the bishop, his two counselors and the ward clerk. She was stripped of her job as Relief Society counselor and forbidden to lead prayers or speak at meetings while she set about repenting her sins.

"The sacrament was what I missed the most," she recalled later. "In our ritual, the broken bread and water are handed along the pew. All I could do was pass it on. Everyone in the church knew why."

Alone at night, she mourned her loss of worthiness. "The hardest part is forgiving yourself, and I couldn't. The whole thing ripped me to pieces. I thought, I'm not a terrible person, I'm a *good* person. I'd wanted to marry the boy, but he told me he couldn't be true. I tried everything in my power to get him to marry me."

She stayed in her room and spurned males. The church court had ordered chastity, and she took no chances. Healing came slowly. She repented publicly at a branch meeting and gave the required talk on modesty. She changed wards and attended youth meetings. She began to speak up at church functions, usually to younger members in need of counsel. She'd been a leader for as long as she could remember, and it was unnatural for her to keep silent. One of the men took her aside and said, "You're a born leader. Why don't you take over one of our groups?"

They were the first kind words she'd heard in months, but she had to tell the truth. "I can't," she said. "I've been disfellowshipped."

His face froze. "Then keep your mouth shut at the meetings," he ordered.

She cried in her room. For weeks she told herself this wasn't happening. She slipped into a melancholia so profound that she would strum her guitar for hours, seeing no one and talking only to herself.

At the end of a year, she was brought before church authorities and asked if she'd stayed "clean"—no petting, no heavy kissing, nothing remotely sexual. Did she feel above reproach morally, back on the true path?

"No," she answered. "I don't feel any different now than I did a year ago. I'm just as repentant now as I was then, but inside I . . . I don't feel different."

One of the brethren smiled and said, "Meg, you won't feel different till you've forgiven yourself. Have you been able to do that?"

"Hunh-uh. I haven't."

The elders huddled and then ruled that she'd made amends to her church and the world.

She began seeing a likable young man. On the night he date-raped her, she couldn't have held him off with a club. She didn't date again for a year.

She earned degrees in speech and theater but still yearned for love and marriage. Twice she became engaged and disengaged, then fell deeply in love with a handsome agnostic and even flew to New York to meet his parents. On the return flight to Utah, she remembered the warmth of her dad's hands on her head as he gave her the priesthood blessing. How could she deny this experience to her own children? Ever since she'd been a little girl, her fondest dream had been to be sealed in the temple with her husband and children and go on to eternal life in the Celestial Kingdom. She loved her irreligious fiancé, but earthly time was no more substantial than a fast paradiddle on her drums.

She waited till his birthday to tell him it was off. He made her promise never to communicate with him again. She felt terrible. He was the first enemy she'd ever made.

5

Minda Brinkerhoff

Introducing the bent handle of a spoon, I saw everything as no man had ever seen before. . . . The Speculum
made it perfectly clear from the beginning. . . . I felt like
an explorer in medicine who views a new and important
territory.

—J. Marion Sims, M.D.,
father of nineteenth-century
American gynecology

BOYS entered Minda's life at fifteen, but she had no particular interest
in sex. Her first boyfriend would put his head in her lap while they
watched TV on the floor. "I didn't catch on," she said in laughing
retrospect. "I never got aroused. I just didn't *know*."

One night when Meg was home from college, she told the young
couple, "I just don't think you should lie around like that."

Minda said, "Like what? Watching TV?"

Inevitably, the boyfriend took her for a drive and tried for a kiss. "I
didn't give anything back," she recalled, giggling at her naïveté. "He
kissed me again and I still didn't respond. He says, 'Are we having a
good time or what?' Then he took me home. Gol, I wondered what
ticked him off."

She fell in with rowdies from Calley, six miles up the Billings
highway, telling herself she was "raising their souls." It was an odd
mix. She'd been girls' president of the Mutual, the LDS young people's
group. Her new friends dubbed her "Little Miss Churchy" because she
attended every Mormon function, neither drank nor smoked, and insisted
on being home fifteen minutes before her father's 10 P.M. curfew. And
she never stopped chattering about the mission she planned and the
souls she would save for her Heavenly Father.

42

In her junior year, she met classmate Scott Brinkerhoff, a devout Mormon from an old Lovell family. He was six feet tall and built like a linebacker, with broad shoulders and a narrow backside. He had liquid brown eyes and a lovely golden tan. He wore his slightly wavy brown hair in a "missionary cut" that she knew her parents would approve. His baby face didn't look as though it would ever support a beard or mustache. She liked his values and his style. He wore cowboy boots to school. He hunted and lumberjacked in the Shoshone, Big Horn, Pryor, and Absaroka Mountains, the ranges that defined the Big Horn Basin. His idea of a good time was rising at dawn and cutting firewood all day. "Scott," she chided him, "you won't quit till you've logged the whole mountain."

"That's my plan," he admitted with a laugh.

He intended to go on a two-year mission and then become a cowboy. He was president of the local seminary, a high honor, but he remained quiet and modest. Like her, he had a zest for work. He left school an hour early each day so he could help his dad build houses.

After Minda and Scott had become friends, he confessed that his parents sometimes griped about "that damn Dean McArthur." Minda was dimly aware that a few citizens resented her dad. There would always be folks who couldn't stand perfection.

Scott recounted an odd story. In the mid-70s the Brinkerhoffs had built Dr. Story's new clinic up near the hospital. The place still smelled of sawdust and fresh paint when the doctor complained, "This examining room door is hung backward. I want more privacy for my patients."

Gerald Brinkerhoff, a wiry little man with a quick tongue, didn't mind making sensible changes, but this door swung inward and leftward against the wall—perfectly standard. If it opened to the right, it would cover the light switch.

"Too late, Doc," Scott's father said. "We've got the wires in."

A few days later, Brinkerhoff heard that Dr. Story was downtown shopping for heavy drapes to circle his examining table. The two men finally settled on a doorknob that could be locked from the inside of the room with a twist. Scott said his father had passed the incident off as an example of Dr. Story's weirdness.

For a long time, Minda loved Scott but kept it to herself. "Then one night he said, 'I love you, Minda,'" she recalled, "but I took Mom's advice and kept quiet. She'd always said, If you ever say I love you to a boy, you'll feel committed to him and you won't know how to get out of it. I loved Scott, but I never said the words."

It almost seemed to Minda that she learned the theory and practice of lovemaking simultaneously. As she wrote later, "I gave something to Scott and it was all I had that was mine and mine alone."

The next morning she wondered if he would speak to her. "I went to school early. Scott walked in and said, 'Good morning.' I was real uncomfortable. I thought, Shoot, what have I done to this perfectly good relationship? He leaned over my desk and kissed me and told me he loved me more than ever. After that, we were totally dependent on each other."

While Minda's parents were on a day trip to Billings, the young lovers considered eloping. She held back. "What about my dad?" she said. "It would hurt him."

Late that night, her mother tiptoed into her room and asked, "Minda, are you awake?"

"Yes, Mom." They often had bedside chats.

Arden said, "I need to ask you something." There was a tremulous note in her voice. "Are you . . . sleeping with Scott?"

The McArthur children did *not* lie. "Yes, Mother," Minda said. "I am."

"How long?"

"Two or three months. Oh, gol, Mom, why are you asking?"

"I don't know," Arden said. "It's just something I had to know." She paused, and Minda didn't know how to fill the silence. "Are you pregnant?"

"Oh, no. Hunh-uh!"

Shortly after her mom left, Minda tiptoed to her parents' bedroom and asked if she could go deer hunting with Scott after her chores in the morning.

Her father said, "Well, I don't think it's a good idea right now. I need to think a little bit more. I'm not thinking real good right now."

She was milking in the morning when he took her aside. He looked as though he hadn't slept. "I can forbid you to see Scott," he said, speaking softly, "but then you'd just see him behind my back." He reached out and took her hand. "If there's anything I can do to help you . . ." His voice trailed off, and he started again. "You know what I think is best, Minda? I don't think you should be sleeping with the young man, but I'm not gonna say you can't. I'll support you. Do you need anything? What're you doing about birth control?"

"We're fine," she said. She felt squirmy talking to her dad about sex. "Gosh, Dad, we're being careful."

He warned, "There's no such thing as being careful."

She didn't tell him that birth control was Scott's department. She knew nothing about it and didn't want to know.

The lovers exchanged the deepest vows short of a wedding ceremony. "We knew dang good and well that they wouldn't let us be married," Minda said, "so we just finally decided to be committed to each other and not to care what our parents thought. We just wanted to be together. Then one night Scott said, 'I'm not gonna be careful anymore.' "

A few months later, in November 1975, she realized that she was pregnant. She hadn't missed a period, but she knew. She even figured the baby's due date: August 20. She was positive.

When she told Scott, he said, "Well . . . okay. Are you gonna tell your parents?"

She said yes.

She told them two months later. Her dad said, "You're *not* pregnant, Minda. Mom told me you've been having your periods. You're just too ashamed and embarrassed about what's going on, and it's getting harder for you to face us."

"No," Minda said. "I'm really pregnant."

Her mom chimed in, "No! You can't be!"

But her father's face showed that he believed. "Well," he said, "what do you want to do about it?"

She knew he wasn't referring to abortion. No former LDS bishop would consider such an offense against the Heavenly Father.

The three McArthurs met with Scott. Her parents proposed giving Minda money so she could give birth outside the range of Lovell's jungle drums. "You can go to your uncle's in Texas," Arden said. "That'll give you time to think, to get a little older."

Scott said, "As long as Minda carries my baby, she's not going anywhere without me."

Her dad asked Scott if he intended to tell his folks.

"I just can't," he said.

Dean McArthur said he would handle that chore, and he did.

At school the next morning, Scott reported that his parents believed he'd been seduced by "that McArthur girl." It was the only explanation the Brinkerhoffs could accept. Their son was still president of the seminary and a shining example for the other Mormon boys. A boy that pure couldn't be blamed for anything.

Minda kept going to class but frequently had to slip into the girls' room to compose herself. Her family was supportive. Sometimes Scott, as manly and strong as he was, cried along with her. To people who ranked immorality just short of murder, the situation seemed hopeless.

Scott filled her in on developments at the Brinkerhoff bungalow on Nevada Avenue. For the first three days after they found out about the pregnancy, he said, his parents refused to speak to him. On the fourth, there were cookies on the table when he came home from school, with "Scott" written in icing. He ate them in his room.

Next came a painful family meeting. Scott said that his mother insisted that he verify the pregnancy because "Minda might be trying to trap you into marriage."

Minda dried her tears and drove up the hill to Dr. Story's new clinic. With her own mother in the room as usual, she underwent her first pelvic examination. It was quick and painless. The family doctor told her she was two months gone.

Years later, she remembered every detail of the events that followed. "We asked our bishop, Brownie J. Brown, to marry us. The LDS church doesn't have a paid clergy. Our high priests can be anything from day laborers to bank presidents. Bishop Brown was a farmer, a school board member, a nice man. He said he'd be glad to officiate. But Scott and I made one mistake. We didn't cry or act ashamed. Shoot, we were all cried out."

A shotgun wedding was arranged by the unfriendly families. After intense negotiations, the date was set: Friday, January 23, 1976. Territorial problems were headed off by scheduling the ceremony in the home of a relative who lived midway between the McArthurs and the Brinkerhoffs. It was agreed that no one but family members would be invited, and publicity would be minimal. "They're treating it more like a spy plot than a wedding," Minda complained to Scott. "The only feeling I have is dread."

On the day of the wedding, a classmate said. "Aren't you getting married tonight? What on earth are you doing at school?"

Minda said, "What should I be doing?"

"You should be home getting ready."

"Oh?"

"Minda, you only get married once!"

The wedding was an ordeal. All four parents looked ashamed. The grandparents stared into space. The little kids paraded in and out of the bathroom and were told to shush. Bishop Brown sounded like a funeral director. The cake was too small. There were no wedding checks or jokes or toasts, no conviviality, nothing to remember with pleasure or joy.

Minda's father took her aside and promised that it would be different when she and Scott were remarried in the temple at Idaho Falls. He said, "We'll have a great big cake, and we'll take pictures and everything. We'll do it up like we should have tonight." Then he cried.

The next day Brownie J. Brown summoned the newlyweds to his office in the big Mormon church that dominated the center of town like a set piece. Even in the dead of winter, flowers lined the walkway from Main Street; they were grown in homes and hot houses and replaced by the women of the stake. The broad green lawn was hidden under an inch or two of gray snow, and the weeping birch at the west end was droopy and denuded.

The bishop smiled and said, "We're here because we need to know where you guys stand on this. Tell ya the truth, neither one of you kids seemed very contrite. Scott, you're seminary president and everybody looks up to you." He quoted one of the seminary teachers to the effect that an example had to be made.

As she listened, Minda thought of three other couples who'd recently been forced to marry. They'd all had big happy weddings and nice honeymoons and their pictures in the *Chronicle*—and not one couple had been admonished by the church. She was too shocked to protest when Brownie J. Brown announced that he was convening a bishop's court.

All Minda remembered about the trial was that the two of them were put on indefinite probation, one step short of disfellowship. "We were ordered to attend all church functions, keep up our tithing, show contrition and *repent*. They told us we darn had to straighten up. We couldn't hold any office or teach any classes, something we'd both always done. Scott was mad. He went to church a couple times and stopped. We'd already been following all the steps to forgiveness, the way you're supposed to. We'd gotten married to make things right, and then they gave us a bishop's court, just because it was Scott and me."

The demoralized seniors returned to high school. "Our friends didn't know us anymore," Minda recalled bitterly. "That's the way Lovell is. We ended up with the rejects, the kids who use bad language and party all the time. They invited us to a kegger out in the hills. Golly, it was such a sad thing to see our new friends drunk, slobbering, mumbling to themselves. Scott and I decided not to try the beer. It would have been a first for both of us."

The two young Brinkerhoffs were only a credit or two away from graduation, and they asked the principal if they could attend class an hour a day to enable Scott to earn money and Minda to run their home. The answer was no. Nine weeks before graduation, they dropped out. "We realized later," Minda said ruefully, "how stupid it was. It was kids saying, 'We'll show you.' But nobody gave a dang. We only hurt ourselves."

Every month she visited the clinic. Dr. Story tried to counsel her and always inquired about her sex life. Scott gave her a hickey on her breast and the doctor demanded to know how she got it. "Oh," she said, "I must've bumped into something." He palpated the discolored area and told her to be more careful.

She wondered why he always put her in the stirrups and examined her "down there." Her mother explained that it was his old thoroughness. He complimented the middle child on how pretty she looked, and sometimes complained that it was unfair for so much of the world's beauty to be allotted to a single family.

The visits began to take more and more of her time. There were days when she reached the clinic at 1:30 or 2 P.M. and didn't get away till the office closed at 5:30. She would sit in the waiting room for ages before the nurse escorted her to the examining room and told her to strip and get on the table. An hour or so later Dr. Story would come in and ask her to scoot down so that two or three inches of her rear end protruded over the end. Then he would poke and probe.

Sometimes he interrupted himself to see another patient. When he returned, he always seemed energetic and ready for action. Sooner or later he would complain, "I can't get it in far enough," and ask if he could "dilate" her to make it easier to insert the speculum. It didn't occur to her to say no. He was the doctor.

She came to know every inch of his ceiling. A sheet was drawn tightly across her knees and kept her from seeing what he was doing.

She didn't want to know anyway. As he manipulated the instrument, the pain made her sweat and turn red. When she cried out, he would complain that they just had to try harder. She knew she had a narrow canal, but he was making her feel like a freak.

She told her mother, "He sure does a lot of pelvics."

Arden said she was lucky to be getting such expert attention.

In July the high-country temperature climbed into the nineties. Minda lifted her blimpish body onto the old tractor and drove into the fields with her dad. Just working with him picked up her spirits. He seemed to be feeling better, too.

"This whole thing's taught me a lesson," he told her in his soft voice. "I thought we were a perfect family—didn't smoke, didn't drink, didn't party, worked hard, obeyed God's laws and man's. I thought we were a little bit above everybody else. But this thing made me realize we're no better or worse'n the rest." He took her hand. "It's made me reach out a little, make a few friends. Feels good, Minda. It's the best thing ever happened to me."

On a scorching day in mid-August 1976, she was driving the tractor when the baby flip-flopped in her stomach. Dr. Story took X-rays and told her that the fetus was in a breach position and wouldn't fit through her narrow canal.

A few days later she staggered the half mile home from church and told Scott, "I've got this water dripping down my legs." Soon she was in hard labor. For a while, the infant was in fetal distress, but Dr. Story's skilled hands delivered a squawling Curtis Scott Brinkerhoff by cesarean.

As soon as her stitches came out, Minda dressed the baby and took him to church alone. Scott was still refusing to attend. She passed the sacrament tray with head held high. Church made her feel good, even without the sacrament. Church was something between her and God. All those staring fools could be danged.

A veterinarian named Ed Lowe became the new ward bishop, and he called Minda to his office. "Well, what do you think?" he asked.

"I think I've been on probation long enough," she answered.

Minda could see that Scott was the bishop's real concern. The church didn't want to lose an active young leader, but Scott's pride presented a problem.

"He's hurt and angry," Minda explained. "He doesn't think this was handled right."

The bishop shuffled some papers. "Look, Minda," he said, "I'm afraid if I don't take you kids off probation, Scott will fall away completely."

Minda knew better—Scott was LDS to his boot tops—but she didn't comment. "And he's too fine a young man for us to lose," Bishop Lowe went on. He shoved his chair back and said, "Your probation is over."

Minda's first thought was, Wait till I tell Dad! She stuck out her hand, and the bishop shook it. Then he said, "Do you want to be married to Scott in the temple?"

She'd dreamed of a temple marriage ever since her first excursion as a child. "Oh, yes!" she said.

The bishop summoned Scott into the office and asked him if he wanted to go to the temple with Minda.

Scott looked at her and smiled. "Well, sure," he said. "Well— *yeah!*"

"Come back to church. If you make yourselves worthy, I'll see that you get your Recommends."

They were married in the Idaho Falls Temple on Minda's nineteenth birthday, March 25, 1977. The relatives attended, McArthurs and Brinkerhoffs united at last. After the rites, little Curtis was carried into the sealing room, all cleansed and anointed—a cherub in white robes. The family was joined together "for time and all eternity." Minda was so happy she couldn't cry.

If there was any question about the prodigals' complete acceptance by their church, it was dispelled by one of the wedding gifts, a book called *The House of the Lord*, by James E. Talmage, which explained why Mormons built temples ("This then is sufficient answer to the question as to why the Latter-Day Saints build and maintain temples. They have been instructed and required so to do by the Lord of Hosts. . . . *Temples are a necessity*"). The book was inscribed in the Lovell stake president's own handwriting, "To Minda and Scott Brinkerhoff and Curtis as they embark on their Journey to the Celestial Kingdom."

Scott hired on at a nearby bentonite plant, shoveling the slick fine-grained mineral that was mostly used as an oil-drill lubricant but also turned up in ice cream, cosmetics and medical products. He hated the job and the product. Bentonite had an extraordinary capacity to absorb water, but it also insinuated itself into the nearest available nose. The plant's informal slogan was "Bentonite builds bigger boogers." Scott swore they bounced.

Minda tried a few jobs of her own but soon became pregnant with Garret Mac (for McArthur) Brinkerhoff, delivered by Dr. Story in another C-section on January 17, 1978. This time the prenatal care was even more intensive—a pelvic per month for eight months, then one a week till she delivered. Dr. Story explained that the extra exams were necessary because of the previous cesarean, and advised her to build herself up before getting pregnant again. She began using foam.

Early in 1979, she stepped on a lag screw and rushed to the clinic. As always, Dr. Story asked about her sex life. "It's fine," she said. "Just fine."

He gave her a tetanus shot and told her to come back the next day to make sure there was no infection. On her return, he remarked that she hadn't had a thorough examination in a year and a half and that he needed to see how her last C-section was healing. "Do you have time for a pelvic?" he asked.

She dutifully took off her clothes, climbed on his automatic table, and lifted her feet to the stirrups. He stepped on a pedal and the table whirred and groaned as it raised her head a few degrees and lowered her bottom half. He kneaded her breasts, the customary first step in his exams, then began his finger work, first one and then two, occasionally asking if it hurt. She confirmed that it did.

After a while, he said, "Minda, maybe if you help guide it in, it would be better. I can feel you're really tight."

She thought, I'm not gonna help him hurt me. What makes him think I can guide the instrument any better than he can? "No, Dr. Story," she gasped. "I don't think I can get it in any easier."

He stepped to the side of the table. Something warm slipped between the fingers of her hand. At first she thought it was the medical instrument and jerked her hand to her mouth, coughing nonchalantly so he wouldn't think she was offended.

My word, she said to herself, that's a penis! Nothing else felt like a penis; she'd known that since age seven.

Then something poked against her bare thigh. It felt like his belt buckle, but it wasn't cold. He stepped back from the table and told her the exam was over.

As she was getting up, he said, "Did you know you're two months pregnant?"

On her way home, she was more upset about the poke in her side than the failure of her birth-control foam. Was the Uncle Bob craziness starting all over again? Was it some kind of bad karma, some unknown signal she emitted? No, she thought, it can't be. Not Dr. Story.

After a discussion with her mother, Minda was sure that she'd misunderstood. You dum-dum, she berated herself, why would you even *think* a filthy thing like that. Come on, Minda, ya know? Are you sick or what? *You're really sick. . . .*

Six months later, when the baby was almost due, she went through the same experience and again jerked her hand away.

When she got home, her mom was serving dinner. Minda went upstairs to her parents' king-size bed and lay there shaking. My land, she said to herself, once was bad enough.

Arden came in and said, "How'd it go?"

"Just fine," Minda said, and murmured, "Oh, yeah, just fine."

"You can't lie to me. I know there's something wrong."

"Nothing's wrong!" Minda said, and started to cry.

Arden climbed into bed and held her daughter tight. Minda flashed on the silliness of the scene—I'm an adult, this is my third child, my mother's comforting me like a baby, and she wants to know what's wrong. When does the middle kid grow up?

At last she managed to say, "I think I felt Dr. Story's penis today, during the pelvic exam."

Her mother pulled away and said, "Oh, for heaven's sakes, you did not. No way. I don't know why you would think that." She didn't seem flustered, just a reasonable woman stating obvious facts. Minda wished she were like her mother—always so *sure.*

Arden was saying, "Nothing like that would ever happen. Dr. Story loves us. We trust him with our lives. He's good, kind, gentle, caring."

"Mom, I know what a penis feels like."

"Honey, you're just blue. Get some rest. When you wake up, you'll feel better. Criminy, he's the only doctor you've ever had! He loves you. He'd never do anything to hurt you. Why would he do a thing like that?"

"Well, I don't know why," Minda said. "I think I felt it once before. But I convinced myself it wasn't."

"Of *course* it wasn't! It could've been an instrument. It could've been . . . anything."

"But Mom—"

Arden hugged her and said, "You're not feeling well. You want this pregnancy to be over with, and you're just a little bit distraught. You need to relax."

Minda thought, She's probably right. Mom knows him better than any of us.

She'd already taken one of the Darvon samples he'd given her at the clinic. She thought, Maybe it went to my brain. She began to feel better, knowing how much her mother loved her. It was so reassuring that her mom had simply corrected her instead of ridiculing or laughing. After a while she dozed off.

Two weeks later, Scott drove her up the hill to deliver. It didn't feel as though her time had come, but Dr. Story had booked the delivery room. She wondered, What makes him so sure of the date? He's never been that sure before. Suppose my baby isn't ready?

They wheeled her into the delivery room and put her under for her third cesarean. The scalpel cut into her old scar and she doubled up. She heard him say, "Give her some more."

Nurses grabbed her legs and tried to straighten her body, but she couldn't help resisting. "Give her *more*," Story ordered in his soft voice. The anesthetist shot her again and again—five times in all—and she could still feel the doctor's hand inside her body. She thought of the Prophet Joseph Smith lying in the grove of trees, unable to open his eyes.

She lost track, then heard Dr. Story say, "The baby's not breathing. There's something in her lungs. She's either swallowed liquid or she has a wet lung."

Minda thought, I'm gonna lose my first little girl!

Dr. Story said, "We've got to take the baby to Billings. I wish Minda would wake up."

She tried, but she couldn't move or open her eyes.

After a while she felt a tap on her shoulder and heard Dr. Story say, "Scott, we've really got to get Minda waked up. That baby has to go to Billings. I want Minda to see her in case she doesn't make it."

She felt Scott's hand in hers and managed to move a finger. "Can you hear me?" he asked.

Her eyes slowly opened. A nurse wheeled the baby in on a table. She was the tiniest person Minda had ever seen. Her black hair was three or four inches long, and dark fuzz covered her shoulders, legs and back.

Minda thought, My boys didn't look like that. They're both so fair. From far away she heard one of the nurses say, "Boy, where did this one come from?"

She stayed in the hospital for a week while her infant daughter fought for her life in a preemie ward seventy miles north (and ran up a bill that would take the Brinkerhoffs seven years to pay). Amber Dawn's birth certificate listed her weight as seven pounds, but to Minda she hadn't looked half that big.

Her mother returned from a visit to the Billings hospital and told about a conversation with one of the pediatricians. He'd said, "These wet lungs often happen in premature babies."

"She's full term," Arden said.

"Her lungs weren't fully developed," the doctor insisted. "This baby is six to eight weeks early."

Amber Dawn Brinkerhoff stayed in the hospital for three more weeks while her mother grieved at home, confined to her bed on Dr. Story's orders. Minda found that the maternal instinct was strongest just after delivery. She twisted up her bedding on the cool fall nights and called for Amber in her sleep. She wished she understood what was happening. Dr. Story had been way off on the due date. Why had he insisted? Why hadn't he been more accurate?

Arden took the baby in for her first checkup while Minda continued to rest up. By this time the fuzz had begun to disappear from Amber's back and shoulders, but her dark skin and eyes made her look different from Curtis and Garret Mac. Several friends had taken notice.

When her mom returned with the baby in her arms, she was chuckling. "What's so funny?" Minda asked.

"When I walked in, the nurse said, 'Oh, grandma's got the baby, huh?' So I just said, 'Hey, take a good look. This is Dr. Story's baby.' We both laughed. It was our little joke."

For months, Minda had realized that her husband was growing restless, but it wasn't his nature to share his feelings. Scott wasn't bookish, but he was quick and bright, and for two and a half years all he'd done to exercise his brain was work a control panel at the bentonite plant.

One night he came home with the usual film of greenish dust in his hair, and said, "I looked at the guy next to me today, Minda. He's sixty, sixty-five years old. I said to myself, Man, am I gonna be pushing these buttons for the next forty-some years? I can't see myself doing that. We're already in debt, and it's just gonna get worse on my salary."

They decided to sell their half-completed new home and their Ford Bronco and do what Mormons had done for a hundred and fifty years— pack up and head out. They both loved their hometown, but Lovell was more of a dead end than ever. The lack of a future was what drove so many of its young people to drink and drugs. One of the town's biggest employers, the Lovell Clay Products Co. (known for forty years as "the brick 'n' tile") was collapsing on its own bricks, a victim of the nation-wide switch to plastic pipe. The annual beet campaign hadn't started; the sugar refinery at the west end of Main Street lay in hibernation. Pumping jacks jerked up and down in the oil fields, but whenever petroleum demand dropped off, workers were laid off. Employers took advantage of the unsettled conditions and paid accordingly. Those who didn't like the low wages could always rent a few hundred acres and sow some beets or barley, but even if they observed the backbreaking Mormon work ethic to the letter, they usually went broke.

Scott decided to break Lovell's grip on his life. He took some tests and won a scholarship to Western Wyoming College in Rock Springs, three hundred miles to the southwest. He didn't know what to study, but it wouldn't be bentonite. When Minda's big sister Marie suggested computer technology, he said, "Sure. Why not?"

Dr. Story seemed upset at the news. "How *can* you?" he asked Minda. "You've got a home here, you've got roots."

"Scott needs to go to computer school," Minda said, feeling defensive.

"Well, that's silly. You were just settling down here. You have a beautiful family. This is a lovely place to raise children. Why, you and Scott grew up here!"

She thought, Is this his idea of counseling? What's he so uptight about? He should be encouraging us. All we're trying to do is better ourselves.

Newly settled in a Rock Springs apartment, she was troubled by a crazy thought: Could Amber be Dr. Story's baby? The idea wouldn't go away. The child was certainly different. And he'd always acted as though she were special to him.

Minda had a hard time sorting out her feelings about this latest squawling Brinkerhoff. She felt resentful when Amber caused prob-lems, and then felt guilty about the resentment. She'd never been a demanding mother, but these days a wet diaper could send her into a tirade.

For a while, she lost herself in hard labor. She took orders at Taco Time, drove a Rock Springs school bus, hired on as a janitor for the Sweetwater County School District. One day she discovered that her throat was sore and her tongue swollen. A female doctor in Green River said, "You're worn out and you're a nervous wreck. Get this prescription filled. You've got to get hold of your life. Do it now!"

Minda ordered herself to stop dwelling so much on Dr. Story and Amber and her other problems. They were probably just a bunch of weird fixations. It wasn't long before she began to feel better. The prescription went unfilled.

Pregnant for the fourth time, she didn't want to make 400-mile round trips on icy roads to return to Dr. Story, but after three C-sections no obstetrician in Rock Springs would take her case. They told her to stick with the man who knew her best.

For the first six months of her pregnancy, she treated herself. Then she drove her children to Lovell and temporarily moved in with her parents. In the last two months of her pregnancy, Dr. Story gave her seven pelvics, each more painful than the last.

She selected Scott's birthday in December for the delivery in Lovell's hospital. At her request, Dr. Story also planned to give her a "bilateral tubal ligation and transection," which translated to "sterilization." She didn't care about the fancy terms; she just wanted to survive this birth and retire from the pregnancy business.

By now she knew the procedure backward. He would scrub her up, numb her abdomen, make his incision and burn away the old scar tissue. At that point her eyes would be closed, but she always smelled the charred flesh. Soon he would say, "Okay, I can see the baby. You're ready to go under." He would have a minute or two to lift the baby out. She would wake up and find out whether she'd had a girl or boy.

This time it was different.

Just as he was getting ready to start, there was a sharp knock on the delivery room door. A voice called out, "Dr. Story, it's an emergency."

Then he was gone. Minda was disgusted. She thought, Can't he ever get his act together? He's delivering my baby; what could be more important than that?

No one explained or apologized. Didn't they know she was scared? The anesthetist and the nurses acted as though she were a dead body at a surgical demonstration. They told doctor jokes, not one of them funny. She thought she would vomit, or die.

Dr. Story returned, sweat gleaming on his wide forehead. "Put her under!" he ordered.

She thought, What about the other steps? Why the hurry? A voice said, "Are you sure?"

"Put her under now!"

The next thing she knew, a nurse was showing her a chubby baby girl and informing her breathlessly that her father had suffered a heart attack. "Don't worry," the nurse told her. "He's out of danger." During the forty-five minutes she'd waited on the table, Dr. Story had been saving her dad's life.

When her head cleared, Minda felt sick all over again about her poor father, but infinitely better about the family doctor. He'd brought beautiful Shanardean (from "Shan" and "Arden" and "Dean") into the world with one hand and saved her dad with the other. Minda, she told herself, how could you ever distrust a man like that?

She decided that the experience with Bob Asay must have warped her mind. Dr. Story was *nothing* like Uncle Bob. He was a healer, not a pervert. The middle child offered up a prayer for her dad and the doctor. Wondrous were the ways of Father in Heaven!

After nine days in the hospital, she drove her baby back to Rock Springs, where Scott was finishing up his computer course, and went shopping for someone to remove her stitches. Once again the local physicians referred her to Dr. Story, but he was too far away and she didn't cherish the idea of a postnatal pelvic.

One of Scott's new friends, a fire department aidman, snipped out the stitches while Minda lay modestly draped in towels on her kitchen table.

A few days later, the incision began to weep, and she sped to Lovell. Dr. Story treated the problem, gave her a pelvic, and told her not to worry.

She said, "I really shouldn't be here, because we owe you a lot of money." The young Brinkerhoffs had no health insurance, and they owed a bundle to Dr. Story and several other specialists and hospitals.

He smiled and asked, "How much do you owe me?"

"Fifteen hundred," Minda said. She felt *so* ashamed. Her parents paid their bills on time.

Dr. Story asked, "How do you know it's that high?"

"I got a bill from Marilyn the other day. It said the bill had to be paid or else."

"Well," he said firmly, "you'll never receive another bill like that. You pay on it however you can and whenever you can. Don't worry about it."

Minda thought, Well, isn't that just like him! No wonder Mom takes him cinnamon rolls on his birthday.

6

Arden McArthur

SHE'D ALWAYS HAD visions and premonitions, and now she saw Dean slipping away. The city shoved a highway through their farm, appropriated some of their land, and clove the rest in two. It wasn't a farm anymore, but it didn't matter. Dean was too sick to work the big spread and tend all the animals, and he began to sell off the rest of their land and take part-time jobs that weren't too hard on his heart. He'd always been a two-hundred pounder, as sturdy as one of his beeves, but with congestive heart deterioration and so much forced inactivity, he soon ballooned up to nearly three hundred.

Dr. Story kept warning that he was eating his way into his family's burial plot. Dean complained to Arden, "I'm not going to the doctor just to be told I need to lose weight. I *know* that already." A few days later he was drawn up in pain, and she drove him to the clinic.

"I'm telling you, Dean," Dr. Story said in his whispery voice, "you have to lose weight." Dean moaned, too weak to argue. A few days later, he was rushed to Billings for open-heart surgery.

Through the difficult months, Dr. Story was always available by beeper or phone call, and Arden thanked the Lord for sending such a paragon to care for her loved ones. She told her children that their dad would already be waiting for them in the Celestial Kingdom if it weren't

for John Story. Sometimes her sick husband awoke in the middle of the
night sucking in air by the teaspoonful, eyes rolling like a tied calf's, his
big hands clenched and clammy. A telephone call brought Dr. Story in
ten minutes with his black bag and his soft voice and his calmness—
always so controlled, a rock for his patients.

Arden had done the Story clinic's washing for years, ever since the town
laundry had gone out of business. Helping a doctor, whether he was
LDS or not, came under the heading of "compassionate service," and
she tried to set a good example as a member of the Relief Society. But
Dean's heart problems were running the family bill up higher than their
cash flow could handle, and Dr. Story insisted that she receive financial
credits for her laundry work. "It's a pittance," she informed Dean, too
sick to respond. "I told him, 'I will do this for you as a friend.' " She
never noticed whether he adjusted their bill. And she still delivered
fresh-baked rolls to the doctor's home.

He'd treated her for arthritis for five or six years, tried several
different approaches to relieve her pain—cortisone, prednisone, hot
wax, sulfa, some drugs she couldn't spell. He told her she might have
rheumatic fever, and promised that he wouldn't give up till he'd made
her well.

The two true believers never stopped debating religion. Sometimes
Arden's half-hour appointment would stretch to two or three while they
worked at mutual conversion. They had a few harsh words after the
daughter of another Bible Church elder talked Arden's daughter Mia
into driving sixteen miles north to Frannie to watch a propaganda film
called *The God Makers*, which was nothing more than a frontal assault
on the Saints. Three hundred and fifty people attended, some of them
hooting with derision at sacred LDS rituals like baptism for the dead
and temple marriage, and Mia had come home upset. Arden suspected
that the Lovell Bible Church had financed the event and told Dr. Story
so.

He assured her that she was wrong. "Somebody wanted to show that
movie in our church and I told them absolutely not," he insisted. "I
knew it would offend my LDS friends." But he never denied that he'd
seen the film himself or approved of it. She suspected that he did.
It was a standard item in the Mormon-bashing hagiography, and she
was sure she'd heard some of its trickiest arguments echoing from
his mouth.

He continued to give her pelvic examinations, and she continued to attend in body only. A friend sitting in the waiting room asked her, "Why do his pelvics take so danged long?"

She thought, What a silly question. "Because he's thorough," she answered.

When others complained about waiting, Arden smiled and said, "This doctor's worth waiting for."

She talked him up wherever she went, even in places like the nearby oil towns Byron and Cowley, the Yellowstone jumping-off town of Cody, and the Big Horn county seat of Basin. She brought him dozens of new patients, including Dean's parents and her own. Once she even considered using him as a family counselor, but the Lord intervened to change her mind. A succession of female problems had diminished her sex drive, and she prayed for a way to be a better partner for the husband she loved. But . . . Heavenly Father was silent.

She thought, If He won't give me an answer, why can't I talk to my family doctor? She was dressing to go to the clinic when a voice spoke in her head: "Do not discuss anything with Dr. Story! He is a man of the world. He doesn't believe the same as you do. Everything will work out. *Don't discuss anything personal with him!*"

She thought, Why, Dr. Story loves us! We've entrusted our lives to him. He's performed surgery on every member of the family. He's keeping Dean alive.

But her "burnings in the bosom" were always on target, and as far as she was concerned, they came straight from Father in Heaven. She told Minda, "Honey, whatever you do, never discuss your private life with Dr. Story."

Minda said, "It's too late, Mother. That's one of the first things he asks. He already knows all about me and Scott."

"Well, don't discuss it anymore." She described the message and the voice, and Minda nodded. Arden told herself it was nice that her family understood her spirituality. Not every family would.

7

Meg Anderson

The psychopath hits upon conduct and creates situations so bizarre, so untimely, and so preposterous that their motivation appears inscrutable. Many of his exploits seem directly calculated to place him in a disgraceful or ignominious position.

—Hervey Cleckley, M.D.,
The Mask of Sanity

MEG THOUGHT, All those years looking for the right man, and he was under my nose the whole time!

She'd fallen in love with the straightest arrow in Lovell, the town milkman, Dan Anderson. She'd known him ever since the second grade, and now he'd been to college for a year and intended to finish up in psychology and police science and become a thinking man's cop. His family dated back to the Utah Mormons who'd come to dig the canals—righteous strong-backed pioneers with names like Heber and Alma and Seth. He'd already been on his mission, two years of pounding on doors in darkest Texas. He made Meg laugh with his description of southern Baptists: "They'd open the door and say, 'Not interested.' Then they'd invite me in for dinner."

Meg dated him a few times on visits to Lovell, and it didn't take him long to confess that he'd loved her for years. She took a good look and realized that he'd grown into a prize catch. He'd always been shy and likable—she remembered that. He kept his hands to himself and didn't try to push through her front door at the end of a date. He seemed secure in his maleness and didn't need to keep proving it, unlike so many of the men she'd met in college. She couldn't imagine him in a police uniform, packing a gun, but that was his decision. She decided it was the influence of his mother, Lovell's longtime police dispatcher. Mrs. Anderson knew all the town secrets. But she also knew how to keep them.

One lonely night in Moab, Utah, where Meg was teaching English and speech, she came back to her apartment and made a long-distance call to Lovell. "Honey," she told Dan, "let's get married and have a family."

"Well, sure," he said in the soft voice that reminded her of her sick father. "That's all I ever wanted."

There was one obstacle. She was twenty-six, and her voluptuousness continued to make her a target of a certain type of man. "I fell back a few times," she confessed to Dan. "I'm a submissive person and these guys kept coming on to me. It's my own fault, but it's long over now."

She explained that she'd moved to Moab from the college town of Logan to make a fresh start, thrown herself into LDS activities, and cried herself to sleep night after night. Sometimes guilt or shame would wake her up and she would grab her guitar for comfort; in troubled times, the McArthur clan had always fallen back on its music. But no matter how many hymns she sang, the message wouldn't stop playing in her mind: You've been with men. You're not worthy. *You're not worthy.* . . .

Dan said he understood and loved her all the more. But she wasn't sure that the church would be as forgiving. It was even possible that she could be excommunicated. She couldn't marry a devout Saint under such a dark cloud.

She asked her ward bishop to convene a church court, and she bared her soul. When she was asked if she felt she could change her life, she answered in a steady voice, "I already have." The high priests wiped her record clean.

In the fall of 1981, she married Dan in a civil ceremony. He helped her to run a children's clothing store bought by her father and mother with money from selling off acreage. Most of the nine McArthur children had left Lovell or planned to—the historical pattern for the region's young people—and Meg suspected that her parents had invested in the store to keep her and Dan in town. That was fine with her; she'd never wanted to leave in the first place.

Soon afterward, Dean and Arden added the dry cleaners on Main Street to their business assets, and sister Minda was summoned home from Rock Springs to run it. The sweat-shop work was perfect for her.

Meg remembered how the middle child had run the family tractor in hundred-degree weather and complained when their father made her stop.

Meg enjoyed having Scott and Minda around; the Andersons and the Brinkerhoffs met each other's needs. Scott had finished his two-year course in computer science and temporarily hired on as an oil company carpenter. Dan ran the Queen of the Valley Dairy and prepared to enroll at the community college in nearby Powell. Meg operated her store, Kids Are Special, and waited for a special kid of her own. After so much misery, her life as an Anderson seemed heavenly. Soon she was pregnant.

In his gentle way, Dan told her one night that he would be happier if Dr. Story didn't deliver their child. His family had broken with Story after he sent Dan's brother Jerry back into a high school football game with a damaged neck. These days the Andersons drove thirty miles to a doctor in Powell.

Meg told her mother, "I don't know what to do about a doctor."

Arden asked. "What's the matter with Dr. Story?"

"Well," she said, "Dan wants me to go to Dr. Haberland in Powell."

"You can't go to Powell," her mom said. "You need somebody here."

Meg hadn't forgotten Dr. Story's busy hands and painful precollege pelvic, but she was reluctant to disagree with her mother. Arden was still the little doctor's biggest advocate. And now that he was treating her father, Meg had begun to see him in a different light. Compared to what he was doing for the McArthurs, her own petty complaints about him were a joke. She was sure she'd overreacted to the pain of the pelvic. And the high school exams—well, maybe he was feeling her spleen or something when he put his hands down her pants. It was so easy to misunderstand a doctor, and so unfair.

So she resumed seeing him, and his pelvic exams hurt worse than ever. Dan would come home and see her sprawled on the sofa, barely able to move. "Oh," he would say. "You've been to Story." Sometimes the pain lasted three days.

Daniel Vincent Anderson arrived on July 3, 1982, but not before Dr. Story had made a radical incision extending through Meg's anal sphincter and part of her rectal wall, a forty-five-minute procedure requiring two hundred stitches.

She kept putting off her first postnatal examination because she was afraid it would hurt. Ever since the pregnancy, sex had been out of the question. Nine weeks after the birth, Dan's lightest touch made her jump. She decided to see if she'd been permanently damaged.

After an hour in the clinic's waiting room, she was prepped by the nurse and left naked under a sheet on the automatic table in Examining Room No. 2. Dr. Story arrived in his loose-fitting lab coat and his pleasant smile, told her how pretty she looked, and asked about her milk supply. She told him she thought she had a lump on one breast; he palpated her and told her she was normal.

She said, "I'm concerned about the way I'm healing. It hurts whenever Dan and I . . ." She let her voice trail off. "I never had an episiotomy before and I don't know how much soreness is okay."

He asked if she'd had the tightness problem before the birth, and she told him that it had always hurt at the start of intercourse—"but not like this."

He said, "You need to be dilated." She remembered that word from giving birth, when she'd needed to be "dilated' to ten centimeters before going to the delivery room. He said, "Let's take a look."

He adjusted the table so that her head was slightly raised, and turned on the water in the sink, an arm's length away. He always ran water during pelvic exams; she wondered what purpose it served, other than to dilute the sounds of Lawrence Welk and Mantovani. Around the house, she'd been overexposed to her father's favorite singer, Johnny Cash, but the clinic's weary music made her yearn for a few bars of "A Boy Named Sue" or even the Lennon sisters.

Dr. Story pulled on a pair of latex gloves, squeezed some gel from the big white tube, and began probing her uterine walls with a finger. "Does this hurt?" he asked.

"Yes," she said.

He pushed harder. "Did that hurt?"

"Oh, yes. It did!"

He tried again. The pain jerked her upward in the stirrups. He stepped back, peeled off his gloves, and left the room without a word. Here we go again, Meg said to herself. Another two-part torture. The discomfort was always worse in the second half, when he stationed himself between her legs.

She glanced at the counter to check out the speculum. Maybe it was a size too big. She'd been shown one in Utah during a pelvic exam; it was shaped a little like a duck's bill. There was nothing on Dr. Story's counter but the open tube of gel. She assumed he'd taken the instrument with him.

She was damp with sweat by the time he returned. He didn't seem to be carrying anything but his clipboard. His white lab smock hung open an inch or two.

He rinsed his hands and stepped to the foot of the table. "Can you move down?" he asked. He helped her slide a little beyond the end, so that a few inches of her bottom jutted into space. She clenched her fists and thought, This *has* to be done. She couldn't put Dan off forever.

She wished she could ask why it hurt so much, but she didn't dare. It was her old submissiveness again. The doctor could have beaten her with a horsewhip and she would have thanked him and paid her bill.

As the pain began, she tensed and twitched and hoped he wouldn't take offense. Salty beads formed on her face and burned her blue-green eyes.

He asked if it hurt. When she answered yes, he said, "Well, we'll just keep trying." She still couldn't bring herself to protest.

Something popped out of her insides and something else slid in. His hips moved closer. She thought, This must be the dilation. "Does that hurt?" he asked.

"Yes, it hurts."

He asked her several more times and she kept saying yes. She counted the squares on the ceiling. "Does it still hurt?" he asked, shoving the thing in hard.

"Yes," she said. "It all feels the same." It hurt the way sex hurt at home, but worse. And it *felt* the way sex felt. She thought, If I wanted to endure this much pain, I could be having sex with Dan. *No! My word, what am I thinking? He's my doctor!*

He probed around for five or ten more minutes, then asked, "Should I go any further?"

"It all feels the same," she repeated. An ugly feeling came over her. Something's wrong, she said to herself. Something's *wrong*. This feels too much like Dan.

She lifted her head to see. His head and shoulders were visible above the sheet that stretched across her raised knees. He was staring at her face.

"How's it feel?" he asked.

She bit her lip and repeated, "All the same."

The dilation went on forever. She didn't know whether she blacked out, but she heard him telling her to come back in two weeks. She looked up to see the tail of his white coat disappearing out the door. She had the feeling that she'd let him down.

As she dressed, she wondered if she had an abnormally low threshold of pain. Or was she just weak? No one else in the family complained about Dr. Story's exams. She wondered if she was just making something out of nothing again. She and Dan planned the traditional Mormon family; there were plenty of pelvic exams in her future. She couldn't turn every one into the last act of *Medea*.

As she left the clinic, she looked at her watch. Her first postnatal visit had lasted three hours.

She tried to erase the scene from her mind. She told Dan that Dr. Story had dilated her so that they could start making love again, but she was still too sensitive. The subject was dropped.

She stayed tender and thought of consulting her mother about postchildbirth experiences. But she could already hear her mom's answer: *If Dr. Story did it, it was proper. You're danged lucky to have him.*

And anyway, the more she thought about it, the more she realized she'd probably overreacted. If he'd used his penis, wouldn't she have heard his zipper? She decided that she'd just been on another flight of fancy—Meg being Meg. Dr. Story was the only person she would trust with her baby's life, and every McArthur felt the same about him.

She reminded herself that she'd been tender long before she'd gone in for the pelvic. She thought, That wasn't Dr. Story's fault, was it? How could he possibly dilate you without hurting you? Of *course* the instrument felt like a penis. Anything that would fill a passageway wide enough for babies would have to be pretty thick. That was the whole point of dilation.

She phoned her sister in Idaho Falls and asked how long a woman should wait to have intercourse after childbirth. It was the first time she'd ever discussed the forbidden subject with any member of her family.

Michele told her, "If you're not healed by four months, you better go in and find out what's wrong."

Meg marked a date on the calendar.

In October, a month before the time was up, she was sealed to her husband and son in the beautiful soaring temple at Idaho Falls. Nothing in her life had prepared her for the majesty of the ceremony or the glow she felt afterward. It was every Saint's dream: the sacred ritual, the music, the flowers, the white-robed Temple attendants gliding in and out of the sealing room, the anointment with oil and the laying on of hands, the bestowal of the secret name. She could hardly breathe for excitement. Six years had passed since her disgrace in Logan; she'd lived through shame and misery to make herself worthy again. She thought, No one can ever take this away from me—now it's Dan and Daniel and Meg Anderson, together for time and all eternity.

She had to face the problem of what to do about wearing the sacred LDS garment on her revisit to Dr. Story. Four months after Daniel's birth, nothing had improved in the bedroom. The few times Dan had tried, gentle and loving as always, the pain had left her breathless. She was beginning to suspect that something was seriously wrong.

She checked around and found that some Mormon women bathed one leg at a time so their sacred garment remained on, but the decision was personal, not a matter of holy writ. That being the case, she certainly didn't intend to wear her garment in front of a Gentile male.

She returned to the clinic with the idea that she would pay close attention this time and dispel her silly suspicions. How stupid it would be to lose the best doctor in the whole Big Horn Basin over a girlish misapprehension!

She noticed two changes at the outset. He didn't run the water and he kept the nurse in the room after she took the gel and the surgical gloves out of the cabinet. Meg guessed he had no hard and fast rules; maybe the nurse stayed in when she wasn't busy and left when she was needed elsewhere. If he was up to something, wouldn't he keep her out every time? Meg thought, One point for Dr. Story!

The finger probing was uncomfortable, but less so than on the previous visit. He asked if sex still hurt and she said it did. "Maybe I sewed you up too tight," he said.

As he and the nurse were leaving the room, he told her, "Don't get up. I have more to check."

Alone on the table, she looked around the small room to see if she could spot the instrument he would be using in the second half. The water was still turned off. Nothing was in sight except the latex gloves.

When he returned, she watched carefully from her supine position. She wanted to see if his fly was open, but it was concealed beneath his smock. He turned on the water and told her he was going to dilate her with a "tube." She wondered where the tube was and felt apprehensive.

Once again he rearranged her so that her bottom protruded. He moved into position at the foot of the table and slid into the V of her thighs. His hands were out of sight. Something pushed into her vagina, and the same dark feeling came over her. She thought, My land, it can't be. *It can't be* . . .

He pressed a finger to her abdomen and kept asking, "Does this hurt? Does *this* hurt? How about here? Does it hurt here? *Here?*"

To herself she said, Oh, Dan, what's he doing to me? She tried to keep up with the questions, but the pain was bad. The worse the pain the deeper he pushed inside her. Sweat made her blink.

"Now I have to dilate you," he said, looking straight into her eyes. "If you let me keep working with you, you'll find you can have intercourse with your husband. You'll get rid of the pain."

She wanted to jump up and run, but he stood between her and the door. She counted the ceiling tiles as he asked again, "Does that hurt?" She tried to answer but couldn't catch her breath.

He stepped to the sink and rinsed his hands. When he turned back to the table, she lowered her head so he wouldn't see her watching. She was sure her life was in danger. If he would do this, what *wouldn't* he do?

He slid back into position. Something brushed along her pubic hair. He asked softly, "Would you like to guide it in?"

She was paralyzed. She thought, I can't believe this is happening, and I can't do a danged thing about it. But oh, how it hurts! Please, Lord, please, *make it be over.* . . .

The "tube" moved slowly in and out for two or three more minutes while he studied her face and inquired about the pain. The next time he asked if it hurt, she managed to blurt out, "No!" If he was the sadistic monster that she now suspected, that might turn him off.

It worked. He stepped back and said, "Get dressed." As he walked into the hall, she saw that his hands were empty.

She inhaled deeply, then searched for a tube to make absolutely sure she hadn't been mistaken. Clutching the upper and lower sheet to her body, she checked out every inch of the small room. There was no tube.

She didn't open the cupboard, but neither had he. A surgical glove lay crumpled in the sink.

She dressed and walked out without acknowledging the receptionist. She hurt so much that she wasn't sure she could make it to her car. Two and a half hours had elapsed. She thought, That's how long it takes him to satisfy himself. I didn't want to believe it, I didn't want to lose my lifelong doctor. What on earth do I do next?

She couldn't bring herself to tell anyone, not even Dan. For days, she went around with her knuckles to her mouth. She asked herself, How could he! After six years of misery I go through the temple and change my whole life, and then a doctor, our family's friend, a man who's supposed to love us, does this . . . this . . . sick, disgusting, *unmentionable* thing.

She wondered what it was about her that drew the sickos. They seemed to sense her vulnerability. What made Story choose her from hundreds of patients? She'd been Uncle Bob's first victim, too. When she thought about the ramifications, she felt as though she were going in and out of shock—rapid heartbeat, fluttery pulse, chills and fever. She thought, I've got a little sister Mia, and he's her doctor. And he's Minda's doctor, and Mom's. If he's turned rank, what might he do to them!

She thought back on his touchy-feely high school exams, and the time when he'd interrupted her pelvic and claimed that he couldn't get it in far enough. Couldn't get *what* in far enough? She realized that he'd been doing it to her for years. She could just die of shame.

She visited with Minda—the two young families now shared a house at 1115 Road 11½—and Meg confided, "This is gonna sound crazy, Minda, but I had a funny feeling at the clinic the other day. It felt like Dr. Story was dilating me with his, uh—penis."

Minda frowned, then laughed and said, "I've seen his penis, too. Four years ago."

Meg said, "Oh, my goodness, no!" She wondered if Minda was kidding. She often deflected touchy subjects with jokes.

Minda giggled and said, "I think he forgets to zip up after he goes potty."

They exchanged nervous laughter and a few more absurdities, and Meg was relieved when the conversation ended. She realized that she'd been looking for approval when she brought the subject up; she needed someone to tell her that Dr. Story was to blame and she hadn't led him on, intentionally or otherwise. But maybe Minda wasn't the right person to grant absolution. Neither sister had ever been able to talk comfortably about sex, and certainly not about this crime of—what? Was it rape? Invasion of privacy? She had no idea what the law would call it. Of course the law would never find out. She could never tell a soul about such a shameful thing.

8

Minda Brinkerhoff

The commonality among pornography, gynecology, and sex crime is further underscored by the shared icon of the *spread-eagled*, i.e. the punished, debased, and defeated female body.

—Jane Caputi,
The Age of Sex Crime

AFTER she finished talking to Meg, the middle child wondered why Dr. Story didn't get it together. Can't he examine people without making them suspicious? Does he have to be so *rough*? He's even got poor Meg upset.

She was glad the conversation was short. She'd stopped worrying about the family doctor and didn't want to revive her fears. How could she explain to Meg that she'd gone over the whole thing a thousand times in her mind and it added up to a big fat nothing?

Now that they were back in Lovell sharing a home with Meg and Dan, the young Brinkerhoffs' finances were improving. With Scott's skills, it wasn't long before he was running his own carpentry crew in the oil fields and bringing home a good paycheck. Minda was making the Lovell Cleaners pay off for her co-owners, Arden and Dean. The $1200 monthly mortgage payment left no money for wages, but the equity was building. Minda knew all about working for nothing. At heart she was a Mormon farmer, an end product of LDS history. Once the prophet Brigham Young had beckoned his wagon train to a halt, looked out on an alkali waste and a fishless lake, and announced, "This is the place!" Other Saints had worked the same miracle in Lovell.

Minda felt she was creating her own version in the family's steaming, scorching cleaning shop. Every day she would tag the clothes, go through the pockets, spray solvent on armpit and crotch, stuff the clothes into the cleaning machine, pull them out and peel them apart, press them in the clamp-down press, then hang them on hangers for Mrs. Kelly, the old lady who ran the front and did the books and had been around for years.

Summer turned the dry cleaners into a hissing blast furnace. Minda loved the discomfort. She'd had arthritis from childhood; the heat warmed her bones and gave her a measure of relief. Not even Dr. Story had been able to do as well. They figured her arthritis was congenital; her mom suffered from it, too.

Scott added a moonlighting job to his work in the oil fields and Minda adjusted her schedule accordingly. She put the four children to bed at seven and dry-cleaned other people's clothes till midnight. The old bills weren't getting paid off fast enough to suit her, so she hired her sister Meg to baby-sit the kids and took a daytime job at the Queen Bee Gardens east of town. From 8 A.M. on, she worked the hives, helped to make honey candy, and built up her immunity by getting stung. At 5 P.M. she sped home to make supper for the kids, put them to bed, and worked till midnight at the cleaners.

The symptoms hit five months later. Her tongue and throat became irritated from the dry solvent in the prespotter. The arthritis in her hips forced a steady diet of Motrin. She had a semipermanent cold and a permanent headache.

Her mother insisted that she see Dr. Story. "Oh, Mom," Minda said, "he always gives me pelvics, and I hate 'em."

"If he gives you a pelvic, there's a reason," Arden said. Minda thought, Gol, Mom, you sound like a broken record.

When her throat was so swollen that she couldn't eat solid food, she made an appointment, canceled it, made another a week later and canceled again, then phoned in to cancel a third. The receptionist, a family friend and Mormon sister named Diana Harrison, said, "Minda, you've really got to get in here and see Doctor." That was his regular name around the clinic: "Doctor," as though it were a proper name.

"Well, Diana," Minda said, "I—"

"Come up right now, Minda, and we'll work you in. It's for your own good."

———

In Examining Room No. 2, Dr. Story squeezed her breasts. "Your children are healthy and beautiful, I'm sure," he said in his soft voice. "Just like their mother. How's Amber Dawn?"

"Fine," Minda answered. She sat on the table and thought, He won't hurt me. He cares too much for me and the children.

She described her symptoms while he studied his clipboard. "It's been eight months since you were in," he said.

"I know," Minda said. She didn't want to admit that she'd deliberately stayed away. It wasn't his fault she was chicken. "My hips hurt," she said quickly. "I think it's from working on those concrete floors. When I get upset, my stomach has fits. Tums don't even touch it."

"You can't be as sick as you think, Minda," he said, smiling. "You look too nice."

He pushed at her stomach and she tucked it in. "Feels good," he commented.

He told her she needed a pelvic examination for her hips. She thought back on all the times she'd been dilated for colds, bee stings, kitchen burns, pregnancies, a nail puncture, sometimes even for vaginal problems. She thought, It's a wonder he recognizes me by my face.

"I've had so much trouble with my tongue," she said. "Is there such a thing as a tongue transplant?"

He laughed with her, and said, "No, there's no such thing."

"The last time my throat and tongue were this sore," she said, "I went to a doctor downstate and she told me I was having a breakdown. Not mentally, but physically. I was just worn down."

"Well, I don't know about that," he said. "Are you taking care of yourself? Maybe you shouldn't be working at the cleaners' if it's too hard on you."

He got up from his stool, took a paper sheet from the closet, and said, "We'll get ready for the exam."

He was just stepping out of the room when she asked, "What about my throat and tongue?"

"Oh," he said, "I forgot."

He made her say "ah" and depressed her tongue with a wooden stick. "I don't know what to tell you," he said. "It looks fine to me."

She didn't understand. The last time she'd looked at her throat in the mirror, it looked like raw hamburger. Her tongue was a swollen lump. Had there been a miracle cure?

He returned in fifteen minutes and turned on the water. He warmed his hands and the speculum, then began probing at her insides. "You've healed very nicely," he said. "You could have another baby."

"Hunh-uh," Minda reminded him, "you tied my tubes."

"Oh," he said. "I didn't remember. You're really pink inside. You look really nice. But I'll have to get in further to see if everything's okay. If I dilated you it would help make things go a lot easier."

Minda mumbled, "Okay."

When it was all over, Dr. Story handed her some drug samples and told her to return in a couple of days, "to see if I can get in further," and then again a week after that.

She walked to her car in a daze and sat for ten minutes trying to decide what to do. Then she headed for her mother's house to sound the alarm.

9

Meg Anderson

MINDA and her four children had been gone for three hours, and Meg wondered what was up. Now that the sisters were sharing the same house, they kept closer tabs on each other, especially with Meg pregnant again.

It was a lovely spring day in the Big Horn Basin. Meg drove to her mother's and found Arden baby-sitting Minda's kids. "Where's Minda?" Meg asked.

"Up at the doctor's," her mom answered.

"For three hours?"

"Well, you know how slow he is."

Meg was just leaving to pick up Dan at the Queen of the Valley Dairy when Minda drove pell-mell into the driveway, slammed on the brakes, and jumped out as though fleeing for her life. Her skin was as white as her mother's summer skirt, and her face was streaked with tears.

"Meg!" she announced loudly. "Dr. Story will *not* deliver your baby!" Then she turned to her mother and yelped, "He's kinky! He's kinky! Don't you dare tell me he's not. *Don't you dare!*"

Meg saw that her sister was trembling. Her blue-green eyes were red, and she teetered on her pumps like a drunk. Arden said, "Oh,

Minda, no! Now didn't we go through this before? Dr. Story would *never* do that."

Minda's skinny arms flopped like broken wings as she stomped back and forth in the driveway. "Slow down," her mom kept repeating. "Let's talk about it." Meg saw that her mother's face was ashen.

"No!" Minda said in a hysterical voice. "I've got to get the kids home." She brushed past her mother toward the house. "My undergarments are full of semen."

Meg didn't want to get into a discussion with her mother about Dr. Story. As she drove away, she thought, He did it to me and now he's done it to Minda! *Why us?*

Whatever had happened, she realized that it couldn't be brushed off. Other female relatives were coming along, including her sister Mia. Someone had to face reality.

When Meg and Danny got home, she phoned Jan Asay, Dr. Story's nurse. As she dialed the number, she said to herself, Jan's married to my cousin. She's family. She'll tell me the truth.

"Jan," she said, "this is in confidence. Listen, what does Dr. Story use that might feel like a penis?"

"During pelvics?" the nurse asked.

"Yeah. It feels like a tube and it's kinda soft and warm and it, uh, fills you up."

"Meg, I don't know," Jan said. She sounded puzzled. "He has a metal tray and it's got the duckbill in it, the speculum. But it clinks around and you can hear it. I don't know about any tube."

"What if I didn't see a tray and there was no clinking?"

"Meg, I don't know."

"Does he use anything that could feel like a penis?"

Jan said, "Not that I know of." She asked why Meg wanted to know, and Meg told her the truth. Jan sounded disturbed. Meg wondered if anyone had ever asked the same questions, but she couldn't bring herself to ask.

After the dinner dishes were put away, the sisters huddled in a quiet corner and shared their stories in voices just above a whisper. Minda said, "There's no way I can tell Scott. He'd kill him."

Meg said, "I don't know how much longer I can keep this from Dan." It made her feel sick to admit that she still hadn't been able to tell her husband. "He knows everything about me except this. But Minda, I was so ashamed."

Minda nodded.

"This is a moral sin," Meg went on, "and a moral sin has to be taken to the bishop." She was thinking, Minda and I both hold Temple Recommends, and that means we have to live worthy lives. Their spiritual futures were at stake.

"I know," Minda said. She didn't sound enthusiastic.

Meg said, "I want to ask the bishop what to do. Do I tell Dan or not? I need some guidance."

She phoned and made an appointment to meet Bishop Larry Sessions the next afternoon at three.

Before she left for the interview, she called upstairs to Minda, "Are you coming with me?"

"I guess I should," Minda said. She sounded uncertain.

"Yes, I guess you should!" Meg said with a big sister's authority.

Meg had known Larry Sessions for years. He worked with his brother-in-law Bob Asay—Uncle Bob—at the furniture store. People said the two of them dabbled in stripper oil wells and other modest enterprises. Sessions was responsible for the moral and religious welfare of some two hundred Mormons in the Third Ward, one of six wards that made up the Lovell Stake. Like most LDS bishops, he was known as a pure and righteous man. This news, Meg said to herself as the sisters entered the store, is gonna knock him off his horse.

Brother Sessions invited them to sit on a couch covered with transparent plastic. "What is it?" he asked. His face showed concern. Meg thought, We must look like we just came from a hanging.

"We have something to tell you that's just gonna floor you," Minda said in her high-speed delivery, "and it's something that's just terrible and it's bad for me to even be thinking about it."

Meg chimed in, "But it's something that we have to tell you to get off our chests. We—"

Minda interrupted. "We think that Dr. Story has violated us."

The bishop listened patiently as they added details, then said, "Girls, I thought you were going to tell me something I didn't know. I've been hearing these reports for over five years."

Meg felt the hair stand up on her neck. She was horrified, then hurt, then angry. She flashed on her little sister Mia, lying on Story's table any day now, losing her virginity and not even knowing it. How many others had he deflowered the same way? She said, "Five years? Then why did I have to go through this? Why wasn't it taken care of five years ago?"

"There's nothing we can do," Brother Sessions said. "We can't prove anything. I just tell the women to change doctors."

"Change . . . doctors?" Meg asked.

"Yes. And you should tell your husbands what happened, too."

Minda said, "I can't. I just can't."

"Well, then, Minda, wait till you're more comfortable about it." The bishop turned to Meg. "I think you should tell Dan right away."

Meg drove to the dairy to break the news. She had no idea how Danny would react. He was a mellow man with a relaxed, forgiving attitude toward people, but he also had a cop's mentality about molesters and perverts.

Meg told the story in an agitated burst, talking almost as fast as Minda. At first Dan didn't seem to react. He turned away and she could see that he was upset. After a while he said softly, "Your challenge and mine is understanding."

She breathed again.

"I oughta do something to him," he went on. His words came out in terse little bites. "Some guys would blow him away. But I won't make that mistake. I could end up in prison. I refuse to risk losing my family for John Story. He's not worth it."

Meg agreed. She told Dan that she'd informed the church.

"That's good," he said. "They'll take care of it." She couldn't bring herself to tell him that the high priests had known about Story for five years.

By the time she phoned her mother, the sun was starting to slide down the back of the purple mountains to the west. "Mom," she said, "we've been to see the bishop."

"Who's been to see what bishop?" Arden asked.

"Minda and I."

"What about?"

"About Dr. Story."

"Meg," her mom said in her stoniest voice, "what are you trying to tell me?"

Meg wished she had better control of her emotions, but she was afraid she wouldn't be able to conceal her anger—toward Story, toward the bishop, even toward her mother. "We visited with him and he said he's been having complaints like this for five years."

Arden sounded confused. "Complaints like *what?*"

"Mom, we've been violated by Dr. Story."

There was a long silence on the phone line, and then her mom snapped back, "What do you mean, 'violated'? Be specific. I don't know what you're saying."

"Mom," Meg said, lowering her voice, "we think Dr. Story has been dilating patients with his penis."

Another long silence came over the line. "Mom?" Meg said. The silence continued till Meg said "Mom?" again.

Then she heard her mother whimpering. "No," Arden said. "No, Meg, *no.*" Wrenching sobs came over the phone. "Don't tell me any more!"

"Mom, the bishop said he'd been having these complaints for five years. And Minda has wondered for four."

"No!"

"He told us to change doctors. There's nothing else we can do about it."

"I can't believe that." Her mother didn't seem to be crying now.

"Well, that's what the bishop said," Meg told her.

Arden insisted that they inform their dad right away. "He has to know. Sick or not, he's our strength."

Dean McArthur's face turned blood-red. Meg worried about another heart attack. He asked some of the same questions her mother had asked, then picked up the phone and dialed a doctor friend in California. "Do doctors ever insert some kind of tube in a woman," he asked, "when they're doing routine office inspections?" He listened for a minute, said "Thanks," and turned back to his wife and daughters.

"No," he said. "They don't. Never. You girls were abused."

10

Minda Brinkerhoff

IT TOOK the middle child six days to get up the courage to tell Scott. When she tried, the words stuck in her mouth. Fingers trembling, she handed him a copy of a long letter she'd prepared in case they decided to go to a lawyer. He frowned and flopped into a chair. She sat on the armrest as he read:

He stood between my legs, looking at my face, and began to dialate me. I was tight, right? I was. He went in further. Tight here also, right? Further he went in. Tight here, right? Yes. Next he pushed all the way in and it hurt me terrible. I turned red and started to sweat. That was what always happened.

Why was he looking at my face? Nowhere else, just in my face. Again. It hurts there? Yes it did.

Then he said, "Let me pull out a little." Very slowly he pulled out and then he said, "Let me try again." He pushed back in. It hurt me. Out he pulled again and asked, "It still hurts there?"

"Yes, it does."

"Well, I'll try one more time and if I can't get in far enough, we'll quit. Do you think it would help if you guided it in?"

I responded, "No, I'm sure it wouldn't."

He pushed in one more time and tears rolled down my face. He turned around to the sink and did something, walked up to the side of the exam table and began pushing on my bladder and what not. My hands were at the sides of the table. Something long and soft slipped underneath the cup of my hand.

I left my hand there. It was poking my side and sliding in and out of my hand. Very slowly I lifted my hand, watching everything I was doing, and underneath my hand was his penis. He didn't care if I saw it.

He continued to push two more times on my stomach, then walked very cautiously back to his sink. I'm sure I went into shock. I couldn't believe it. It was true and I was back in there for more. What was I thinking of?

At this point I should have up and left. I don't know what happened to my senses. I just laid there. It was unreal.

He turned around and asked me to stand up with the paper sheet held in front of me. I did so. He then said he would see what was wrong with my hips. He asked me to squat with my legs together. I did and as I did I could feel his clothes up against me as he squatted with me. Now right arm touching left shoulder and squat. Legs together, legs apart. Then left arm up over to right shoulder. Squat; legs together, legs apart. And then, the killer. "Minda, do you think it would be easier if I went in from behind?"

"No, Dr. Story, I think you have gotten in as far as you are going to get." How stupid of me. I can't believe what an idiot I was. I should have said something—done something. How could I let this happen?

He left and I got dressed. When I was getting dressed, I took the paper sheet and wiped so much crap from between my legs it wasn't funny. I looked at it, felt it, let some dry on my fingers. It looked just like, felt just like and dried just like male discharge that I'd wipe from myself after having intercourse with my husband.

The letter fell from Scott's hands. He shut his eyes so tightly that squiggly lines formed on his face. "Did you lead him on, Minda?" he asked. "Is this something you brought on yourself? Why didn't you—"

"Oh, Scott, how can you ask?"

"—come to me first? Why would Dr. Story do a thing like that in his own office?"

He couldn't seem to picture the gymnastics on the automatic table. Minda had to remind herself that her husband was a Lovell Mormon; he'd never discussed sex with anyone. He had no idea what pelvic exams were or why they were necessary. He seemed hurt that Minda hadn't let him in on the information years ago.

No explanation satisfied him. "How could he do this without you knowing?" he asked more than once.

It seemed to her that he was being plumb obstinate. Maybe it was because Story had delivered him and he'd never been to another doctor. Or maybe it was because he'd helped his father build the Story clinic and felt loyal. It was Scott who'd lovingly crafted the artistic wooden placard and burnt in the words "Lovell Medical Clinic." The senior

Brinkerhoffs, Dorothy and Gerald, still owned 40 percent of the building. The family had a big interest in John Story.

Scott drove off to work in a squeal of rubber and didn't speak when he returned.

Meg phoned to remind her that they had to see the stake president to "make things right." He'd approved their Temple Recommends, and moral matters concerning those who'd been through the temple had to be resolved at the highest local level, not by the ward bishop alone. Minda was sure that the brethren would take steps to protect their women; the church had majesty and power behind it, and members in high places. Dr. Story was just a sick little weirdo.

She counted back and realized that he'd probably been violating her for six or seven years. She told herself, I let him get away with it for so long that he probably thought I don't mind! Maybe that's why he turned so bold. *Minda, do you think it would be better if I went in from behind?* What would the stake president think about that?

President John Abraham, spiritual leader of two thousand Mormons in the Lovell stake, was a middle-aged farmer who lived in an old ranch house near Byron, twenty miles west of Lovell. As a child, he'd been so close to her mother that Arden still thought of him as kin. Whatever he'll do, Minda said to herself as she stepped into the cavernous, empty church, it'll be in our interests.

At first, the old friend of the family seemed sympathetic as he sat with fingertips touching in his church office, but as soon as she mentioned Dr. Story, she noticed a change. The stake president was a nice man, a pleasant man, not at all stern or schoolteacherish, but his face showed disbelief. "Dr. Story violated you?" he asked. "*Dr. Story?*"

"Yes."

After she'd finished with the details, he asked, "Why didn't you jump up and leave?"

She tried to explain. He let her finish, then said, "Look, there are certain questions I have to ask you, because I have to find out where you stand in the church. Did you have an affair with Dr. Story?"

"No."

"Did you ever meet him outside his office—"

"No!"

"—for a drink or something?"

"Absolutely not. I'm sorry you asked me that. He was my family doctor since I was a baby."

"It's not you," the stake president said apologetically. "I have to ask these questions. I *have* to. You could lose your membership over this."

"I understand," Minda said. She thought, I've come to my church for comfort and reassurance, and my own stake president makes me feel like Jezebel. She started to cry.

He asked, "Has anything like this happened to you before?"

She gave him a brief rundown about Bob Asay, and he looked shocked. "That happened before I was stake president," he said, almost as though he were apologizing. "This is the first I've ever heard."

Everyone in town knew that Uncle Bob was going to be married in the temple, which meant that the ward bishop and President Abraham must have signed his Recommend. Asay also had influence in Salt Lake City; a relative sat in the inner councils of the church. Minda wondered if any action would be taken against him this time. She certainly didn't want to run into Bob Asay in the Celestial Kingdom. One McArthur or another had brought the matter to the church's attention at least three times now, but Asay was still a Saint in good standing.

The stake president acted as though he'd heard enough history. "Let's get back to Dr. Story," he challenged her. "What in the world made you think he wasn't using an instrument to dilate you?"

"I saw—"

"But you said you couldn't see past the sheet."

Tears choked her voice as she realized she wasn't reaching him. He asked her how high the table was, and how far her buttocks had pooched out. She stood alongside his table and held her hand about three feet off the floor. "It was about this high, and his coat fell in front so I could only see one end of his penis, and—"

The president's face was a mask. She had the feeling she could have drawn him pictures, could have climbed up on the table and performed a demonstration, and he still wouldn't have believed.

"My wife goes to Story," he mumbled. He talked about his wife for a few minutes. She'd had ten children, but it sounded as though she'd had very few pelvic examinations.

Minda tried to bring him back to the subject. "What do I do next?" she asked.

He paused. "Drop it," he ordered. "Don't ever go back to him."

"What about the other sisters? Isn't the church gonna protect them?"

"We can't take a stand against Dr. Story. It would cause too many problems. There's no proof. It's your word against his. This isn't a religious matter anyway."

Minda thought, Of course there's no proof! How could we prove it unless we brought a camera to the danged examining room? "But he did it to Meg!" she said. "And the bishop said he's been hearing these stories for five years."

"Well I haven't."

She asked if she should go to the police or the state medical society, or maybe get a lawyer and sue. "Drop it, Minda," he repeated. "You're just asking for trouble."

After forty-five minutes, he warned her that she could be excommunicated if she returned to the clinic on the hill. Then he smiled and said, "I'm glad you came in and straightened things out."

She thought, Straightened *what* out? I wish I'd stayed home. She left sobbing.

Her silent Scott was no comfort. When she reached out for him in bed, he pulled away. She knew what he was thinking: *Why should I touch her now that Story's touched her?* She was hurt, but she understood. Scott was hurt, too. She wished she knew how to regain his trust.

11

Arden McArthur

ARDEN couldn't shake off feelings of guilt and shame. Talking about it later, she was harder on herself than anyone. "Instantaneously, after all those years," she said, "I knew that Minda was telling me the truth. But I wasn't composed enough to know what to do. I was ignorant."

She moped around her house, provided no comfort to her daughters or her husband, made no decisions or plans. Remorse disabled her brain. She prayed that she would wake up and find that Dr. Story was still her friend and her daughters were still bound for the Celestial Kingdom, pure and undefiled in their flowing white robes.

A few times she almost talked herself into believing her own fantasy, but too many images flooded back—the girls coming home upset, the complaints by others, the persistent rumors, the way Story's exams took so long and hurt so much more than other doctors'. As president of her ward's Relief Society, Arden wore the mantle of truth, like a bishop. She was dumbfounded that Minda had gone in with a throat problem and ended up in the stirrups.

An unsettling thought began to flicker across her mind like a ghost image on TV. Had Story abused her, too, in between the talks about God and the sugary compliments? She thought, *Did he do it to me all those times I was off in space?* At the very least, he'd set her up, won himself a prominent LDS supporter who ran around town like a danged fool telling everyone what a good man he was while he was raping the danged fool's own children.

She felt like a coconspirator. She tried to imagine who else might know the truth. Maybe Diana Harrison, his receptionist. There'd been a phone call from Diana minutes after Minda had left for home, still half hysterical. "We've got laundry up here," Diana had said.

Arden had gone dead on the line. "Ard," Diana had asked in her sweet voice, "are you still there? You *will* pick up the laundry, won't you?"

Arden had choked back tears. "Yes," she'd said. "First thing tomorrow morning."

Diana looked concerned. "There's something wrong," she told Arden as she handed over the bag of soiled sheets and smocks. "What is it?"

Arden began to cry.

"Tell me!" Diana insisted. She was a petite, pretty woman, mother of a child whom Story had treated from birth for a serious urethral blockage. The two Mormon sisters often sewed together, and they'd been working on a junior prom dress, a darling little thing made out of gunnysack fabric that cost twenty-five cents a yard, for the McArthurs' youngest daughter, Mia. Diana was now in her late twenties; she'd been Story's receptionist off and on since high school. "There's something wrong," Diana repeated. "I could tell it on the phone yesterday. Is it about—Doctor?"

Arden nodded.

Diana took her by the shoulders, squared her around, and said, "I have a right to know! I work for him. *I have a right to know!*"

Arden couldn't bring herself to respond. It was just dawning on her that she could have shut Story down twelve years ago, when she'd refused to listen to Dottie Parry, or three and a half years ago, when Minda had voiced her first complaint. Neither of her daughters would have been violated if it hadn't been for her own mulishness.

Diana said, "It has to do with Minda, doesn't it? I thought there was something wrong when she left yesterday. She was white as a sheet."

Arden shouldered the laundry bag. The receptionist was still chattering as she left, something about other complaints against "Doctor." She
couldn't bear to listen.

Sometimes Arden didn't get around to the laundry for two or three
days, but she did up this load right away and headed back to the clinic.
She'd expected to see Diana again and brought along Mia's prom dress.
Instead, Marilyn Story answered the back door.

Arden tried to act nonchalant. Weren't wives always the last to
know? She showed Marilyn the dress and asked what she thought of it.
The two friends chatted until the door of Examining room No. 2
opened and Dr. Story strolled out with a woman. Both their faces were
flushed. His smock rustled as he brushed past without even saying
hello. "Where've you been" he asked his wife in a compressed voice.
"What've you been doing?"

Marilyn looked shocked and said, "Why, I've been standing here
visiting with my laundrywoman." Arden was baffled. The three of them
had been close for years; when had she become "the laundrywoman"?
The day he attacked Minda?

He issued some orders and spun away, still avoiding her eyes. Arden
thought, Well, if I had any doubts, they're gone now. Usually he
falls all over me. What could this coldness be but a blunt admission
of guilt?

When she got home, Dean was sitting in the living room, breathing
hard. Since hearing about Story and the girls, he'd gone downhill. His
life was bound up in his nine children. Some of the townspeople
thought he was uppity because he didn't bother to make friends, but
every friend he wanted lived in his own house.

He bemoaned the potential scandal, the notoriety. In both looks and
attitudes, he favored his mother, Zilla Harris McArthur, whose patri-
cian face seemed copied from a carved cameo brooch. Dean's mother
was of the opinion that a person's name should be in the newspapers
three times: at birth, marriage and death. Old-time Mormons avoided
public strife or confrontation. Dean had torn up accounts receivable
rather than make a fuss about nonpayment.

When Arden described the latest incident at the clinic, he said,
"Ard, you want to remember, if we do anything about this, we're gonna
lose our business." He was talking about the dry cleaners and Kids Are
Special. The farm was already lost, and the two downtown businesses
were their only source of income.

"Well, Dean," she said, "I'm just plumb stupid, and I'm gonna do something about it."

She wished that the bishop and the stake president were more encouraging. They kept repeating that John Story wasn't LDS and therefore their hands were tied. She thought, I've always had the false idea that if something goes wrong in my life, I can go to the high priests and they'll help make it right. She thought back on the time she and Dean had reported Bob Asay to the bishop. Come to think of it, nothing had been done about that, either.

More than ever, she realized that her spiritual life was strictly between her and Father in Heaven. The elders listened to problems but solved nothing. From here on in, she would deal with the Lord one on one. She was glad that it didn't take Him long to make contact.

A seventy-year-old member of the church phoned and asked for the president of the Relief Society. She told a loose-jointed, pathetic tale about Dr. Story's abuse years before.

A few hours later, another sister called to say that she'd gone to the police seventeen years back, after Story raped her daughter, and they'd refused to touch the case.

The next day, there was a similar call, and then a fourth. Not for an instant did Arden entertain the possibility that the women were merely reacting to Lovell's traditional jungle-drum gossip. "The Lord put me in charge of the Relief Society for a reason," she explained to her daughters. "I have a hard time running my own life, let alone an organization of a hundred and fifty women. You tell *me* why I got those calls!" It could only be the hand of the Lord.

There were also several calls from the clinic. Diana Harrison would say that Doctor wanted to meet with her, and Arden would reply, "No, Diana. Not just yet."

She sought divine assistance with prayer and fasting. She'd always been able to see the bright side; if the family had a Pollyanna, she wasn't ashamed to be it. But the hopelessness of the situation was wearing her down. She looked tired, defeated. Another woman stared back at her from the mirror. Her finely articulated features were the kind that could turn craggy in old age; she hoped John Story hadn't hurried the process.

She took Minda aside and confessed, "I never told you before, but your dad was molested as a child. And I was, too. So we wanted more than anything else to protect you children. And now—" She couldn't finish.

Before Arden and Dean turned in that night, he comforted her with a priesthood blessing. "Listen, Ard," he said gently, "we'll handle this. You can't let it consume you."

It was obsessing her poor daughters, too. Meg and Minda were spending most of their time fasting, praying, singing hymns, looking for signs. Minda was the first to observe that Dr. Story might be crying out for help. "That's why he was so open about what he did," she theorized at a family breakfast one morning. She wondered aloud why she hadn't complained on the examining table—"I'm usually so mouthy."

"I don't know," Arden replied. "But down the road, Father in Heaven will give us the answer."

Meg had studied psychology in college. "Minda's onto something," she said. "He needs help and he knows it. But he can't come right out and ask."

"He has to repent first," Arden said. "There's no repentance without confession. Christ was crucified so we could all repent, but first you have to recognize what you did wrong."

Arden knew about repentance; she'd been repenting her own existence ever since she'd learned what Story was doing to her daughters. For the first time in her life, she sought help from a counselor. He told her she had to take the transgressor to court.

"But we don't want to ruin him," she said. "We just want him to stop what he's doing."

"You've got to go all the way," the adviser told her. "You can handle the problem spiritually, but unless you handle it legally you'll never be able to live with it."

Arden phoned the North Big Horn Hospital and asked the name of a medical organization that would consider a complaint against a doctor. Story was well connected at the hospital—the administrator, Joe Brown, was active in the Lovell Bible Church, and so were some of the other functionaries—and she wasn't surprised when no one was willing to help. She tried two local doctors and got the same runaround. She called telephone information in the state capital of Cheyenne and found out about the Wyoming Medical Society.

When she gave the address to Meg and Minda, her adventurous

middle child said, "Mom, I've got a better idea. Why don't I go back for another pelvic, and when he rubs that big ugly thing against my hand, I'll grab it and scream and drag him into the hall."

Arden forced a smile. "Hunh-uh," she said, "But it might've been better if you'd done that before."

12

Minda Brinkerhoff

MINDA wrote a dozen different drafts to the Medical Society before settling on a short note saying that Dr. John Story had been the family doctor for twenty-four years and had been "dialating" her with his penis for the last seven.

When she mailed the letter, she thought, Nothing'll come of this. But she received a reply from the executive director saying that he'd referred her letter to the society's Committee on Professional Conduct. He thanked her "for giving the Wyoming Medical Society this opportunity to investigate . . ."

She thought, At last.

Then she received another letter and found that the medical society had kicked the case to the Wyoming Board of Medical Examiners, a public agency. She was advised to contact the executive director, Dr. Lawrence Cohen, in Cheyenne.

On June 17, 1983, two months after the last ordeal in Story's office, she wrote, ". . . I have doctored with him since I can remember. He has delivered four children of mine, and I trusted and believed in him. I trusted my life to him—and he has violated my body."

She told Cohen about the numerous "dialations," and how Story kept instructing her to come back so he could "get in all the the way."

She told about seeing and touching his penis in her last examination—"it was hell—I am still living with it—hoping to cope soon."

She thought about what her mother had told her and wrote that Story had been abusing women for at least twelve years; "I hate to see all the women that he has violated during his practice." She said she felt like an idiot and wondered how she could be so stupid—"I feel like I could crumble."

Dr. Cohen put her on the defensive. "Do you know what you're doing?" he asked her on the phone. "Do you understand that this could ruin this man's life?"

He dragged her through the pelvic exams in detail. Was she sure about this, certain about that? How did she know it was a penis? Couldn't it have been an instrument? In the end, he announced that her word wouldn't be enough to support a Medical Board investigation. Five witnesses were needed, and their evidence would have to be solid, not a hodgepodge of intuitions and guesswork.

For the first time, Minda saw what was coming—not the ruination of Dr. Story but the ruination of his victims. She visualized herself in the witness box, being asked about penises and vaginas and other personal stuff and how he'd made her scoot down so her bottom hung over the edge of the table, and all the while reporters would be taking notes and TV cameramen shooting away. Every sordid detail of her life would be recounted in the Lovell *Chronicle*—the ugliness with Bob Asay, her high-school pregnancy, the hurry-up wedding, the "court of love." *Everything*. She thought, It'll kill my dad. It'll wreck our lives, all of us—Mom, Meg and Danny, Scott, Scott's mom and dad. They'll say, It's those danged McArthurs again. . . .

She couldn't sleep.

13

Arden McArthur

ON A HUSHED FRIDAY MORNING a few weeks later, Arden was in Idaho Falls, helping a group of young people perform ordinances for the dead. Temple excursions were planned a year ahead, and to her great joy, Dean had felt well enough to make the long drive and was serving as a recorder. There were hundreds of details to jot down. He'd always been good at keeping track.

It was 5:30 A.M. and the chapel was silent when she stepped inside. As she meditated, she felt moved, raised, prompted, lifted—she was never sure later how to describe the strange feeling. She rushed over to a matron and asked directions to the prayer roll for the sick and afflicted.

As fast as she could scribble, she found herself writing the names of Dr. Story and his family, Meg, Minda, Scott, everyone involved. Certainly they all came under the heading of "afflicted." The morning prayer was scheduled for 7:30, two hours later. Then she resumed her duties for the dead.

When she returned to Lovell, Diana Harrison called. "Listen, Ard," her Mormon sister said, "Doctor's got to talk to you."

"I don't know what to say to him."

"Well, he's about to drive me crazy, making all these phone calls for him."

"What can I do? It's out of my hands."

An hour later, Dr. Story phoned. "Arden, we've got to talk."

"Yes," she said. "We do."

They met the next morning at 9:30 in the doctors' lounge at the hospital. When she first walked through the emergency room entrance and saw the familiar wispy figure standing alone, she had an irrational urge to hug him and say, Why, Dr. Story? *Why?* Some part of her still saw him as a pathetic figure, crying for help. And her daughters, when they weren't overwhelmed with anger and hurt, seemed to feel the same.

Later, she recounted the conversation:

"Arden," he began, "I'm beside myself. I'm appalled."

"*You're* appalled," she said. "I can't believe that all this has happened."

"Who started these rumors? Dr. Welch's office?" Dr. Welch was Story's main competitor. He was staunchly LDS.

"No," she said, looking straight into his brown eyes. "It had nothing to do with Dr. Welch. It came from me. You violated my daughters. Why did you do it?"

He gave a meandering denial: he was a good Christian, a family man, a leader in the community. He loved the McArthurs, every one of them. His life was dedicated to medicine and he would never violate the Hippocratic Oath. How could she even entertain such dreadful ideas?

Arden said, "When Minda told me it happened three and a half years ago, I said the same things. 'No, he wouldn't do that to our family. He carries us in high esteem.' But then when she came back and told me the second time, and then Meg told me it happened to her, I said, 'I have to believe it. I don't have any choice.' "

In a calm voice, he asked, "Do you realize what I'm being accused of?"

"Yes."

"Well, it's satanic."

She didn't disagree. Both their churches perceived the devil as real—Satan is "the author of all sin," said the book of Helaman. "And behold, he doth carry on his works of darkness and secret murder. . . ."

Arden said, "It's not only satanic. It's criminal."

"But it didn't happen," he insisted. "I didn't do it."

He looked steadily at the floor. He reminded her of a naughty boy in the principal's office. She said, "When word first got out, I had four women call me and tell me that it also happened to them. So you see, it *happened.*"

He sat back in his soft chair and cupped his chin in his hand. "All weekend long," he said, "I've been trying to figure out who would hate me so bad that they'd want to do this to me. And I made a big long list."

Arden was surprised. "I can't imagine you've got an enemy in the world."

He gave her a sardonic snicker and said, "I've got a list like you wouldn't believe." He paused, as though recollecting. "Alma Kent. Do you know her?"

Arden nodded.

"Twenty-four years ago," he said, "I had to kick her out of my office." He gave the impression that she'd made sexual overtures.

Arden thought, I'm glad Minda didn't make a scene. So this is how he handles the problem! Throws the victim out and pretends it was *her* fault? Why, Alma Kent is so straitlaced she puts the prophet to shame!

They parried for another hour. "Well, Arden," he said, smiling at her, "how're we gonna stop this talk?"

She wasn't out for blood. "The only thing the girls are asking is that you have a nurse in that room with you at all times."

He seemed surprised. "You mean that's all they're asking?"

"Uh-huh."

He seemed to think it over, then said softly, "Nobody's gonna tell me how to run my practice. I've taken a survey and found out that women don't want a third party in that room. It's embarrassing to them."

"It's embarrassing even *being* there," Arden put in. "Just having a pelvic's embarrassing."

He frowned and looked sharply at her. "What are you saying, Arden?"

"I'm saying that I have yet to ever go in for a pelvic and feel comfortable."

"Not even with me?"

"Absolutely not."

He seemed surprised. Arden thought, My lands, does he think his pelvics are fun and games? The poor man was definitely sick.

He repeated. "Well, what can I do?"

"I told you. Have a third party there."

"I can't do that. But I can cut my examination rooms down to one, and I'll quit examining women under fifty. And I'll have only one counseling room."

Arden thought, What silly ideas. "That won't work," she said.
"Why not?"

"Because four of your victims are over fifty."

He insisted it couldn't be true and she argued back. Then he said,
"What about Marilyn?"

Arden thought, Yes, what about her? Your poor wife didn't abuse
anybody. "That's one reason this has never been brought out in
the open," she said, "because of my concern for Marilyn and the
children."

"Just how far have you gone with it?"

She wondered if she should tell him, then realized that he would
know soon enough through official channels. "Minda and Meg have
written to the Medical Society," she said.

He acted relieved. "Oh, well," he said. "That's no problem. Somebody else made a complaint like that twelve years ago. I took care of it. I
can handle that."

She wondered what he meant. For weeks she'd been feeling pangs of
guilt about Dottie Parry, the woman who'd tried to complain to her
about Story's pelvics years ago. Had Dottie taken her case to the
Medical Society? She tried to pry the name out of him, but he refused to
reveal it.

She looked at her watch. They'd been talking for two hours. He
asked, "Do you think Minda and Meg will see me?"

"Minda maybe. Meg's crushed."

"This'll kill Marilyn," he mused.

Arden said, "You should've thought about that before you ever
did it."

"What's gonna happen to her?" he asked in a woeful voice. "This is
the end."

"If you won't have a nurse in the room, then something has to be
done," she said. "I'm sorry, but that's the way it is."

She asked when he'd found out what was going on. He said, "At a
quarter to eight last Friday morning. The hospital administrator, Joe
Brown, knocked on my door. It spoiled my weekend."

She told him she'd put his name on the prayer roll at Idaho Falls at
5:30 that same morning and the prayer had been at 7:30 She didn't
tell him that she viewed the timing as another sign of divine intervention. As Marilyn had pointed out long ago, they didn't believe in the
same God.

When she stood up to leave, he said in his Mr. Peepers voice, "Arden, if you ever need anybody to talk to, just call me. Any time of the day or night."

"Thanks," she said, and left.

It was still a few minutes before noon on a hot summer day. Lately the earth had seemed bursting with life, and on the way down the hill she spotted Dorothy Brinkerhoff, a short, well-nourished woman of fifty with a frizzy cap of brownish hair, weeding her garden. Arden pulled alongside and mentioned that she'd just talked to Dr. Story.

Scott's mother turned away. When she looked back, Arden saw the tears. It made her feel weepy herself. She thought, Well, we in-laws have had our troubles, but we're all together now.

When she got home, she told Minda, "Now we know why you didn't speak up when Dr. Story abused you. He would've kicked you out and then turned the whole thing against you. He did it before. The hand of the Lord shut your mouth."

She told her daughter that Story wanted to talk to her and Meg. Minda said, "I'll go if Scott'll go. But I'll never be alone with that man again."

14

Minda Brinkerhoff

SHE WAS SURE Scott would say no, but he surprised her. He seemed to welcome a showdown. Her husband had lightened up in the two months since learning about the incidents, but he still gave the impression that he was offering her forgiveness instead of belief. "I need to see Story face to face," he said. "I have some questions." She thought, Gol, what if Story convinces him? What'll happen to our marriage? She had to take the chance.

She called Meg and reminded her that the doctor wanted to meet with her, too. Meg said, "I already feel scummy enough. I'm not going to give him any satisfaction, you know, to sit there and call me a liar. That man, he—he raped me! And he wants to keep on raping others."

"How do you know that?" Minda asked.

"Because he told Mom he wasn't gonna have anybody in the room." Meg advised her sister to take a tape recorder to the meeting. Minda wished she had one.

They waited in the hospital while Story finished with a patient. He led them to a back room, sat down, and began twisting in his chair. He wouldn't look at her. She thought, This is a first. He's nervous and showing it. He said, "There's some problems. We all know why we're here tonight."

Scott nodded.

"This is all rumors," Story said. "Rumors and stories."

Minda drew her strength from Scott and spoke right up. "I'm not a rumor. I am firsthand. I was in your office and I experienced this—and that is *not* a rumor."

Story looked at Scott. "I don't know where your wife dreamed this up," he said, "but I have definitely not violated her. You can't believe that." He interrupted himself with a dry laugh. "I don't know what she's talking about. I want you to know I've never done anything that would hurt your wife or family."

He went on for five or ten minutes in a whiny voice, frequently repeating himself, sometimes talking so weakly she had to lean forward to hear. He said something about having a nurse in the room from now on—apparently he'd softened on that point—and how he would have to "live with that for the rest of my life."

Minda spoke up. "Look what I have to live with for the rest of *my* life."

"I could limit my exams to women over sixty. Would that strike you as fair? I want to make things right with you kids."

Minda thought, You want to make *what* right? Are you admitting your guilt? But she kept quiet. Scott was looking impatient.

Story said, "If there's anything I can do to work this thing out, get ahold of me and let me know. Anything. You let me know what will make this thing better and calm this thing down, 'cause you know how rumors hurt people."

She hoped Scott recognized that they were being offered a bribe. "Uh, what thing are you talking about?" Scott asked in a voice as flat as the doctor's.

Story mumbled something about rumors and innuendos, then said, "I don't want to have to take legal action."

"Legal?" her husband said sharply. "You wanna go legal? I'll take it as far as you want."

"No, no," Story said apologetically. "I was thinking about your bill." They owed eighteen hundred dollars.

"Bill?" Scott said. Minda reached for his hand. It was squeezed into a tight fist. "As far as I'm concerned, we don't owe you a cent."

"Well, I've worked that out and you don't have to pay," Story said. "We'll go ahead and wipe that clean." He leaned forward. "You know, Scott," he said just above a whisper, "if I thought anybody did to my wife what you're saying I did to yours, I would feel the same way. So don't think I don't understand. But—I didn't do it." He sounded so misunderstood, so sincere. Minda figured he'd played the same role before. "I wish you two would tell me what you expect me to do," Story went on. "What do you want?"

Scott said, "Give up your practice. Retire. Just walk away. Then nobody has to do anything or know anything."

"But . . . why?"

Scott stood up. He was a half foot taller than Story. "You know why," he said. "If I was in my right mind, I'd throw you against that wall."

Minda nudged her husband toward the door. "By the way, we've referred it to the Medical Society," she called over her shoulder.

She thought she heard Story say that he could handle that.

As they drove down the Nevada Avenue hill, Scott apologized for ever doubting her. "He gave it away himself," he said excitedly. "What a little liar! That's what made me mad at the end, the way he could sit there and smile about it."

Minda dropped Scott at work and turned off Main Street toward the little bungalow where her husband had grown up. Now that she'd written to the Medical Society, there was a chance that the Brinkerhoff name would be made public. She wanted to bring her in-laws up to date so they wouldn't say, Look how Minda's dragging us through the mud again, and she didn't even give us any warning.

She was met at the door by Dorothy Lindsay Brinkerhoff. Minda had always suspected her mother-in-law of being the force behind the difficulties at the time of the teenage marriage. The two of them had made peace since then, but Minda still felt a trill of tension.

Dorothy beckoned her to a seat at the dining room table and Minda talked fast, as she always did when she was nervous. "I've written to the Medical Society about Dr. Story," she said. "I guess Scott's mentioned it?"

Dorothy bit her lower lip. "Don't worry," Minda said. "I'm okay."

Dorothy wiped away a tear. Criminy, Minda thought, she's sure emotional. "We're getting over it now, Dorothy," she said consolingly. "You don't have to cry."

The mother-in-law poked at her eyes with a table napkin. Minda thought, At least she's sympathetic. That's an improvement.

Dorothy said, "I'm crying for me, Minda. Dr. Story did it to me, too. I've never told a soul. Not even Gerald."

They talked for an hour. Scott's mother admitted that she'd always been backward about sex. "I didn't even know what my period was when it started. We didn't talk about those things. When I was fourteen, my girl friend asked me if I'd ministrated yet, and I said no. She said, 'You haven't had your monthlies?' I said, 'Oh, yeah, I do that.' "

She told Minda that Story had abused her five years before. He'd been dilating her with a large instrument and asking her to work her vaginal muscles. When he stroked her clitoris with his finger and asked if it felt good, she wrenched away. He stepped to the washbasin and announced that the exam was over.

Dorothy said she hadn't been afraid, because Story was a doctor and part-time preacher at his church. And it hadn't felt like rape because she'd known him for so long. She said it felt more like incest. But it had shattered her faith in doctors.

The two women agreed he had large equipment.

Minda swore Scott to secrecy and repeated his mother's story. She'd never seen him so angry. She thought, Who can blame him? Story's abused his wife, his mother, his sister-in-law, maybe even his mother-in-law (although Arden still refused to discuss that possibility).

They sat up late trying to imagine what smoldering animosities Story might be trying to settle with his penis, but nothing made sense. He was still partners with Scott's father in the medical building, and the two men were friendly. Nor had there been bad blood between the McArthurs and the Storys.

"Maybe it's not us," Minda suggested. "Maybe it's . . . everybody."

Scott said that Story's motivation really didn't matter; he was a rotten son of a bitch and had to be stopped, whatever the cost.

15

Arden McArthur

ARDEN discarded plan after plan. She quickly learned that the musty old Wyoming laws were skewed against medical-rape victims, and state officials were scared to take on doctors. She burned up the wires to the attorney general's office, cried and railed and cajoled and pleaded for justice. One public servant insisted that Meg and Minda take lie detector tests. "Not unless Story takes one," Arden replied. Then she realized that a medical man could probably beat any lie test ever devised. He would know exactly what drugs to take and find them in his sample drawer.

The bureaucrats kept her off balance with legalistic doubletalk. "Mrs. McArthur," one said at the end of a long phone conversation, "your problem is that you think Dr. Story's done something criminal. But under our statutes, he hasn't."

Arden knew better. She said, "Sexual abuse isn't criminal? Doctor rape isn't criminal?"

"Your daughters were in his office of their own free will. And the law says they can't testify for each other."

"Do you mean to tell me that if I invited a man into my home and he violated my family members, it wouldn't be criminal? And they couldn't witness for each other?"

"That's different," he said, "because he's in your home."

"But I invited him in!"

The stubborn lawyer said, "Mrs. McArthur, you're wasting your time and ours."

Tears of frustration filled her blue-green eyes. "And there's not one danged thing we can do?"

"You can do what we've suggested," he said impatiently, and repeated the Medical Board's tired old formula.

Arden asked, "How'll I find five victims? I'm a housewife, not a detective."

"I'm afraid that's your job," the lawyer said, "not ours."

She remembered how everyone in Lovell had rallied behind the beloved town doctor when his daughter Annette was killed. Why, there'd almost been fistfights over which church would get the funeral! She thought, He's one of our two or three most prominent citizens. If I go up against him, we could lose everything. Dean's right. We could get ourselves run out of town. . . .

Minda kept talking about action, but most of her ideas were on a par with her plan to go back and grab Story's penis. The middle child was still too upset to make much sense.

Meg was sunk in depression. Ever since the childhood trouble with Bob Asay, she'd suffered from deep-seated fears. "Lovell was my oasis, my paradise," she complained to her mother, "and Dr. Story's stolen it from me. I don't know why we don't all pack up and leave." Sometimes she didn't even answer her telephone.

Arden consoled herself that the McArthurs didn't have much more to lose. The clothing store and the dry cleaners were slumping, and the farm was gone. Dean, now under another doctor's care, had had open-heart surgery and several seizures, each more intense than the last. Every night she propped him up and prayed he would last till morning. She thought a lot about the Celestial Kingdom.

For weeks she'd expected her own anger to subside. She prayed and meditated but was rewarded with no burnings in the bosom. Every day she grew more upset. She thought, What kind of Relief Society president am I if I let that sick man abuse more women? The Lord has given me the job of solving the problem.

But how? The four women who'd phoned after Minda's rape had spoken in strictest confidentiality. She wished she'd paid more attention to the jungle telegraph. People had been trying to tell her the truth about Story for years, and she'd turned them off.

She remembered some scuttlebutt about a member of the Bible Church who'd threatened a lawsuit against Story for bothering her daughter. At the time, Arden had disregarded the tale as typical Lovell gossip.

In a phone conversation, the woman said, "Arden, are you trying to destroy this man?"

"I'm trying to help him," she said nervously. "He can't be helped if he doesn't admit what he did." She described what had happened to Meg and Minda, and said she'd heard that something similar had happened to the woman's own daughter.

"Absolutely not!" the woman exclaimed. "Dr. Story is a fine man. My daughter just came back to town with her baby, and they went straight up to his clinic for a checkup. How can you say a thing like that?"

Arden felt like saying, Woman, I remember when I was as stupid as you. She also thought, Strike one.

She chewed on her pencil and tried to recall Story's words back in the doctors' lounge. Who was it he'd kicked out of his office twenty-four years ago? *Alma Kent.*

En route to Sister Kent's house, she spotted Aletha Durtsche crossing broad Shoshone Boulevard in her brisk stride, delivering the mail. Arden admired the letter carrier. She had a nicely chiseled face, butterscotch hair in a neat pageboy, and a laugh that rang up and down Main Street as she delivered to the storekeepers and matched them quip for quip. Raised on a farm, she shared Arden's directness and open manner— neither had ever been at home with euphemisms. Aletha was an active Saint, but she wasn't a stick about it. She directed the choir, played piano and taught in primary, coached boys' baseball, worked as a lifeguard and was raising three fine kids.

As Arden put it later, she was "prompted" to pull over. "Aletha," she called through the car window, "do you still go to Dr. Story?"

Aletha started to cry. It was so out of character that Arden jumped from the car to comfort her. "Aletha," she said, "he violated Meg and Minda. Has he ever done anything to offend you?"

She wiped her eyes and nodded.

Arden asked if she would be willing to file a complaint.

"Yes," she said, "I would."

She seemed to want to say more, but Arden interrupted. "I don't want to know the details. That's not my place. Please, Aletha, just write a letter. I'll call you later with the address."

The mail carrier nodded, and Arden drove off.

"I'm sorry, Sister McArthur," Alma Kent said as the two women sat in her front room under a photo display of her family tree. "I don't have the slightest idea what you're talking about. He said he did *what?*"

Arden repeated Story's claim that he'd kicked her out, stressing that she herself didn't believe a word. Could it be that he'd made advances?

"No," the woman said nervously. "Nothing like that ever happened."

Arden didn't believe her and said, "Did you know that if this goes to court, you can be called in?"

"Yes," Alma said, "and all I'd have to say is, I don't remember."

"But you'd be perjuring yourself!"

"I've already talked to a lawyer," the woman said. "All I have to do is deny it. I don't have to admit a thing."

"Well, if you can live with it," Arden said as she got up to leave, "I can too."

Strike two.

Driving west toward the sugar factory, she saw herself falling short of the Board of Medical Examiners' demand. Presuming Aletha added her complaint to Meg's and Minda's, the total was three and not likely to go much higher, judging by the reactions so far. The letter carrier had been a breakthrough, but how many more victims would Father in Heaven send her on the street?

She dropped in at the frame house of a widow she sometimes visited on rounds of compassionate services. The old lady required frequent dialysis. As they talked, Arden asked, "Didn't you used to doctor with Story?"

"Yes," the woman said.

"What did you think of him?"

The woman shook her head.

"Did you quit him?"

"Yes."

"Why?"

The woman shook her head again. Arden asked, "What does that mean?"

When the woman started to cry, Arden said, "I'm looking for people who've been offended by him." She described what had happened to Minda and Meg.

The old woman threw her arms around Arden and began to sob. "How did you find me?" she asked.

Arden said, "I'm . . . not sure."

"Only my husband knew. I went to Story for twelve years before I realized what he was doing to me." Arden held the upset woman till she stopped trembling. She couldn't bear to ask her to write a letter. Maybe if her health improved. But that was so unlikely.

The sun had gone down by the time Arden pulled into the driveway of her last prospect. Years before, she'd overheard Story's name in connection with a child abuse case and dismissed it as gossip. The victim's name had been "Jean Anderson," but she wasn't sure if she had the right Anderson.

Jean Anderson's mother answered the door. She said the incident had happened eighteen or twenty years before, when the child was nine. "He took out his penis and told her he was gonna put something under her to make her feel better," the woman said with no sign of reluctance. "He made her lay naked on his table. She said his penis looked brown. He told her to lift up and then slid it under her hips while he was giving her a hypodermic in her bottom. I went to the police and they said they couldn't do anything. I wrote a complaint to the State Medical Board, but nothing came of it."

"Did you keep a copy?"

"I was so angry, I kept it for years," the woman said. "Let me look." Ten minutes went by before she returned. "I can't find it. I'll look later."

"Would you mind writing another letter to the same people?"

Mrs. Anderson said she would discuss the matter with her daughter, now married and living in West Jordan, Utah. As Arden drove off, she thought, At least it wasn't strike three.

16

Aletha Durtsche

Physicians are created as much by their patients as by
their training, and most patients want to give up all decisions to the omnipotent father figure.
　　　　　　　　　　　—Bernie S. Siegel, M.D.,
　　　　　　　　　　　　　Love, Medicine & Miracles

ALETHA drove to her home on Carmon Avenue and told Mike about
the meeting on the mail route. "Don't get involved," her husband
warned.

"I've got to," the letter carrier said. She was still choked up by the
unexpected meeting with Arden McArthur. "No matter how hard it is,
I've got to go through with this, or the guy's never gonna be stopped."

Mike asked if she wasn't afraid of the consequences for the five
Durtsches. "Yes," she said, "but I don't care. When the time comes
that I meet my maker and he says, Why didn't you stop this? I'll have
no excuse other than that I was afraid."

As she sat down to write her letter, the memories flooded back. At
fifteen, she'd been a virgin undergoing her first pelvic exam. Dr. Story
told her he had to dilate her and inserted something warm. The examination lasted for about a half hour. That was all she remembered except
that she'd wondered if sex felt like that. Then she'd put it out of her mind.

By 1970, she was seventeen and pregnant with Mike's child. Dr.
Story examined her and kept complaining that he couldn't get the tube
in far enough. She thought, Whatever he's doing, it sure feels like me
and Mike. There was a knock on the door and the nurse called out,
"Doctor, we need you right now."

"What do you need?" he said crisply. For just those few words, he didn't sound like Dr. Story.

"I've got these papers for you to sign."

She could feel the tube slip from her body as he stepped backward. "Just a minute," he said, and then more smoothly, "Just a minute."

He sat on his stool with his back to the door and said, "Put 'em on the table by the door."

Aletha was perplexed. His behavior was so out of character. And that tube felt *exactly* like Mike.

After the nurse left, he resumed the procedure. Good grief, Aletha thought, can it be?

Mike was waiting outside in his pickup. In her usual direct way, she said, "I think maybe Dr. Story just screwed me."

"You mean on the bill?" Mike asked.

"No. I mean really."

"Dr. Story? He'd never do anything like that."

Aletha thought about it and said, "Naw. I guess not. It must've been something that felt real."

They'd married and traveled in the Air Force and come back in 1980 to be sealed in the temple at Idaho Falls with their three children. The church taught that Satan worked extra hard on Saints who were on a course for the Celestial Kingdom, and the warning seemed to apply to the young Durtsche family. Mike was a saloonkeeper's son, a Methodist who'd converted for Aletha. He didn't drink. She wouldn't even sip iced tea; hot, cold or strong drink were forbidden by church law, and she took the admonition literally. She told her husband, "You drink too much pop, and one of these days the promise of the word of wisdom's gonna hit you hard."

Her prophecy was fulfilled and then some. Mike got drunk and had a one-night stand. He told Aletha, "I don't give two whoops about that woman," and confessed to his bishop and stake president. They scheduled a high council court, and when he ignored its summons, he was disfellowshipped. He told Aletha he was sick of being ordered around by ordinary men posing as high priests. "Tell ya the truth,'" he said, "I'd rather be excommunicated." It seemed to her that he was forcing her to choose between him and the Saints.

But the church was her life. She asked herself, How can my own husband do this to me? We've been through the temple. By golly, he's hurting me, so I'm gonna hurt him.

She swallowed thirty aspirins to shock Mike into getting straight with the church. At the hospital, Dr. Story gave her a drink that made her throw up. Then he sat at the foot of her bed and asked, "Why'd you do it, Aletha?"

"Mike doesn't love me."

He listened as she sobbed out her story. "I want Mike, and I want my church," she said, "and I can't have both."

"Well, you come to the clinic tomorrow," he said. "You're gonna have to have something to relax you a little bit."

The next day, he led her to a chair in his private office and told her he would return. The place looked decorated by Norman Rockwell. An antique brass balancing scale was next to a set of tiny weights. A collection of old-time remedies filled a glass case; she saw Calomel, strychnine sulfate, Asthamador cigarettes, belladonna, syrup of this and elixir of that, sulfur and molasses. An open leather pillbox held crumbling pills in faded colors. Three boxed sets of books adorned a shelf: the four-volume *The Wisdom of Conservatism*, by Peter Witonski; a collection of patriotic biographies of early Americans; and a set containing de Tocqueville's *Democracy in America*, *The Federalist Papers*, a work by Edmund Burke, and Adam Smith's *The Wealth of Nations*.

Aletha turned to the framed documents on the wall. One confirmed that John Huntington Story, M.D., age thirty-two years, a graduate in medicine and surgery, had been admitted to practice in Wyoming on Oct. 6, 1958. She admired the family pictures of Marilyn and the separate ones of their three daughters, including the little lost Annette, and the framed layout showing the eight or ten sets of twins he'd delivered through the years, and the print of a vessel under full sail. There was a picture of a tiger, but she was disappointed to see that it wasn't the stalking beast she'd painted for him on black velvet after he'd cured her son Justin of the croup. The office smelled like baby powder. A Rubik's Cube lay on a shelf.

Dr. Story came back in and sat behind his messy desk. When she'd finished telling her story, he counseled her, "Maybe you'll have to stay away from your church awhile. It might save your marriage."

He'd delivered two of her children and treated her and her family most of her life, so she didn't tell him that she had no intentions of taking his advice. Nor did she inform him later that his free samples hadn't worked out. The first one made her dizzy, and she capped the bottle and decided to let the Lord do her healing.

The next time she went to the clinic, Dr. Story gave her a pelvic exam, and more in the following months. He told her she needed counseling, but he seemed more interested in hearing the intimate details of her life than in providing advice. One day as he was dilating her with the tube, he asked, "Do you have intercourse very often?"

"Probably once a week," she said. It felt strange, making conversation flat on her back.

"Have you ever had an orgasm?"

She thought, Gee, what's this got to do with anything? "Well, I don't know," she said.

"One thing that would make it more enjoyable for you," he said, "is to change positions. That would pretty much make sure you'd have an orgasm and be satisfied."

She thought, Gosh, who brought this up? And who says I'm not satisfied?

On the morning of her thirtieth birthday, Saturday, February 12, 1983, she was lazily tying a quilt. Mike wanted to drive her to the new Kmart in Cody to pick out a present for herself, but she'd had pneumonia recently and felt as though she might be relapsing. Her chest burned, and when she checked her temperature, it was 101. She made a call. "Dr. Story's so nice," she told Mike when she hung up. "It doesn't matter, day or night. He always accommodates us."

She drove herself up the hill. Somewhere in the back of the clinic, she heard a man and woman talking. After a while Dr. Story installed her on the automatic table in Examining Room No. 2 and checked her eyes, ears, nose and throat. "I can't see anything," he said. "Maybe you're coming down with a virus. How long has it been since you've had a pelvic?"

She thought, A pelvic for pneumonia? He looked at her as though reading her mind and said, "You might have a low-grade kidney infection."

She thought, Well, yeah, I guess so.

He told her to undress, handed her a sheet, and left. She heard the other people say good-bye and the front door shut. The place was silent.

He returned and turned on the water. In earlier pelvics she'd noticed that he always warmed his instruments under the faucet. Some doctors used cold speculums, but Dr. Story was concerned about his patients' comfort.

He asked her to slide to the end of the table till her backside touched his hands. He inserted the speculum and said, "This is awfully uncomfortable, isn't it?"

"Yes," she said, "but it always is."

He told her he would dilate her with the tube. She felt uneasy as he laid the plastic speculum on the sink and returned to his position at the foot of the table. Something slipped inside and it felt exactly like Mike. She thought, This can't be true. Dr. Story wouldn't do that to me.

She noticed a rhythm to his motion. When the tube was far inside, his body was close, and when he stood back, the tube slid back with him. She thought, Oh, my, this can't be happening.

He paused and asked, "Can I get in farther?"

She didn't know what to say. "Yes," she mumbled.

She closed her eyes and prayed, O Heavenly Father, please don't let this be happening to me.

Again he asked if he could get in farther, and this time she said, "I guess." She couldn't decide what to do. Should she jump up and yell? But they were alone. She thought, He could kill me. He could inject me with a shot, make it look like a heart attack. He could tell Mike that I'd died of pneumonia.

He pushed back and forth, slowly and steadily. She remembered an admonition in the Book of Mormon to guard your virtue with your life. She thought, Gosh, I shouldn't just lie here. But when he asked for the third time if he could get in farther, she heard herself say "I guess" again.

Tears slid across her temples and into her ears. He stared at her boldly, a look of triumph and dominance in his flat brown eyes. She thought, He knows I know—and he's not stopping. Ooooooh, this is terrible.

At last he stepped back. "Well," he said in his normal soft voice, "I can't find anything, and—I don't know, you might be getting a virus or something. I'll give you a prescription."

She heard the sound of his zipper. He scribbled something on his clipboard and left the room.

Driving down the hill, she thought, I'm going to the police. She looked at her watch. It was noon; she'd been gone two hours. She decided she'd better tell Mike first.

As she walked in the door, she heard his anxious voice. "Is it pneumonia again?"

She thought, How can I tell him? He'll shoot Story like a buck deer. She tried to sound unruffled as she said, "He didn't find anything."

"Did he give you a prescription?"

"Yeah, but I'm not gonna get it filled."

"Yes you are."

"No I'm not." She tried to decide how to put it and finally said, "Dr. Story didn't know what he was doing today."

Mike drove downtown and filled the prescription, marked "for misery," but she refused to touch the pills. She moped around all day. Her best friend brought her a lovely blouse; Aletha mouthed a joyless thanks. Mike peered at her several times as though to ask what was wrong. All she could see was the face at the top of the sheet. And all she could think was, Oh, you dirty thing. I know what you've been doing all these years. You dirty, dirty thing . . .

At I A.M. that night she lay listening to her husband's breathing. She thought, I can't handle this alone.

She nudged him and said, "Mike, are you awake?"

"I am now," he growled.

"Can I talk to ya?"

He raised up on an elbow. "Yeah," he said. "What's wrong?"

She said a few words and began to cry. When she recovered her composure, she started again. "You know, uh, this morning? At Dr. Story's office?"

That was all she had to say. He put his arms around her. "All those years ago," he said gently, "when you thought that's what had happened—that was true, wasn't it?"

"Yes."

They rocked in each other's arms. After a while he said, "What should I do?"

"I was gonna go to the police this morning."

He hesitated. "It'll be your word against his. They're not gonna believe you. The only thing you can do is get another doctor."

"But Mike, I feel like I've got to do something. I feel like . . . I've got to go to the stake president."

"What can he do? Story's not LDS, and you didn't do anything wrong."

"I feel so dirty. I feel like I allowed him to go on. Is there something about me that makes men come on to me? I mean, why did he pick me out of all the women in Lovell? There's a couple of older guys on the mail route that're trying to get friendly, too. Why, Mike? Do I ask for it?"

"You're just nice." He squeezed her hard. "Don't change."

"Well, gosh, I'm gonna have to start being not so friendly, but I hate to be that way because that's not me, ya know?"

She decided to be more formal on her route. It might help head off more misunderstandings.

On Monday, two days after the incident, she had to deliver a registered letter to the clinic. It made her nervous. She was confused by her own feelings. She thought, *I still like him!* She tried not to let it show.

To make matters worse, she kept running into him downtown. Each chance meeting made her more upset.

When she broke out with bad eczema, she went to Story's fellow churchman, Dr. Douglas Wrung. He asked her to show him the rash, and she had to take off her blouse and pants. He prescribed an ointment, and asked a few routine questions. As she was leaving the office, she said to herself, No way I'm coming back. He didn't do anything wrong, but I'm not taking any chances.

Spring runoff filled the canals with yellowish-orange snowmelt. She couldn't chase the rape from her mind. Playing the piano at primary or leading the choir at church, she would fight back tears. She didn't know what bothered her more, that she'd been abused or that she'd let it happen. Who would understand? She lectured herself by the hour: *Aletha, this guy raped you, and if you don't do something, other people are gonna get raped, more and more and more. They're gonna go through what you went through, and it'll be your fault.* She prayed, O Heavenly Father, please help me to know what to do. Help me to know where to go. Help me to do . . . something.

She listened as Stake President Abraham counseled her Relief Society on virtue. He reminded the women to allow no one but their husbands to touch their private parts. "And be careful about doctors," he warned. "Just because somebody's a doctor doesn't mean that you need to let them violate you. If you know a doctor's doing something improper, stop him! Make sure you're not one of the unworthy who are taken advantage of. Make sure there's a nurse in the room. And don't let a doctor give you a lot of pelvic examinations. They're not that necessary. My wife bore ten children and she hasn't had ten pelvic exams in her life."

Aletha listened and thought, He's talking about Story! How did he find out? He's talking about . . . *me*. I've got to do something. But what? Months ago, Mike had predicted that the police wouldn't believe her. Were they any more likely to believe her now?

By Memorial Day, she hadn't seen Story as a patient for three months, but she took her daughter in because the child was afraid of other doctors. Story treated her strep throat and gave her a painless shot and smiled at both Durtsches as if they were his favorite patients. Aletha hated herself more than ever.

By the end of June, four months after the birthday trauma, she'd begun a fast for guidance. She'd been on the second day, walking a double route to help out another carrier, when Arden McArthur's car pulled over and stopped.

It took three hours to compose the letter to the State Medical Board. A few days later, she was sorting mail in the post office when a call came in from a man who identified himself as Dr. Lawrence Cohen of the Medical Board. He said, "I hope you realize that these are very serious charges to bring against a doctor." He didn't sound friendly.

"I do," she said nervously.

"I hope you realize that if this goes to a hearing, you'll have to testify. Are you willing to do that?"

"Yes," she said, "I am."

By repeatedly stressing the gravity of her charges, Cohen gave the impression he was trying to frighten her off. "We have two other letters," he said in his stern voice, "but that's not enough. And they're both from the same family. Did you women get together on your stories?"

She assured him that they hadn't. Her palms were wet when she hung up.

She phoned Arden and learned that the Medical Board had demanded the names of five victims. She remembered a remark that her friend Irene Park had once made: "I wouldn't go to Story if he was the last doctor on earth and I was dying. Not after what he did to me."

She called the Park home and briefed Irene on the situation. "Would you be willing to write in?" Aletha asked.

Irene said she would take the address and think about it.

———

The stake president phoned. "I've been hearing rumors about you," he told his choir director. He asked if she'd made an official complaint against Dr. Story.

"Yes, President Abraham, I have."

He expressed his sympathy, but reminded her that the prosecution of medical rape was not the church's job. He mentioned that there was strong LDS support for Dr. Story. "Personally, I'm sure he's guilty," he confided. "I've heard from so many women."

She breathed a little easier. At least he knew. In all of Big Horn County, there was no more important ally.

17

Arden McArthur

ARDEN prayed and meditated and exercised her brain, but she couldn't change the arithmetic. If every one of her prospects wrote in, they would end up one victim short of the Medical Board's magic formula.

She dredged up an old memory and phoned Sister Dottie Parry. Arden had hardly started speaking when the excitable Dottie began bellowing into the phone. "I tried to tell you about Dr. Story twelve and a half years ago! And Arden, you dang thing, you wouldn't listen!"

"You're right," Arden answered calmly. "You're absolutely right. But this is important, Dottie."

"It was important *then*, too. Now you're asking me to write a letter to somebody?"

"Only if he did something that was against your principles."

"I'll think about it. But . . . don't count on me."

Arden thought, Well, that's the end of the line. I'm a dollar short and a day late. And that creature can keep right on abusing women, by approval of the state's numbers game.

She called Meg and Minda and asked if they could remember any random criticisms of Story by friends. They repeated some high school gossip. "People didn't talk to us about him," Meg reminded her mother.

"We didn't let them." Yes, Arden said to herself, and what fool taught you to do that?

She'd given up trying to remember patients who'd quit him. She tried to recall his ex-employees. They might know some dirt. Who'd he ever fire?

The only one she could think of was Ina Welling, sixtyish, an LDS convert from Methodism who combined the stern moralities of both religions. She was a tall, stately woman, married to McKay Welling, the best heavy-equipment blade operator in Wyoming. Every time Arden saw Ina in church, with her tinted stepdown-frame glasses and her thick black eyebrows and wiry graying hair, she was reminded of an old-time school principal.

Arden reached her on the job at the sugar factory. "Ina," she said, "I need to talk to ya."

Ina drove down after work. It turned out that she knew a lot.

18

Ina Welling

"I WORKED for him from sixty-five to sixty-seven, near two and a half years," Ina Welling repeated later. "He saved my son's leg after a motorcycle accident, and we owed him six hundred dollars. I paid it off fifty dollars a month out of the two hundred he paid me. When I left I was making two eighty a month, but Story had a lot of little angles to cut down on the take-home.

"He had everybody's day blocked into hourly squares on a sheet of paper. If I worked late, it didn't count. He'd work me on my afternoon off and not pay overtime. I got docked for every little thing. He said we were all professionals and he would expect to be treated the same.

"He was so cheap—well, I guess some folks would call it frugal. In those years, Marilyn came down to do the bills. He always kept her separated from the rest of the staff. Whenever she got in a discussion, he found something for her to do. She was frugal, too. She used to separate the Kleenex leaves that we gave the patients. She used scraps of paper or old envelopes for our pay slips. Here, look! I've saved a few.

"Women in jeans or pants, he'd tell me to give them a used sheet. At the time, we were paying ten cents a sheet to have 'em laundered. Patients in nylons and a dress got a clean sheet. Some of the high school girls got no sheet at all. He'd let 'em sit there bare to the waist till he was good 'n' ready.

"He'd have the nurses turn the disposable rubber gloves inside out, wash 'em and autoclave 'em and use 'em over and over. And the throwaway plastic speculums, he'd put 'em in a strong disinfectant for reuse. Two drug detail men asked one day how come he didn't need more speculums.

" 'Well,' the nurse, 'we use 'em over again.'

"Those two men were just horrified! Then they found out about the rubber gloves. They said, 'That's one of the worst things a doctor could do! What if he had a hole in one?'

"But he had a fixation about neatness and the way things looked. He'd find a piece of tape on the floor and yell, 'Get that filthy thing outa here!'

"He always had Marilyn handle the collections, and she could be pretty blunt. One morning he grabbed me and said, 'Someone stopped Marilyn downtown and jumped all over her about the note on his bill. From now on, if somebody comes in and complains, don't tell 'em Marilyn writes the notes. Tell 'em it's you. No one talks to my wife like that.'

"He didn't want welfare patients. One of the first things I learned was I'd get in trouble giving an appointment to 'them'—Mexicans, Indians, blacks, any different race. Didn't like Germans either, or folks with German names. He'd say, 'I do not want *them* in this office.'

"Once I made a phone appointment for a very sick man, and the man's wife brought in his welfare papers. I went back to the lab and told the nurse, 'Boy, I'm in trouble. They're on welfare 'cause the husband can't work. You know how *he* feels about that.'

"Dr. Story grabbed the papers and took the couple into his office, and he was really nasty to 'em. Then he came out and lectured the nurse and me about welfare patients. He said the government was wasting *his* money. He said he had to take some welfare patients, but keep it to a minimum.

"He'd get a year behind with his welfare papers. He hated medical insurance, Blue Cross, Social Security. One time he had me fill out papers for twenty-some welfare people and mail 'em to Cheyenne, and he had me put every one of their names for a return address. He wanted the clerks in the Lovell post office to see who was on welfare.

"One night I had to leave for Mutual at seven-thirty, and the next day he told me I couldn't hold any LDS position as long as I worked for him. He despised the Book of Mormon, the *Doctrine and Covenants*, everything about our church. All I had to do was quote, 'As man is, God once was, and as God is, man may become,' and he'd turn red. I'd ask him, 'Don't you think you've progressed in life?'

"He'd say, 'Yes.'

" 'How'd you get your medical degree?'

" 'Somebody taught me.'

" 'Don't you think maybe you'll progress some more?'

" 'Well, I never thought of it.'

" 'If you keep on progressing,' I'd say, 'don't you think you might progress toward godliness?'

"He'd say, 'That's blasphemy!'

"After a few conversations like that, he began to get on me about every little thing. He'd tell me to change a procedure. A few days later he'd bawl me out for changing it and deny that he'd ever mentioned it. Everything had to be perfect. If I drew a dividing line across the typing paper, he'd say, 'Who did this? Look at this.' He cut me to pieces with that soft voice, a terrible look in his eye, never cussed but made you feel like he was educated and you were nothing. Then he'd open the door and see a patient and his whole personality would change. 'Well, how are *you*, Mrs. Mayes? And how are those *beau*tiful children?'

"I'd go home and tell my husband the things that went on in that office, and he wouldn't believe me. I'd say, 'McKay, why would I make it up?'

"It got so the nurse and I couldn't do anything right. He was polite to men, but women were dirt. One day our pharmacist said, 'Ina, has Dr. Story made you cry yet?'

"I said no.

" 'He will. That's one of his things. He has to make his women cry.'

"Well, that man knew what he was talking about. I was in the office alone one day, and Dr. Story was so vicious that I started to cry. I said, 'Well, Doctor, I didn't know I was so terrible.' When I started to tell him I quit, he took out the door and wouldn't listen. I swore to myself, You'll never do that to me again! Of course, Dr. Story never apologized.

"By that time I'd begun to notice a few things. The way some of the ladies looked when they came out of the examining room, flushed, flustered. He was very particular about having the music on and the water on. I couldn't figure out why. We weren't allowed in the room when he did a pelvic. When he did a Pap test, we'd hold the slide, then spray it with fixative back in the lab. After that, we weren't supposed to go back in. And we weren't allowed to knock on the door unless it was an emergency or a phone call from the hospital. He had the nurses so scared, they'd ask me to knock. He'd say, 'What do you want?' as if he was annoyed.

"Sometimes after pelvics I'd find spots on the floor at the foot of the table. I used to wonder why his examinations took so long, but then he was slow about everything. Some women used to get longer appointments than others. One morning he had Wanda Hammond come in when he had no other appointments. The nurse was gone and he asked me to prep her for a pelvic. I went in and told her to undress, and Wanda grabbed me and said, 'Ina, don't leave me!'

"I kidded her. 'Oh, Wanda, what's the matter? You've done this before.'

" 'No, no, Ina, don't leave me. Stay in here with me.'

" 'Wanda, you know I can't.'

" 'You can ask Dr. Story's permission.'

"I said, '*You* ask his permission, Wanda.'

"She said, 'I can't.'

"She had ahold of my arm and was hurting me. 'Wanda,' I said, 'what's the matter?'

"She said, 'I think he's gonna do something he shouldn't.'

" 'Wanda, what do you mean?' I was shocked.

"She mumbled, 'Well, things that he shouldn't do.'

" 'Wanda,' I said, 'don't tell me that. You're married and have six children. You should know—'

" 'Ina,' she said, 'I'm telling the truth.'

"She seemed *so* upset, I said, 'Well, you ask him if it's okay, Ina, and I'll stay with you till he's done.'

"I went back out front. Wanda came out an hour or so later and she looked awful. She whispered to me, 'It happened.'

"I guess I was dumb. I thought, *What* happened? But it never occurred to me it was sex. I thought maybe she was just afraid of the pain, or upset about taking her clothes off, some little embarrassment. LDS women are very straitlaced about things like that.

"After that, I watched more closely. Wanda came back a few months later and he locked the door again. And I noticed a few other things about other women. You could tell by their faces that something was going on. I mentioned to a couple of my friends, 'Dr. Story has problems. Don't go to him.' And then I quit.

"Later on, he put out word that he fired me because I was too dumb, and I heard tell that Marilyn was saying the same thing. After I quit, he called my house and begged me to come back—I guess I didn't turn dumb till after I quit."

19

Arden McArthur

AFTER Arden heard Ina Welling's story, she phoned her friend Lanita Thompson, "Grandma" Thompson to her sisters in the church, a wise matriarch who knew everything that went on in town.

Grandma revealed that her daughter Wanda indeed had been abused by Story and that she knew of another young female who'd been induced to undress and "bounce around" for the doctor when she'd come in with a sprained ankle in the seventh grade.

Arden knew Wanda Thompson Hammond as a gentle, friendly woman in her fifties, not five feet tall, as solid and round as a garden turnip. She worked as a checker at the Rose City Food Farm on Main Street, smiling and beaming at her clients. Everybody kidded her because her nose turned red when she smiled. Arden couldn't imagine terrorizing such a dear person.

She'd caught a hint in Grandma Thompson's voice that Wanda might be willing to help out, so she addressed an envelope to the Medical Board and took it with her to the Hammonds' one-story frame house across the street from Aletha and Mike Durtsche's home on Carmon Avenue.

Wanda cried from the minute Arden entered till she left. The little woman played with her stubby fingers and looked everywhere but into Arden's eyes. Arden thought, I've never seen anyone so anguished.

"I'm sorry to upset you, Wanda," she said, cutting her visit short. "If you have something to tell the Medical Board, would you mail it in this envelope?"

As she drove off, she saw Wanda at the front window, poking at her eyes with a handkerchief. My laws, Arden said to herself, I'm making folks plumb miserable. It was one more burden to carry.

20

Wanda Hammond

IT TOOK Wanda hours to stop shaking. Now there would be more nightmares, just when they'd about ended. She looked at the envelope on the table. It was addressed to an office in Cheyenne. She couldn't imagine why anyone would want her to repeat such a shameful story.

She'd been brought up in rural poverty ten miles east of town. As a child, she'd warmed herself by a wood stove, read by kerosene lamp, cut thick slices of sugar beet for candy. For the Thompson children, popping corn and toasting marshmallows doubled as snacks and entertainment. For years the family had no electricity or radio, car or tractor. The barefooted kids hooked horses to a wagon and rode to the Shoshone River bottom to gather wood. They thought they were having fun.

The farm work was mostly stoop and crawl. They had a few milk cows and raised cattle, pigs, chickens, hay and barley. The cash crop was beets. They planted the tiny seeds, thinned the shoots on hands and knees, separated the rows, irrigated, and chopped out redroot weed, sunflower and bogweed with short-handled hoes. They worked till the last shadow disappeared. By the end of summer the fat beets would lie on their sides under their thick scratchy leaves. There were beets so big it took two hands to carry them—eight-pounders, ten-pounders. The biggest were shown to their parents for praise. Wanda had her own beet knife with a nick in the end for pulling them up by the tops. She slashed off the greens and threw the beets in the wagon for the ride to the sugar factory. She and her brother and three sisters thought that was fun, too.

All social connections were through the church. Sex wasn't discussed. Lanita told her children they would learn when they were old enough. Looking back, Wanda said, "I guess fifty-five isn't old enough 'cause she still hasn't told me. I spent my whole life with one man. You don't need sex education for that."

No one in the Thompson family went undressed. Wanda avoided taking showers at school because she was embarrassed. One day the gym teacher forced her to disrobe; forty years later Wanda still considered it an act of unreasonable cruelty. She taught her own children to shut the bathroom door during potty training. "We LDS folks talk about our bodies being a temple," Wanda explained. "Nobody watches you naked. Nobody touches you . . . down there. That is your private parts."

She married Charles Hammond when she was eighteen. They rented a small farm three miles out in the country and contracted ten acres of river bottom in beets. Her life was still stoop labor, but with variations. Charles, as shy as his wife, worked on farms and repaired cars, and the two of them spelled each other driving the school bus for extra cash.

Dr. Story delivered the last two of their seven children. Wanda found him an odd duck but skilled. When she suggested that her infant son's diarrhea might be caused by teething, he said, "What gives you the authority to be the doctor? I'm the doctor here."

He kept good track of her plumbing, and her daughters', too. Right after she started seeing him around 1962, he began talking about doing a "full-length." She told Charles, "I don't know what he means by a full-length. He's checked down my throat as far as he can look. He's examined me in every way."

In those years Wanda was firm and tanned from her long workdays in the sun. Every time she went in for a pregnancy checkup, Dr. Story gave her a pelvic, and some of them lasted a half hour. "He sure watches closely," she told Charles. "The other doctors just felt around a little bit."

In the fall of 1969, she finally realized what the doctor was up to. She had a 1:45 P.M. appointment for a sore throat. He let her wait till he'd treated the other patients, then ushered her into an examining room at 3 P.M. After he looked at her throat, he said, "Now we'll do that full-length."

"I've got to run the school bus at four," she said.

"We'll have time."

At three thirty she was still waiting, and she called Charles to take over the run. Dr. Story came in, arranged her knees in the stirrups, and stretched the sheet across as a drape. Then he inserted something that felt like Charles and started pushing it in and out.

She didn't know how to react. He said, "Would you like to help me guide it in?"

"No," she gulped.

"Well, it certainly would be easier if you did."

"No!"

When his pubic hair tickled her thigh, she exclaimed, "Dr. Story!"

He pulled away and she heard him zip his pants. "That'll be all," he said, and left the room.

She dressed and stepped into the hall. The waiting room was dark. She let herself out the front door. It was 5:30.

She thought about going to the police chief, LaMar Averett—a nice man, a retired farmer, strong LDS—but she realized it would be her word against the doctor's. She thought of telling Charles, but she didn't want him in prison for murder. She felt dirty, unworthy. She lay in bed and told herself, In our church, you do *not* commit adultery. I should go to my bishop.

For the first night of hundreds to come, she cried herself to sleep.

She never returned to the clinic, and when she saw Story on the street, she would cross to the other side. For a while, she vented her rage on Charles. He would look sad and she knew she'd hurt his feelings, especially after she pushed him away in bed.

After a few weeks she told herself, You can't do Charles that way. He's the finest man in the world. He's not the one who hurt you.

When one of their children fell ill, Charles said, "You better get him to the doctor. That croup don't sound good."

Wanda said, "Well, I guess I'll take him to Dr. Christensen in Powell."

"How come you're wanting to change doctors?"

She started to cry. "Because Dr. Story took liberties that he had no right to."

At last they had their talk. Charles said, "I oughta go up there and knock that little shit on his ass. I oughta black his goddamn eyes for him." Wanda had never heard her husband cuss. She patted his hand and begged him not to get himself in trouble. When Charles finally cooled down, she thought, I'm glad I waited.

Dr. Ray Christensen asked, "Who was your previous doctor?"

"Dr. Story," she said apprehensively.

"How come you're not doctoring with him anymore?"

She groped for the right words. "He was, uh—he was getting too personal."

Christensen shook his head and said, "That man needs help."

She still owed Story $407. The bills arrived with neatly scripted memos on the face: "This is long overdue." "Can this be paid in full?"

She paid the debt off in six months. She thought it would make her feel less ugly about herself, but it didn't. She'd never known anxiety, but now there were times when she was afraid she would never draw another breath.

She added the checking job at the Rose City Food Farm to her chores. She thought, Good hard work takes a person's mind off their troubles. As the years passed, she began to feel less unworthy. Then the McArthur woman knocked.

She picked up the envelope. She wondered what the Wyoming State Board of Medical Examiners was up to. Whatever it was, she wanted no part of Dr. John H. Story. She ripped Arden's envelope to pieces.

21

Arden McArthur

DRIVING toward home, Arden remembered something that Story had said early in their showdown in the doctors' lounge. "Who started these rumors?" he'd asked. "Dr. Welch's office?"

The more she thought about it, the less sense the accusation made. John Welch was a devout Mormon descended from a pioneer who'd arrived with the first LDS contingent in 1900. A professional like Dr. Welch would never stoop to nasty rumors or backbiting, least of all in his own home town.

Arden wondered if Story might have had someone else in mind. She remembered that Caroline Shotwell, wife of a former LDS bishop, had once worked for Story and now worked for Welch. Like a detective scratching for leads, she made a short detour to the Shotwell home.

Caroline Shotwell gave the impression that she was holding something back. She haltingly recalled that a woman had come to her husband John when he'd held the bishopric and claimed that Dr. Story had abused her. She didn't know the details, and John was forbidden to talk about it.

"Would you be willing to write a letter about what you know yourself?" Arden asked.

Caroline whimpered and turned her head. Arden thought, There's something here. This is a bright, level-headed sister and she doesn't show emotion over nothing. "Well, it's confidential," Caroline said. "Will you let me think about it for a while?"

"Of course, Caroline," Arden answered. "But please—if you know something, don't wait too long. There could be more victims every day."

Caroline chewed her lower lip. "Okay," she said slowly. "Maybe I can do it without using the woman's name."

22

Caroline Shotwell

HOW CAN I USE the woman's name, Caroline asked herself, when the woman is me?

She'd been one of Dr. Story's charter patients. He'd seemed competent enough except for a few quirks. He talked so softly that she had trouble hearing him. He always carried a clipboard or a towel in front of his open smock. He prescribed hormones and gave her a pelvic exam before each injection "to see if you still need your medication." He kept trying to talk religion and politics, but she steered him away; the pelvics took long enough. She was raising a family and working as a gray lady at the hospital, and she had no idle time.

His office staff seemed to have a high turnover, and in the spring of 1972 he offered her a job. Her Mormon sister Ina Welling warned, "He's really got problems." Caroline felt like saying, Ina, if you'd just left religion and politics alone, you'd probably still be working there.

She'd barely started work when the doctor grew fangs. While patients sat in the waiting room, he delivered instructional lectures to the slaves, then later denied his own words. He never admitted a mistake; it was always someone else's fault. His rules varied from day to day; only a mind reader could have followed them. No male patients were to be scheduled before 4 P.M. Whiny children, ethnics and welfare cases were to be discouraged. Patients were never to approach him in the hall. "Caroline," he warned her in his gentle voice, "if you ever let a patient talk to me in the hall, I'll really be nasty to them, and it'll be your fault."

His examining room and office were out of bounds except by personal order. He conveyed the impression that she would be burned severely if she touched the controls on his automatic table. The trash can was to be left open all night to dry and the contents incinerated in the morning. Kleenex boxes were kept half full. The music wasn't turned off till he said so.

He had fits about the Mormon garment. One of his nurses warned, "He's got a hang-up there. He told me, 'I'm not gonna monkey around with someone's underwear.' He said if these people have an aversion to removing the garment, you tell them if they could remove the garments for a Mormon doctor, then they can remove them for me.' "

In front of his staff, he railed against blacks, Latins and what he called "Germans," although Caroline realized that he really meant German-Americans. When a longtime patient's wife spoke up to him, he said, "Oh, that damned German!" Caroline suspected that he felt the same about Mormons, but didn't dare alienate so many patients.

He made frequent cracks about the obese. When the florist Beverly Moody would leave, he would tell the others, "She's just fat!" When Caroline reached a well-proportioned 150 herself, he summoned her to his office. "Mrs. Shotwell," he said, his brown eyes half-closed behind his big glasses, "do you realize you now weigh more than me?"

He seemed to enjoy controlling and bullying women. He ordered Caroline's elderly mother-in-law to walk home and change her blouse because he couldn't roll her sleeve up for the sphygmomanometer. He dominated his wife and frowned when she fraternized with others. Caroline felt sorry for Marilyn. The sad-faced woman complained that her love life was limited "because Doctor's always tired when he gets home." She took his withering sarcasm with a smile, but there were times when she seemed jealous and forlorn. She paced outside the door during one of his lengthy premarital exams. No one dared knock, and he offered no explanation when he finally came out and strode briskly for the bathroom.

After three months on the job, Caroline prepped an especially big-busted LDS woman for an examination. "Please," the woman asked, "can I keep my bra and garment on?" Caroline didn't have the heart to say no.

Dr. Story took one look and snapped, "Mrs. Shotwell, this patient is supposed to be undressed. She'll have to come back tomorrow. You have wasted *her* money and *my* time." When Caroline began to cry, he led her to his private office and lectured her till she cried harder.

She staggered to the reception desk and wrote a note on a prescription blank: "Dr. Story, it's obvious I'm not doing this job the way you want it done. Here's my key."

He called her at home that night and asked her to return. She responded, "I don't have to eat that bad."

"But Mrs. Shotwell," he said, "we need you." She noticed that the situation turned on *his* needs, not on the hurt he'd done to her. It seemed to epitomize his employee relations.

"I told you," she said, trying not to lose her composure again. "I'm not that hungry."

He suggested that she wasn't being fair and asked her to sleep on her decision. "You're very valuable around here, you know." He called with the same message the next day, and the next. In all his importunings, there was no hint of apology.

She saw no reason to drop him as her doctor. Everyone agreed he was the best around. He'd been treating her for fifteen years and had all her records. When she arrived for an appointment, he greeted her with a big smile, and the succession of pelvics resumed.

In the winter of 1974, six months after she'd quit the job, she realized that he was dilating her with his penis and probably had been doing it from the beginning. She kept the secret to herself. Her husband John, the former bishop, had long experience in granting dispensations, but she was ashamed to tell him and worried about what he might do. She knew that sooner or later she would have to warn another Story patient, her married daughter Mae Shotwell Fischer, but she held off for a while. She assumed that Story raped only older women; maybe it was because they couldn't get pregnant.

Six weeks later, her daughter entered the Shotwell home, her face pale and drawn. Caroline made her sit down and brought her a glass of water. Mae said she'd just had a pregnancy test and Dr. Story had dilated her. The tube felt so much like her husband Bill that she pulled the sheet aside for a look and saw his erect penis. "Oh," Story said, "didn't you know?"

When John came home from work that night, the shaken Caroline stopped sobbing long enough to say, "Dr. Story took liberties with Mae. I think something should be done."

She provided no details, and John didn't ask. He arranged to see Story and returned in less than an hour. The doctor had denied any wrongdoing and said, "I'm sorry if that's what Mae imagined. I guess I'll have to have a nurse in the room to avoid misunderstandings." John told Caroline that it sounded reasonable to him.

She thought, I should have told John everything. I should have told him what was done to me, not just what was done to Mae. I didn't give him enough ammunition, and Story gave a convincing explanation. It's too late now.

She advised Mae to forget what had happened. "If you don't, you'll never get over it." She didn't know what else to say. She felt as though she'd arranged her daughter's rape.

At 3 A.M., she was still thinking about Arden McArthur's visit. She'd had nine years of fitful sleep. The memory of how she'd failed her daughter crept up on her when the lights went out and sometimes stayed with her all night.

I was too late then, she said to herself, and it's still too late. If I was guilty then, I'm more guilty now for keeping it a secret.

She brooded for a few more days, then took the boldest step of her life. She wrote the Medical Board but warned that she could never go public, even under subpoena. Neither John nor Mae's hotheaded husband Bill could ever know the truth. She had enough on her conscience. She didn't want to be an accomplice to murder.

23

Meg Anderson

ON A WINDY NIGHT in midsummer, at about the time of the second hoeing of the beets, Meg McArthur Anderson found herself at a class reunion with her childhood friend Susan Story. Nursing school hadn't changed the older daughter. She was friendly, but she retained something of the somber air that the McArthurs had always noticed in the Story females.

Meg was apprehensive when the two of them were assigned to the same table. As they "vizted," it became clear that Susan was unaware of her father's perilous situation. The realization made Meg feel like a hypocrite as she talked about old times and tried to pretend that nothing had changed between them.

For several weeks after the reunion, she met Susan in dreams and guiltily assured her that she treasured their friendship. She explained that Dr. Story was sick, not evil, but that he was hurting defenseless people and had to be stopped for everyone's good, including his own. In each dream, Susan listened understandingly and gave her a friendly hug.

When Meg was awake, she felt like a traitor.

24

Aletha Durtsche

THE LETTER CARRIER kept bumping into the Storys. It was spooky, especially since she'd sent off her complaint to the Medical Board. One day when she was delivering mail to the clinic, Marilyn Story called out "Aletha!" as though greeting an old friend. Her eyes looked so inflamed that they appeared to be infected, and Aletha figured she either had an eye disease or she'd been crying for days. "Look here!" Marilyn said with an enthusiasm that seemed put on. "We've finally got your picture framed."

Aletha looked at the stalking tiger she'd painted six years before. Why were they just getting around to framing it? She was afraid she knew.

Oh, Marilyn, she said to herself, you found out about my letter. I'm the one who ruined your eyes. How could I be so cruel to such a nice lady?

After her shift, she went home and cried herself.

BOOK TWO

The Law's Delays

25

Marilyn Story

Whatsoever house I enter, there will I go for the benefit
of the sick, refraining from all wrongdoing or corruption,
and especially from any act of seduction.
—The Oath of Hippocrates

MARILYN knew who was behind the trouble. It was the McArthurs, with help from Caroline Shotwell. John had made the mistake of telling Caroline she was overweight, and the silly thing had been ticked off ever since. As for the McArthurs, Marilyn had been warning him about Arden for twenty years. "Why do you spend so much time talking to that woman?" she would say. "You're getting farther and farther behind."

John always shrugged. He talked religion and politics with everybody. And Arden—well, she could talk the spots off an Appaloosa. Marilyn had laughed when Arden sent in the Mormon missionaries. Who did they think they were dealing with, a Unitarian? John had studied Scripture since the age of twelve, and it wasn't something forced on him by fanatical parents, either—it was his own free choice. He'd spun the LDS missionaries' heads.

Marilyn wondered why John stopped talking about the silly charges against him. She wished he wouldn't shield her from his problems. Except at the very beginning of their courtship, they'd never talked much. By the time he came to bed at night, she was usually on her second or third dream. He read Scripture, medical books and bulletins, books on religion, patriotism, conservative politics, U.S. history. If he was scheduled for surgery in the morning, he would bone up on the procedure till long after midnight. Sometimes he studied in the doctors' lounge till it was time to scrub up. He'd always been painstaking to a fault.

But Marilyn had learned early that medicine was his true love. "It's been a lonely life," she reflected later, "especially now that my girls are grown and gone. Sometimes I feel sorry for myself. I'm alone most of the time, but I guess that's true of any good doctor's wife. At the end of the day he doesn't want to rehash everything that happened—he's too tired. Even when John's home, I'm alone, because he reads medical books constantly. We have a garage full of them. He delivers a lot of babies, and that means we can never schedule a vacation. I don't know how many times the girls and I have driven to family reunions by ourselves. He'll fly out later—or not come at all."

Marilyn consoled herself with the thought that she'd never expected to marry so important a man. As a child in the Rockies, she'd considered herself ordinary.

She was born in 1930, one of seven children of a well-to-do Colorado rancher. "My childhood would have been perfect," she said, "except for horses." Even full grown, she was only three and a half inches over five feet, and when she was a child, every horse on the Taussig spread looked liked a Clydesdale. "Dad put me on a horse when I was a baby," she said with a grin. "It bucked me off and he caught me in midair. My stirrups were always too long, and when I was a kid the cowhands were too busy to shorten 'em for me. I've been thrown off, run away with, scraped off on trees, whipped by willow branches, bumped and bruised over every inch of my body."

Luckily, she enjoyed her family's other animals, especially the six hundred registered Herefords. During World War II, when her brothers were gone, she worked side by side with the buckaroos. She rode fence, checked gates, roped calves, helped brand. Sometimes a dogie would wander off, and she would find herself riding among hundred-year-old junipers, three feet tall. In summer, when the herd followed the freshly greening grasses up the mountainsides, she bunked in a log cabin without running water or lights. In that male society, she was no stranger to privation or fear and no quitter, but when her father's favorite saddle bronc, part quarterhorse and part Thoroughbred, flipped her into a herd of cows, she vowed never to ride again. She was fifteen.

She grew into a fine-boned handsome woman, a perfect size four, with a dazzling smile, long black hair, and strongly chiseled features that displayed her part-Indian ancestry. After a year of business school in Denver, she took a job as a secretary, and hated it. "I guess I missed the cows," she said.

One Christmas she visited her brother and a cousin at Wheaton College ("For Christ and His Kingdom") and enjoyed the school and the maple-lined Illinois town so much that she got a job and planned to stay. Then she met a young premed student. Nearly forty years later, the memory still excited her.

"John was four years older, handsome, very mature, and eligible. He showed some caring. He was a 'Christian.' He had black hair and deep-set brown eyes that kind of sloped; we called them triangle eyes. He was a charmer, a tease. When I found out that his mother was Inez and his aunt was Lola, I asked him where those names came from and he said his grandpa's name was Ferrero and they were Mexicans. That's still a family joke!

"He asked my dad for my hand, and we were married in the little Parshall Chapel near our ranch. My head was in the clouds. I looked forward to a lovely life as a doctor's wife. We honeymooned in Yellowstone in Dad's big old Oldsmobile because John didn't own a car. That was a rude awakening—the first time I'd ever had to worry about money. I was such an airhead!"

When John was in medical school and money was still short, he would take her to the Omaha Stockyards on his nights off. "I was working full time as a secretary, putting him through school, and Omaha was a tough adjustment. I missed my cattle. We'd walk on the stockyard overpasses. What a sight! I just like watching 'em bawling and carrying on. I like their sound, their smell." The familiar white faces took her back to the Indian paintbrush and columbines in the high pastures around her childhood home.

Except for the stockyards tours, she seldom saw her studious husband. "It was a bad way to start a marriage," she admitted later. "I didn't discover till we were married that he's a night owl. If he wasn't working late, he was reading till all hours. When he interned in Omaha, he worked thirty-six hours on and twelve off, and I was really alone. I about died in Omaha. All I remember is the heat. We had to live in low-cost public housing without air-conditioning. John was embarrassed about living in a subsidized setting. He didn't like public handouts; that was his main topic of conversation with everybody. But we weren't gonna make it otherwise. We were thrown in with black people and cockroaches. I hadn't seen either one in Colorado.

"We moved to Ogden, Utah, for his surgical residency. Mormons were all around us. That's where I first heard the expression 'secret and sacred.' One day I got into a backyard argument with a Mormon man about the trinity. I found out they just don't understand it and there's no use trying to explain. Their heads are set hard against the trinity and the cross, and they speak of Jesus as their 'brother.'

"One day John came home all red in the face. He said, 'Do you know what a Mormon nurse told me? She said, "As we are now, God once was. As God is now, we will become." ' He said, 'Why, that's blasphemous!' John never trusted Mormons after that."

She saw the Mormon religious garment hanging on a clothesline and asked him to find out about it. John reported that ultrapious Mormons insisted on wearing the protective underwear till death. During surgery some of the doctors would let it dangle from a wrist or an ankle. Others would remove it and slip it back on before the anesthetic wore off. Both Storys thought it was a silly charade.

After Susan was born and John completed his residency, they moved back to his hometown of Maxwell to share the big old gabled home with his mother and sister. "John sat up till all hours talking to Gretchen or reading," Marilyn remembered. "I went to bed alone every night. They'd talk about the good old days. I couldn't handle it."

Through the medical grapevine, they heard that an ailing physician named Dr. Ben Bishop needed someone to help with his practice for $1,000 a month. John accepted the challenge and moved his wife and baby into an upstairs apartment in the Nebraska panhandle town of Crawford. Eight months later Marilyn spotted a newspaper ad saying that Lovell, Wyoming, needed a doctor.

"I was pregnant with Linda," she recalled, "and we drove up to look the town over, me and John and baby Susan. John likes big cars. We had an old tan Lincoln Continental, a four-door sedan, with the fanciest inside you ever saw—electric windows, leather, the works."

The drive was an education. After crossing the wet green prairies of Nebraska and the undulating antelope plains of southeastern Wyoming, the northern part of the Cowboy State looked lunar: brown scorched land littered with geological rubble and screes, slashed and pocked with gullies and caves. Salt sage and greasewood dotted the escarpments and the flanks of the mountains, and cottonwoods crowded the twisting river bottoms, but little else seemed to grow except on irrigated benches and hardscrabble patches of farmland. They could see ten miles ahead on the highway. The wind blew constantly, stirring up grit. They passed fumaroles puffing like volcanoes. Phosphates, bromates and chlorides had pushed up to the desert surface along with other ates and ites and ides, giving the countryside a thin frosty coating. Pumping jacks dipped and raised and dipped and raised, but the oil fields looked marginal.

It was a relief to cross the last thirty miles of desert and drive under the trees of Lovell. For an hour or so they just rode around town. Magpies fluttered on Main Street. A cloying smell reminded them of rotting hay; John was usually tolerant of such things, but he said that this particular smell would take some getting used to. They found out that the aroma came from hot beet pulp in the sugar refinery at the west end of town. As they drove past, they heard the whir and hum of the machinery and saw the white plume flowing heavy from the stack.

On balance, the place made a pleasing impression. "We saw a nice little town with wide streets and irrigation ditches running along the gutters," Marilyn recalled. "The Mormons watered their lawns and gardens with it. Quaint. The town needed a doctor desperately, and they treated us like royalty. So we decided to help out for a while. We didn't intend to stay. We found a house up on Nevada Avenue—it was a dirt road then—and I didn't even buy new curtains. John set up in that little building downtown but refused to sign a five-year lease.

"It was exciting to think that my husband was starting his first full practice. Dr. Croft was phasing out. Dr. Horsley, the Rose Doctor, had a limited practice at home—there was some kind of scandal about him.

"People liked John. Within months we were swamped. The mortician's hearse was the town ambulance, and John would follow along on the accident cases. There were no EMT's in those days and he had to do both jobs.

"For a long time we didn't make much money. John always undercharged, and a lot of people never got a bill. He cared about his patients but not about money. It reached the point where the insurance company wouldn't pay one of the claims because he turned it in two years late. It was a mess!

"We had to take trades. An old couple brought in some packaged frozen meat. I thought it was a gift, but they said to apply it to their bill. It was goat—not tender young kid but tough old grandpa. Sometimes we got paid in services: repairs on the car, housework, yardwork. It cut down on our income tax.

"John treated a lot of migrant workers, mostly Mexicans. Two or three hundred came to town every spring to thin and weed the beets. They lived in shacks and saved their medical problems for John. He refused to bill welfare like the other doctors. He'd tell his patients, 'Just pay what you can.' He didn't think the taxpayer should have to reimburse him for treating the poor. So he ended up doing a lot of charity work. If he'd billed welfare, we'd be millionaires.

"After a while, we began depositing money in the bank and making our house payments on time. In 1962 John saw this ad in a medical publication: 'For your ease and comfort as well as your patient's, new Ritter "75" universal table. . . . Gynecological position, a new and exclusive innovation—offsetting the lowered leg section behind edge of table—provides much needed additional legroom for physician. . . .' He had to have one, and we bought it for $1,792, ten dollars down and $148.50 a month for twelve months. It was real nice. But we still didn't consider ourselves permanent citizens of Lovell. The Mormon influence was so heavy. We thought about our kids going to school and maybe marrying a Mormon. It was a constant fear.

"Our daughters, Susan and Linda, were more or less ostracized. Susan had a good Mormon friend from kindergarten till the first day of junior high. Then the friend dropped her because that's when the Mormon church groups got more active with kids. Susan was hurt. From then on she never had a close Mormon friend. It was a real heartbreaker.

"There's always been a certain monotony to Lovell, especially if you aren't in with the Mormon clique. The women's lives revolve around food, putting it up, raising and preparing it, and above all eating it. My, how they eat! There's not much else to do except talk about who was born, who died, who's been disfellowshipped or excommunicated.

"When I asked John why we didn't leave, he'd say, Well, I can't leave till so-and-so dies, or I'm committed to taking care of so-and-so, or so-and-so hasn't had her baby yet. Pretty soon I stopped talking about it.

"There were times when he was the only M.D. in town. A lot of doctors set up practices here and left. They didn't like house calls, they didn't like going out on emergencies. But John said he'd chosen a small town for a reason and we had to take the bad with the good."

Marilyn learned early that malicious gossip was the downside of a life in medicine. Physicians were easy targets of sexual complaints; it seemed to her that John had no more problems in that area than might have been expected in a busy family practice. Of course, he didn't bother her with every little thing. Now and then a high school kid would put in a gripe about a Girls Athletic Association exam. These were mostly Mormons, backward as dirt; they'd never been examined by anyone as thorough as John. Once a new friend told Marilyn, "My daughter says the girls are talking about something going on in your husband's office, but Marilyn—I *know* it's just gossip." Well, of course it was! The mothers all knew John; they came in for examinations themselves.

Ten or twelve years after he set up his practice, a woman named Annella St. Thomas lodged a silly complaint with the state, and he had to drive all the way to Casper to straighten things out. Then Caroline Shotwell stirred up more trouble—something about her daughter Mae, another famous nerve case. Caroline's husband came snorting into the office, which could have been a problem. He was a former high priest, and it wouldn't do to get crosswise with the Saints in a town that was half Mormon. John cooled him off with some facts about hysteria.

Marilyn remembered a few other complaints, par for the course. There was a medical name for the phenomenon: the de Clerambault Syndrome. Sufferers operated under the delusion that authority figures were in love with them; if denied, they were capable of violence. Marilyn had seen more than one candidate flounce in and out of the clinic, but nothing serious had ever developed.

Until now.

The first hints of this latest trouble appeared in the clinic's appointment book. Certain regular patients weren't returning, and Marilyn had been asked to make copies of at least a dozen charts and forward them to Dr. Welch or Dr. Wrung in Lovell or Dr. Christensen over in Powell. The McArthurs were the most prominent deserters.

At first she'd thought the problem might be financial; all told, the McArthur clan owed $4,000, and Dean's heart problems were only driving the bill higher. He'd been coming in once a week, and the female McArthurs were always showing up for one reason or another, even if it was just to pick up laundry or argue Scripture.

But now they were all missing. So was the Storys' old baby-sitter, Lanita "Grandma" Thompson, along with most of her widespread brood, and that nice letter carrier, Aletha, and quite a few others.

"What *is* this?" Marilyn asked her husband. "Something's fishy."

"Oh, that's kind of a natural thing," John assured her. "People want to try greener pastures. It's no problem."

One night he came home and told her he'd listened to a whole set of crazy complaints from Arden McArthur and her daughter Minda, and no explanation seemed to placate them. Then the mail lady, Aletha Durtsche, delivered a certified letter ordering John to appear at an informal hearing in Cheyenne.

"No problem," he repeated. Marilyn wasn't worried. The Medical Board members were practicing physicians. They knew about de Clerambault.

On July 20, 1983, two days before the scheduled hearing, Marilyn wrote in her journal: "Annette was born sixteen years ago today." As usual the scene played back: the crumpled form, the screams, the crowded services at the Lutheran church, the long drive with the tiny casket to the family plot in Maxwell.

How John's family had fussed over the lost child! Back home in Colorado, the departed were put in the ground quickly, but the Storys almost seemed to savor death and burials. John's chipper old mother, Inez, who closely resembled Marilyn in face and stature, often talked about relatives who'd died in her arms, how nice they looked, how the undertakers used to pack the bodies in ice, and other morbid details. The Storys enjoyed wandering around cemeteries. John once said, "I'm a graveyard person. I frequent them, look for the old names. It's a history lesson." Marilyn respected his attitude, but she preferred her history in books.

After Annette's death, John had wanted to take long walks and chew over incidents from her twenty months of life. "Those talks were hard," Marilyn told a friend. "He wanted to keep all his memories alive. That wasn't my way or my family's way." For years afterward, he liked to talk about his dead baby, pull her picture out of his wallet and show it around with pride.

When John left for the Medical Board hearing in Cheyenne, Marilyn ordered herself to stop worrying. He'd been persecuted before; it was no big deal. There'd been talk among friends of bringing a slander suit against the McArthurs, but he said he would never dream of suing a patient.

She couldn't wait for the scandal to recede. In the fall, John would be going to Jamaica on his second Christian medical mission, and this time wives were invited. Marilyn was in her early fifties, but she still had muscle tone and a firm figure, and she would rather ride waves than horses.

26

MINUTES OF SPECIAL MEETING
WYOMING BOARD OF MEDICAL EXAMINERS
(Condensed)

Dr. John Story appeared before the Board of Medical Examiners on July 22, 1983 at 10 A.M. for an informal interview as requested by the Board. He was advised that a formal hearing might be required. It was emphasized to Dr. Story that the purpose of the informal interview was to allow him to participate as fully as possible and to talk freely.

Dr. Story was informed that the Board had received five separate complaints from female patients who described sexual advances made during the course of pelvic examinations. It was emphasized to Dr. Story that the purpose of the informal interview was to investigate the complaints and that it was not a disciplinary proceeding.

Dr. Story was advised that the letters of complaint would be paraphrased since the individuals had requested that their names not be disclosed. However, if there was a formal hearing he would be given the opportunity to confront the witnesses. He was provided with the substance of the five complaints. He responded, "What I think as I listen to this is that I wouldn't do those sorts of things in my office. I have friends that have recommended that I take a hard reaction to this. One friend said I should sue."

Dr. Story felt most of the complaints were the products of an ex-employee who is a friend of the mother of one of the persons he suspects is a complainant. He stated that the daughter of one of the families he believed to be involved had used sim-

ilar accusations to "get a coach out of town." He said of the complainants, "It would take dwelling on it to build up these details. . . . It would take visualization . . . a lot of thinking and dwelling to think up these details." He alluded to the instability and psychological problems of the people involved and to incest in the community.

He stated he has confronted one or two people about these complaints. He further stated that he would not use his office in "that'" way, and that he suspected there were two people involved: middle-aged ladies who were rather "vicious." He explained that one worked for him at one time; his wife told him the other woman had also worked for him, and that half of "this" came from one family.

In response, parts of the letters were read. One complaint stated, "I have no reason to discredit Dr. Story. . . . I dearly love this man and I don't want to ruin him." Dr. Story stated the portions of the letters read to him sounded "compassionate." He said that he is aware of innuendos regarding two family households, marginal information about life-styles, and that he is trying to get some perspective as to what controls the mind.

He was asked if the charges were made because they are true, and he answered that the charges were not correct and that he would not use his office for such a purpose. He was asked if he meant that he was not adverse to using other places. He responded, "I haven't always been as I am now," and that the office was not used for such purposes. Continuing, he stated that to guard against "this" happening, a physician should never be alone in the office. He said that is now his practice and he has decreased the number of pelvic examinations by one-half.

Dr. Story was excused at this point. During the discussion the attendees took into account the fact the Board had received five complaints, and that Dr. Cohen had spoken with the complainants to confirm their identities. There was no reason to suspect the five complainants were lying about such a sensitive subject. On the other hand, Dr. Story had offered little more than a flat denial and the suggestion that he was being victimized for some unstated reason. At this point, the Board members concluded, the investigation would not be dropped.

Dr. Story was invited back into the room, and the following options were reviewed with him: 1) voluntarily agreeing to take some form of action such as relinquishing his license, or 2) proceeding to a formal hearing if an investigation so warranted. If the matter is not settled at the informal interview stage, Dr. Story was advised that there is an obligation on the part of the Board to further investigate the allegations.

He stated, "After twenty-five years in the community, that means the end for that, doesn't it?" At this point, he was strongly advised to obtain legal counsel before he made a decision.

Dr. Story told the Board he felt his choices were to either leave the state or to have all the accusations come out in the open. He was asked if he had any ideas on how to resolve the problem. He responded that the only thing he could suggest would be a requirement that he never examine a female patient without a nurse pres-

ent. Assistant Attorney General Kathleen Karpan responded that this type of dis-cipline would be difficult to enforce and would not address the problem of past misconduct. Dr. Story replied he would respond to charges of past misconduct by calling witnesses where there had been witnesses. He repeated his belief that there are two persons who have helped fan the accusations, and that they have histories of unreliability. He was asked, "Is there absolutely no foundation for the com-plaints, and are the women who have written these letters liars?" He responded, "Yes."

Dr. Story was asked if he has a temporal lobe seizure disorder which would ac-count for otherwise inexplicable conduct. He replied, "No."

He remarked he felt the Board had made a final decision. Dr. Story was in-formed that the majority of the board was not even aware that an informal inter-view was being held, that the informal interview was purely investigatory, and that his blanket denial would force the Board to investigate further.

Dr. Story again said the accusations were a product of sexual fantasies. He asked if the only way he could prove his innocence was by using character witnesses. He was told to consult an attorney regarding his defense.

Dr. Story was asked again if he could explain why anyone would make such an accusation if it were not true. He said, "I am beginning to make connections." One person he suspected of complaining is a member of a family he claims has practiced incest. Another suspected complainant, he said, was involved in making an accusation at a public meeting against a high school coach. The third person Dr. Story suspected of complaining is an ex-employee who was related to a "peep-ing Tom." No names were mentioned.

Dr. Story also said he suspected two of the complainants were patients who owed him quite a bit of money. One patient has a $1600 bill. She and her husband con-fronted Dr. Story regarding sexual conduct. Dr. Story said he lost his temper when the husband said what he would think every time he sent Dr. Story a dollar. Dr. Story told the husband he didn't want to accept any money. Dr. Story said the other patient owes him several thousand dollars.

Dr. Story was informed that the investigation would continue and would require personal interviews with the complainants and other patients. He was reminded that his attorney should feel free to contact Ms. Karpan at any time.

27

Minda Brinkerhoff

MINDA felt more antsy every day. On the phone, the Medical Board kept turning away her questions. Had the necessary five letters reached Cheyenne? That was confidential. Would action be taken? They weren't at liberty to say. Would the victims get a chance to testify? There were no such plans at the present time. The middle child told her mom that making an accusation against a doctor was like throwing a stone into Devil's Canyon. You never heard it hit.

The telephone was in Meg's lower half of the house, and Minda's arthritic hips throbbed as she hobbled down and up to answer. A few people entered complaints ("What are you McArthurs trying to do to Doc Story?"), but most of the callers were victims or friends of victims. The repeated message was, Hang in there. We're with you.

On the street, she was stopped by women she hardly knew. Some stressed that nothing had happened to them, but they had girl friends who'd gone to Dr. Story and . . . on and on. Minda suspected that they were really talking about themselves. The conversations were a constant reminder of how stupid she'd been, all the way back to Uncle Bob. As she drove past the sugar factory one day, a radio station reported on a woman who'd been raped by a dentist, taken him to court—and lost. Minda turned the radio off. Money and power usually prevailed; she didn't need a newscaster to tell her that.

Lately her physical problems had been worsening. The Lovell Cleaners had edged into the black, but the spotting fumes burned her throat worse than ever and her hips were inflamed from dragging around on the concrete floors. Any day now she would have to tell her ailing dad that she couldn't hack it—another Minda screw-up. She dreaded the confrontation; her parents had $100,000 invested, most of it from the sale of the farm. Meg's and Danny's shop, Kids Are Special, couldn't meet its overhead. They'd combined the store with the dry cleaners to cut expenses, but the local demand for modish junior styles proved limited. "What are we doing in this business?" Meg complained one day with her typical straightforwardness. "We're farmers." Yes, Minda thought. Without a farm.

Her biggest worry was so painfully personal that she couldn't discuss it. Amber Dawn was almost four now, a beautiful child with tawny skin and big brown eyes. She'd looked different from the other Brinkerhoffs from the beginning. And from the beginning, Minda had clashed with her.

Years later, she was harshly self-critical as she thrashed around and tried to explain the problem. "I still hated myself. After two boys, I didn't want a child who could grow up and be like me. I resented everything about Amber. She wasn't a baby you could hold and cuddle. The boys melted into your arms, but she was long and skinny. It felt like she was stiffening against me. Folks would say, She's a gorgeous baby. Oh, isn't she beautiful? She had blond hair with so much curl in it that people thought I'd had it layered. I was too hard on her. I expected her to be older than her years." She looked down. "I, uh—I wasn't a good mother."

Whenever Minda snapped at the toddler, Arden said things like, "Minda, if you don't do better by that li'l girl, I'm gonna take her away from you. Let her be a kid. Don't expect her to do things perfectly all the time."

At three, Amber trailed Minda like a pup, trying to please. She yelled, "I hate myself! I hate myself! I'm so ugly!" Minda thought, It's me all over again. My worst fears! I acted the same way after Uncle Bob. My mother was always trying to build up my self-esteem. Maybe it's in the genes. . . .

After her final ordeal in Examining Room No. 2, Minda leaned toward the belief that the child had been conceived during a pelvic exam. She remembered how insistently Story had set the due date, and how he'd taken the baby prematurely and caused her to have a "wet lung," and how he'd always given her extra attention.

The deepening suspicions drained her. She wondered how Scott would react if he knew. He was dewy-eyed about "Daddy's girl." Would he turn against Amber if he knew the truth? Turn against Minda? He was still bitter about Story. If she confided her suspicion, would he attack Story and end up in jail?

When weeks passed and nothing was heard from the Medical Board, the middle child showed her husband a copy of a letter she'd written to the famous Wyoming lawyer Gerry Spence, trying to enlist his help. The letter went into detail about Amber's origins. Scott read the letter and said, "It's okay, Minda." She was surprised at his calmness.

"What do you mean?"

"If Amber is Story's, it just means she's something special. It means we're supposed to have her. And we'll love her that much more."

She was relieved. It was one more secret she didn't have to guard like a hen on eggs. But she still wondered if she would ever be able to treat John Story's child with love.

28

Arden McArthur

ON SEPTEMBER 1, Arden came across an ad in the Lovell *Chronicle*:

Friday, September 9,
5 to 8 P.M.
(6 to 7 P.M. will be a special program.
All are encouraged to attend.)

At the Senior Citizen Building
the hospital will host a
25-year anniversary for
DR. STORY
for his association with
the North Big Horn Hospital

We would ask those who wish to send letters of appreciation to Dr. Story for this occasion to send them to the Personnel Department at the hospital so they can be included.

Arden realized that an instant publicity campaign was being generated by the doctor's admirers. If Dr. Story ever had to go before a Big Horn County jury for violating the fifteen or twenty women she'd now heard from, some of the jurors would surely be from Lovell. What pleasant memories they would have of this "spontaneous" tribute as they sat in judgment on the honored guest!

She went to see her fellow churchman and state senator, Cal Taggart, the most influential man in town. Cal was vintage Lovell, the grandson of one of the first settlers. He owned the building where the McArthurs operated the two stores, and she'd always found him fair and reasonable about rents and other sticky matters. She strongly suggested that he use his power to get the anniversary dinner called off and help run Story out of town.

Taggart reminisced that a hospital manager had come to him in the sixties or seventies with the claim that "Dr. Story's putting his weenie in his patients." He hadn't believed it then, he said, and he didn't believe it now.

"Well, take my word," Arden said. "He hasn't changed."

"You take *my* word, lady," Taggart said with his usual friendly smile. "If you have evidence, you better act on it. Otherwise you better just shut up."

The argument heated up. Taggart's main point was that his family had "doctored" with Story for years and the little man had never made the slightest move on the beautiful Mrs. Taggart or anyone else they knew. "Also," Taggart said, "he's a fine physician and surgeon. One of the best."

"Cal," Arden warned him, "don't help these people cover up."

"Damn it, Arden, you've got a short memory. Wasn't I the mayor when we got rid of Horsley?"

Arden preferred not to think about the Rose Doctor scandal. She knew a set of brothers he'd corrupted. One of them now strolled the streets of Lovell in a funk, his eyes rolling up in his head when he tried to carry on a conversation. Arden suspected that Bob Asay had also been a Horsley patient. She wondered if that was where Uncle Bob had developed his sexual tastes. She and several of her friends were convinced that Horsley had helped create the atmosphere in which behavior like Story's could flourish. There was an awful lot of kinkiness for such a small town.

"What did you do about Horsley, Cal?" she asked. She'd genuinely forgotten.

"Bill was my neighbor and friend. We went duck hunting every morning with my Labs. He got caught with that young fellow at the hospital and we barred him for good. I was on the hospital board that booted him out. I'd do the same to John Story in a second."

"You didn't do the town any favors, Cal," Arden said. "Horsley just kept right on abusing boys in his office at home." She paused. "Now you've got another doctor that's just as bad or worse. What are you gonna do about *him*?"

"Well, this case is different," the senator insisted. "Bill Horsley was guilty."

Still trying to head off the anniversary dinner, Arden called on Joe Brown, who'd come down from Miles City, Montana, to run the new North Big Horn Hospital three or four years earlier. Along with Dr. Story and three others, the fundamentalist Brown was an elder of the Lovell Bible Church.

"Why'd you wait till now to have this dinner?" she asked. "You're being plumb unjust to a lot of women."

Brown said he'd been about to get in touch with her. The hospital board had asked him to look into the Story rumors, and he would appreciate a meeting with her and her daughters. "If there are problems," he said in an earnest voice, "I'd like to know what I can do to help."

When Arden put down the phone, Dean warned in his weak voice, "Don't meet with that guy. You're asking for trouble."

She said that a meeting might help to head off that danged dinner.

They talked for an hour and a half. Minda came along and helped flesh out some of the details, dating to her first complaint and Arden's refusal to listen. She talked in her usual *prestissimo*, not wanting to leave anything out, even her confidential talks with the bishop and the stake president.

The hospital administrator asked a lot of questions about John Abraham's reaction. "It was hard for him to believe it," Minda explained. "Shoot, he didn't know where I was coming from. He'd never been confronted with anything like this. I all but had to get up on his table and show him what happened."

She cried as she described what Story had done to her and Meg. Arden listened and thought, Dear Father in Heaven, how many times will my poor babies have to repeat this story?

Brown seemed concerned. Arden said to herself, Why shouldn't he be? Story is the hospital's big surgeon; he keeps the beds filled. If he's abusing women in his clinic, he's abusing them in the hospital. Unless Joe Brown wants to risk a pile of money in lawsuits, he should be the first to take action, whether he shares Story's pew on Sundays or not.

That night, a distressed Minda phoned. John Abraham had just dressed her down for claiming that she'd demonstrated a pelvic exam on the table in his office. "President Abraham was upset, Mom," she said, speaking faster than ever. "I told him I didn't say any such thing. He told me to be careful of what I say and how I say it. He said, 'Watch your step!' Gol, Mom, I'm in big trouble, and I don't even know why."

Within a few days Arden heard other revisionist versions of the private conference at the hospital. In each playback, the McArthur women were cast as buffoons.

By the time she talked to the hospital administrator again, she was as hot as the presser at the cleaners. "Joe Brown," she said, "I am *so* disappointed in you. We came out there in good faith to give you honest information, and you're trying to use it to destroy us. You really don't want to know the truth, do you?"

Brown said something about rumors and gossip; he'd started hearing scuttlebutt about Dr. Story in his first weeks on the job. Arden jumped in, "And you didn't investigate? Did you ever hear that where there's smoke there's fire?"

"Not always," he said smoothly. "Not always." He suggested that she visit his office for some inside information. His tone made it clear that he considered his fellow Bible Church elder a victim, not an offender.

Arden thought, You've been listening to that little geek's stories about the women he threw out, haven't you?

"I have nothing to say to you, Joe Brown," she snapped. "I've talked to you for the last time. You didn't want information, you wanted ammunition. Well, you'll get no more from us."

29

Marilyn Story

*"In them days you had so much love for your husband
that anything he does, he could never do no wrong. I know
that my own husband, nothing he could do would be no
sin to me because I worship the ground he walks on."*
—quoted by Peter Matthiessen,
Men's Lives

IT WAS SUPPOSED TO BE a high point in their married life, but
Marilyn felt uneasy through the dinner. The affair was Joe Brown's
idea, a way to quiet some of the rumors, and he'd made lavish prepara-
tions in just a few days. The Senior Citizens Center was jammed with
John's admirers—Mayor Herman Fink, State Senator Cal Taggart,
Reverend Kenneth Buttermore of the Lovell Bible Church and three or
four other preachers, plus loyal patients of all denominations. Fresh
flowers graced every table. Six courses were beautifully catered, including nonalcoholic drinks for the Mormons. A big "25" rode the ten-
layer cake.

The hospital's chief of staff, Dr. John Welch, told the crowd that
Lovell was lucky to have a physician with John's skills and dedication.
Joe Brown seconded the motion. One of John's nurses drew laughs
when she noted that Dr. Story had delivered both her and her baby
"and we'd do it all over again." John accepted a watch, a doctor doll
complete with glasses, a hospital smock with his name on it, and a book
of appreciation signed by his admirers. He mumbled his thanks and sat
down. Marilyn thought, He can sew up a chain-saw wound without
a trace of nerves, but if you put him in front of an audience, he
turns puce.

She wished she were enjoying herself. As she looked from face to face, she wondered, Do you know what's going on? Do *you*? She was afraid they all knew. That was why so many were here—to show support. She was properly appreciative, but she wondered if their support would influence the bullheads in Cheyenne. Why, they could void a license with a nod of their heads. Bureaucrats hated mavericks— that had always been one of John's favorite themes—and they'd been after him for years. He opposed Medicare, Medicaid, Social Security, all the giveaway state and federal medical plans. He returned the free immunization drugs like MMRs and oral polio that the Wyoming Medical Board had tried to shove on doctors. He refused to take part in any of their programs and plans, even the ones he approved, because he considered them a form of creeping socialism. He was an old-fashioned independent physician, responsible only to God and his patients, and no state could abide such individualists.

As she looked around the party room, Marilyn's eyes fell on Inez Lewis Story, John's sturdy little eighty-three-year-old mother. She'd driven up from Maxwell with Uncle Howard Story, an octogenarian bachelor with the cutting voice and brisk manner of Dwight D. Eisenhower. The two of them looked so happy and proud. Marilyn said to herself, If you only knew. . . .

Neither Marilyn nor John had mentioned the charges. There was always the possibility that the clouds would pass as they'd passed before, and the Nebraska folks would never need to know. Still, it felt disloyal to withhold information from two of the people who loved John most.

That night, Marilyn sat up late as her chatty mother-in-law recounted the sagas of the Storys and the Lewises, the Merricks and the Huntingtons, John's illustrious forebears. With her precise command of language and her colorful locutions, the good-natured Inez ushered the wraiths of John's ancestors into the living room one by one. As usual, she brooked few interruptions and thoroughly dominated the conversation.

With the passing years, Marilyn had noticed an almost ethereal peacefulness in the woman she called Mom. After a stern and difficult childhood, Inez had seemed to bypass the usual vicissitudes. Until she was in her seventies, she would challenge anyone to a footrace—and usually win. She still broke into lighthearted old songs while doing the dishes:

Every fish and worm began to twist and squirm
And the captain and the ship does a corkscrew turn . . .

Inez had taught Scripture for forty years and still attended Bible Study class in Maxwell. For years she'd exchanged verses with John by mail. As a teen, he'd personally converted his family from Christians to *Christians*, and she still sought his counsel on spiritual matters. "He gives me verses to look up, like the ones in First Peter where it talks about the fiery trials we're all gonna go through," Inez told her daughter-in-law. "John seems to like those verses."

The sweet old lady avoided any mention of sex; the subject was forbidden in her home. She'd had a female operation but never mentioned it to her doctor son or her other two children. Years later, when she'd needed John's expert opinion, she asked Marilyn, "Do you think it would be proper to tell John?"

Inez never said much about her late husband William. Marilyn had always admired the old man and found him interesting. "Dad Story was a wonderful man," she told a friend. "Good-looking, with white wavy hair, a marvelously intelligent man. So *neat*. When he died in 1971, we looked at his desk in the Story general store and it was perfect, everything ready for his death.

"Dad Story was a godlike figure to his children. He flew in the Army Signal Corps in World War I and he liked to take the kids to the sandbars in the river and march them up and down like soldiers. On rainy days they drilled in the house with broomsticks for rifles. Dad Story could be stern, and they really snapped to.

"For a while, he made his own kids speak German around the house. No one knew why; it was just an interest of his. John ended up taking German in school, and his brother Jerod taught it in college. Somehow John ended up disliking German *and* Germans. Isn't that natural for Englishmen? Germans have certain personalities that John doesn't like—he says they're too much followers; they don't stand on their own feet. I always have to remind him that I'm a kraut myself. I'm the only German he likes!

"Maybe it's his rebellion against his dad. I don't know; I'm not a psychiatrist. Dad Story didn't hug his kids or act affectionate toward them. You never heard the word 'love' on that side of the family. Dad Story was a fine man, but he seemed a little overcontrolled, distant. The family would go to visit friends and he'd sit outside in his car reading the market reports. Everybody said, 'Oh, that's just Bill's way.'

"We saw him kiss 'Mom' once. My daughters and I were getting ready to leave Maxwell after a visit and we all lined up so Dad Story could come down the row and give us a kiss one by one, and Inez slipped into line behind us and he kissed her by mistake. She said 'I fooled you!' It's a family joke."

The first issue of the Lovell *Chronicle* after the twenty-fifth-anniversary dinner pictured John in his polyester suit and his brushed-down graying hair, making his shy thank-you speech. "The present was traditional," the caption read, "but the package wrapping was not when Dr. John Story was honored for twenty-five years with the local hospital Friday. The gold pocket watch he is holding came wrapped in bandages."

Several friends called to say how good he looked in the picture, but John said he would be perfectly happy if he never saw his name in the paper again.

As the uncertain days passed, Marilyn couldn't shake her fears. John kept assuring her that every doctor had the same problem and he'd handled it well. A few weeks after the anniversary celebration, she wrote in her journal: "Dreamed several times in one night of being on a high bluff and realizing at the last moment that it had only a crest—the rest being entirely undermined. This morning the verse: Ps 94:18 'When I said, my foot slippeth; thy mercy, O Lord, held me up.' "

She was relieved when it came time to fly to Jamaica. They landed at Montego Bay and enjoyed a week's vacation in Ocho Rios with their good friends from Lovell, the Shumways. Then they were driven to Black River to begin John's second mission for the Christian Medical Society. En route, Marilyn tried not to think of his first. It had been to Honduras, and while he'd been gone, Annette had slipped from their hands.

This time he was the only surgeon on the trip and it seemed as though he never took off his blood-spotted smock and latex gloves. The locals streamed toward the camp for herniorrhaphies, C-sections, appendectomies, tonsillectomies, tumor excisions, wart removals, ingrown nails, even counseling. John was a one-man "MASH." For once in his life, he couldn't spend three hours with his nose in the manuals before every operation. On a sightseeing drive in the mountains, he wound up sewing an auto victim's gashed arm.

She told herself. This is how I always thought of medicine. She felt a soaring pride. Even on the most hectic days, John never forgot his

Christianity, dispensing Scripture along with prescriptions, and Bibles along with drug samples. She thought, How can anyone accuse this man? What kind of satanic fiends would mount a poison-tongue campaign against a man whose only purpose in life is to praise God and help his fellow man?

They returned to Lovell to find his name on everyone's lips. The *Chronicle* had run a long article under a six-column headline:

LOCAL DOCTOR CALLED BEFORE STATE MEDICAL BOARD

The paper reported that investigators were looking into the case and "a dozen letters against Story were received . . . [and] about 30 letters supporting the doctor." A formal hearing was scheduled for mid-November but would probably be postponed.

Marilyn wrote in her journal: "Back from Jamaica to be met with more of our troubles—even more serious and public than before. Brothers and sisters here have been fasting and praying for us. Our hearts are warmed and blessed. But Lord, suddenly I am angry—angry at the so-called professional people in Cheyenne who have become judge and jury and obviously decided on a guilty verdict at the very first (and only) informal visit. Help me to believe the verse you gave me yesterday—(Ps 50:15 + 23) and claim it as your promise to us, Father. Jesus, you were falsely accused. May we model our lives after you?"

30

Minda Brinkerhoff

MINDA AND SCOTT decided to settle the question of Amber Dawn's parentage. They'd been assuring each other that it didn't matter, but it did.

The little Brinkerhoff family had switched to Douglas Wrung, M.D., another member of the Lovell Bible Church. Story had been instrumental in bringing him to Lovell, but the new man had an excellent reputation and the children seemed to like his style.

Minda asked him for a lab slip authorizing blood tests. When she got back home she told Scott what happened next.

"Dr. Wrung said, 'What's this all about?' I said, 'We really don't know if my daughter is Scott's or Dr. Story's.' He told me that was the stupidest thing he'd ever heard. How could I take a perfectly fine doctor and run him through the wringer like this? I told him I wasn't leaving the office till I got the form. Then on the way home I ran into one of my cousins and she said, 'What are you doing to Dr. Story? This is crazy, this is stupid! I can't believe you're doing this.' "

Scott slowly shook his head. She could see that he was sick of the whole affair.

The lab reported that the tests couldn't be 100 percent conclusive without a blood sample from Dr. Story, but it appeared almost certain that Scott was the father.

The news was welcomed, but it didn't solve other problems. Lovell, the town of Minda's birth and life, was becoming enemy territory. After Story's anniversary party, people crossed the street when they saw her coming. A grocer cracked smart. Her children were bullied at school.

As long as they stayed in Lovell, she never knew when she might drag her arthritic bones home from the dry cleaners to find her husband being led away in handcuffs for taking after Story with his deer rifle. Scott was still working in the oil fields, but the job was petering out now that winter was coming. She persuaded him to send out some résumés, and he was offered a junior computer programmer's job in Gillette, 100 miles to the east.

Her mother agreed to take over the dry cleaners, and a week later, the Brinkerhoffs moved. As they drove into Gillette, they were tempted to turn around and go home. The coal-mining boomtown was dreary and dispiriting. But it had one charm: its citizens knew nothing about Minda Brinkerhoff or a weird sick doctor in Lovell. Gillette would be a perfect place for licking wounds.

A few weeks later, Minda underwent her first session of gestalt therapy. The counselor told her to pretend that she was talking to Story. "You're real angry at him, Minda," the therapist instructed her. "Now what do you have to tell him?"

Minda thought, I came to this town to get away from Dr. Story— and now he's in this room? "Huh?" she asked.

"You're angry, Minda! This man raped you! You're—*mad*! Now tell him how you feel!"

Minda thought, I'm *not* angry. At least right now. Sometimes I want to wring his neck, but most of the time I just feel sad.

She took a deep breath and addressed the empty chair. "Gosh, Dr. Story, I'm disappointed in you." She felt stupid. "I mean, I *really* am. Gol, we trusted you all those years." She thought, How embarrassing! "We *loved* you, Dr. Story."

"Minda," the therapist interrupted, "it's okay to yell."

"But I don't hate him. I—I wish I could help him."

The counselor said she was supposed to be helping herself, not the rape doctor. "You're suppressing a lot of anger, Minda."

"Yep," Minda said. "I'm angry about my arthritis. I'm angry about my throat and my tongue and my mouth. I'm angry about a lot of other things. But . . . I feel sorry for Dr. Story."

The psychologist suggested that the angers might be connected.

At the next session, they rooted around in her past. That night Minda told Meg on the phone, "The idea is to put all the blame on Mom and Dad and my crummy childhood. We didn't have a crummy childhood, did we, Meg? Gol, I enjoyed it!"

Her highly educated sister assured her that they'd had the most wholesome childhood since *National Velvet*. Minda dropped the shrink and made an appointment for a checkup with Clinton Hartman, M.D., a young Mormon with a family practice. Her blue-green eyes rolled with fright as she walked into his examining room. "Look," she told him, "I've had some real problems with a doctor and I don't want any kinky stuff. Just tell me what you're doing before you do it and we'll both be happy."

Dr. Hartman looked puzzled, then sympathetic. "Okay, Mrs. Brinkerhoff," he said. "First I'd like to check your heart with my stethoscope." She started to unbutton, after all the years with Story, but he listened through her blouse. "Now I'm checking your knees for reflex. Now I'm taking your blood pressure. . . ."

The examination was thoroughly professional, but she never really relaxed.

One day a State of Wyoming attorney and two lawyers for Dr. Story met her in a conference room and asked a million questions about the case. She'd never heard of a "deposition," but Assistant Attorney General Kathleen Karpan, representing the Medical Board, explained that all she had to do was tell the truth. She explained that Story's lawyers had requested the session to assist them in preparing his defense, which was their right under the law.

Minda gulped when she was introduced to one of the opposing lawyers: William Simpson, son of the U.S. senator from Wyoming. She thought, A senator's son questioning *Minda*? She gulped harder when she noticed that Simpson sat silently while a young woman named Loretta Kepler asked the questions. Dean McArthur's children weren't accustomed to such role reversals.

Kathy Karpan had advised that the Story lawyer might take any of several approaches to pry out information. She might act dim-witted, like Columbo on TV; she might stroke Minda with friendly phrases and compliments; she might play word games to catch her off guard; she might even be abrupt and hostile.

It didn't take long to find out. The first few questions came like
birdshot: What's your name? What is your address? When were you
born? Where were you born?

Minda thought, Can't somebody smile around here? Her tongue and
mouth still hurt from the spotting fluid. She kept trying to remember
Kathy's advice, something about listening to the question and thinking
carefully before answering, but her old compulsion to be heard and
understood *right now* soon took over. The official transcript caught
her tone:

Q   And then you lived in Lovell from 1982—
A   1982 till three months ago I think because Scott graduated. Gosh, he
graduated in college in '81, '82, I don't remember. Shoot, it's been so long
ago. Anyway, we were in Lovell I think nine months so it was a year and a half.
I lied. Gosh, I don't know, golly . . .

Minda caught a look from the assistant attorney general and throttled
down till she was asked to describe what Dr. Story had done to her.
Even at her usual speed, her answer took ten minutes. When she was
finished, the court reporter sighed and looked at the ceiling.

In the next siege of questioning, Minda remembered something that
had slipped from her mind. Talking about one of the incidents in
Story's office, she said, "I went home that time with pen marks up and
down my legs."

Q   Pen marks?
A   Pen marks.
Q   What color ink?
A   I don't remember what color.

She knew it was an odd memory, but she supposed he'd kept his pens in
the waist pocket of his smock. The defense lawyer didn't look too
pleased that she'd remembered a detail like that.

The questioning by Kathy Karpan was more congenial, and Minda
slowed down a little. The state's lawyer asked why she'd tried to keep
her blouse on during Story's examinations:

A   I hated laying there without any clothes on. That is the most horrible
feeling. And I figured that he could either reach up down through the top or
from below because for the amount of time that he spent with my breasts I was
very much uncomfortable laying there without anything on.

Q Did you feel that his examination of your breasts took longer than it should have . . . ?

A That's the only guy that ever did it. In Rock Springs they didn't even check for it, so never—

Q How long do you think it took him? Was it a matter of a minute or two minutes or three minutes?

A Oh, he made sure he felt around real slow and pushed and I don't know how long it was.

She was asked about her earlier years with Story.

A . . . I had an open relationship with him. We talked, we laughed, we joked. There wasn't anything, ya know, that I couldn't ask him about and, ya know. . . .

Q Would you say it was flirtatious on your part or his part?

A I never thought it to be that way on his part. And he would comment, "Oh, you came in. You sure don't look sick." And I never thought, I always thought it was because he cared. . . .

Toward the end, some of Karpan's questions turned speculative:

Q Is it possible again, Minda, and I'm trying to be most generous, is it possible that Dr. Story could have thought, "Well, you know, Minda has touched my penis a couple of times and didn't run screaming out of the room. Maybe I can try something kinky?"

A That's exactly what I thought: he was a kinky dirty old man, and when I think about it, I think that's what it was. He figured, "Well, I haven't scared her off because she was so naive." And she was. She's not anymore. . . .

Q In retrospect, is there anything you would have done differently?

A Yeah. I wish I would have grabbed it and hauled him out in the hall and asked him what he wanted to do now, and I didn't. I won't ever trust anybody like I trusted him. It's hard for me I think now as I go to the doctors, this is terrible. I take my kids into Dr. Setliff. He's very nice. And I think, Gosh, I wonder if he's like Dr. Story. . . . And every doctor I see I think that, and I think that's awful, how terrible, but I won't ever send my kids in. Oh, I don't care if they're eighteen or nineteen. Their mom's coming with.

And so he scared me away from doctors. I don't trust and I won't believe. It's kinda like he's been on a God's pedestal in Lovell. With most of the people that I know in the group we're with, he could do no wrong. And that's why he was defended so much and it's like I've been asked, "He's a God-fearing man. Why would you do this?" And I thought, "Why would he do this to me?" You know. I will not put another doctor in that position again.

Q   So it's had quite an impact on your life?

A   Yeah. When I make love with Scott, I think of that last exam I was with him, you know, and Dr. Story was in and out real slow, and I think—anyway . . ."

The court reporter's transcript noted, "Witness shakes head from side to side."

31

Meg Anderson

MEG felt better after the two investigators interviewed her at home in Lovell. It was the first official confirmation that the case was still alive.

In the long weeks of silence, she'd suffered from her old self-contempt. She took the blame for the scandal, told herself that she should have done something, screamed, jumped up—anything but lain there like a lump. She'd allowed it to happen, and wasn't that just about the same as encouraging it to happen?

She couldn't sort out her feelings. She still felt love for Dr. Story. He'd done so much for her family. She could still see the intensity on his face as he listened to her father's heartbeat through his stethoscope. She could still hear him in the delivery room. "Push, Meg. That's it! Oh, you're doing fine. . . . You've got a beautiful baby boy."

Sometimes she told herself she must have dreamed the incident on the examining table. She'd never seen his penis. Sure, a woman could tell, but could she be certain enough to destroy a doctor's life? She'd learned in college how tricky the mind could be. Was the whole thing an exercise in self-hypnosis?

Impossible, she told herself. I know what I felt.

But if she ever had to go before a judge or jury, would they understand? Or would they just snicker about her "black feelings" and intuitions? Sure, women knew—but did men? Wouldn't Story be judged by men?

Every day she talked long-distance to Minda. The middle child had been wise to exile herself to Gillette. The tension was building in Lovell, and the mercurial Minda might have ended up in a fistfight on the street. *Don't mess with Minda.* Meg remembered her family's watchword.

Even in church, old friends were going out of their way to show their contempt for the Brinkerhoffs and the McArthurs and the Andersons. It was the cruelest blow. She told herself, When we went into this I never thought that my own people wouldn't believe me. Why, I've never lied in my life!

She stayed home and locked the doors.

A week before Christmas, Meg and several others were deposed in a Lovell office by Assistant Attorney General Kathleen Karpan and three defense lawyers. The female of the trio, Loretta Kepler, got Meg to repeat her story as she'd told it times before. All she could remember later was that the Kepler woman wore no makeup.

DEPOSITION OF MEG MCARTHUR ANDERSON
(Excerpts)

Q (By LORETTA KEPLER) Did you say anything to Dr. Story about it [the second] time?

A No, I did not.

Q Why not?

A Would you?

Q Yes.

A Well, I congratulate you. I didn't want to be there. I didn't want to believe what was happening and I certainly didn't want Dr. Story to be the one I was thinking about it.

Q Say that again.

A I didn't want Dr. Story to be the one I was thinking it about. . . .

Q Who delivered your second child?

A Dr. Wrung.

Q Did he give you a pelvic examination?

A Uh huh.

Q How did his pelvic examinations differ from Dr. Story's?

A It only lasted for two minutes maximum. He would insert a finger to see if the head was floating, and that was all.

Q And that was it?

A That was it.

To Meg, the rest of her testimony seemed like a thricetold tale. How many times would she be expected to go over the same set of facts? Did they expect the truth to vary?

As she was leaving the building, Kathy Karpan told her that many others would be deposed, but their names couldn't be revealed. It seemed that the case against Dr. Story was ballooning.

32

The Record

DEPOSITION OF JOHN CHARLES WELCH, M.D.
(Excerpts)

Q (By LORETTA KEPLER) You have said that you believe Dr. Story is a good doctor. Do you believe he's capable of doing these sort of things?

A I think you're asking me to make a judgment that I really can't make, Mrs. Kepler.

Q You mentioned once that he had a split personality.

A No, I didn't say that. I said, my statement was that if he's guilty, then it has to be something like that. I don't believe he had a split personality, okay? Don't misquote me. . . .

Q Do you always have a nurse present when you do [pelvic] examinations?

A Always . . . except when I do one on my wife. Every other time, yes. Never have I ever done a pelvic examination or even continued one if [the nurse] has to leave the room. I stop and leave with her. . . .

Q (By KATHLEEN KARPAN) . . . Is this a policy you adopted as a result of your education at Colorado University?

A Yes. . . . We had a lecture by a physician who was, I think, also a lawyer. . . . He made the statement that the coming thing is medical-legally you have to protect yourself. That even in the case of a physician, if a woman were to holler rape, I didn't have a leg to stand on if I was alone during a pelvic examination. . . .

Q Doctor, aside from this practical concern about potential liability, do you believe there is an ethical aspect, too?

174

A Absolutely. . . .

Q . . . How would you define that ethical responsibility a doctor has towards a woman patient during a pelvic examination?

A It has a lot to do with my religious upbringing, I'm sure. That is, I never see a patient totally naked, if I can help it. There's always a drape or something on her. I am very uncomfortable if I have to see a patient totally naked. I just am. . . .

Q Can you envision a circumstance where it would be appropriate for a doctor and a woman patient to engage in sexual relations in the doctor's office during a pelvic examination?

A No. . . . There is medical ethics among psychiatrists and psychologists wherein they prescribe sexual therapy. I can't fathom it doing anything but harm. . . .

Q In your opinion, as a small town doctor in Lovell, is that a desirable therapy?

A Not only in Lovell, but anywhere, I can't see where it is. . . . There is a very special relationship a physician has with his patient. I am sure you have heard, and it's true, that women fall in love with their doctors. . . . There is no question that the doctor is allowed to do things that no one else on earth could do to them, sometimes even including their husbands. And that would be the greatest abuse of that trust, and that's what it is, that I can imagine. First of all, because a woman who comes to a doctor with a problem is vulnerable because she has a problem in the first place, be it physical, be it sexual, be it emotional or whatever, and . . . the only way it can be is damaging. . . .

Q What type of implements or instruments would you use in conducting a pelvic examination aside from your own hand?

A Okay. I expect the way to make you understand this would be—a pelvic examination means that first of all you feel abdominally, see if you feel any lumps or masses in the lower part of the abdomen. Then the patient is put in the stirrups with the nurse in the room. She scoots clear down to the end of the table or as near as she can get. Sometimes physically it won't allow them, then I use a plastic speculum with a disposable light attached to it. . . .

Then I always tell the patient I'm going to be touching you, and because it has been, in my experience, a big shock to touch that area first, I always touch with the back of my hand on the side of her. Then we manipulate the labia, insert the light. If I need to do the Pap smear or any other kind of things where I have to look and examine, that takes . . . thirty seconds to sixty seconds. Then I withdraw the speculum. Then I do a bimanual examination wherein I insert the left hand, two fingers, in the vagina, put the four fingers on the lower part of the pelvis and then between the two fingers feel all the organs inside. That usually, I would say, almost never takes more than three to five minutes. Three minutes, I would say, is most. . . .

Q During the course of a pelvic examination, if a doctor said, I think I better dilate you, what would that mean? Why would he do it and how would he do it?

A The only reason that one would need to dilate would be because the opening to the vagina for the pelvic examination would be too small, and when it's too small, it hurts like blazes. . . . I never use the word dilate. . . .

Q Have you ever had a patient come and say, Doctor, that pelvic was so painful I hurt for three days? I was very uncomfortable for three days?

A Patients don't come back to you if they do that. I'm sorry to be a little flippant. I have had examinations that are painful. But no, not for three days. If they are having three days of pain, then something's wrong.

Q . . . Would you ever attempt to insert the speculum from the rear?

A Rear of what?

Q Come in and have her turn around and see if you can get it in from behind? . . . Have you ever had to have the patient turn over on the back or squat on the floor, doctor?

A I have never done it. There may be some value gained from that, but I can't imagine what it might be.

Q . . . Is there anything else, doctor? . . .

A No. I just hope it's not true. I really think he's a good doctor. . . .

Q (By LORETTA KEPLER) Did you ever ask Dr. Story whether he had done any of the things that rumors had said he had done?

A No, I have not. I basically am a coward and I was afraid of the answer.

Q Okay.

A A man is still innocent until proven guilty.

DEPOSITION OF JOSEPH C. BROWN
(Excerpts)

Q (By KATHY KARPAN) When you took over in 1979 as [hospital] administrator, did you receive any files or any written or unwritten complaints against Dr. John Story that would involve sexual misconduct?

A I had no transmission of any complaints in writing.

Q Is that true to today? Have you at this point in time ever received—

A I have never received a written complaint on Dr. Story.

Q . . . Have you ever carried out an investigation, formally or informally, about Dr. John Story and allegations of sexual misconduct?

A I have carried out a formal—informal complaint at the request of the board. . . . Prior to this time I had no complaint except hearsay. And so there was no reason for me to follow up anything. . . . [I met with] Minda and Mrs. McArthur.

Q Did you contact anyone else?

A . . . No.

Q The September First meeting was the sole investigative work you did on Dr. Story?

A . . . Well, I couldn't tell you it all because it's kind of been kind of informal, just assisting people with names or with possible questioning that might come up. I can't—it's—you know, if you ask me a specific question, I might be able to answer it. . . . I gave a report verbally.

Q   At a board meeting?

A   At a board—at—I can't remember if it was a formal meeting or it was kind of a—I really didn't say much because it was sexually oriented. We have men and women. And I merely gave my feelings as to the board's—what I felt was the case.

Q   And what were those feelings?

A   My personal feeling was that [Minda] was not a reliable witness. She evidenced other problems. I am not a psychologist nor a psychiatrist, so I can't say. I can only say my own personal observation, my own personal feelings here. But having had many years of experience in the field of health and dealing with mental health situations, I felt that she was unreliable as a witness and she was somewhat—her character was somewhat questionable. . . . And the mother was also fairly contradictory in her statements.

Q   . . . You had doubts about [Minda's] credibility or her reliability because of possible mental problems, and?—

A   No, I didn't say mental problems. . . . Don't say mental problems because I am not a psychiatrist.

Q   . . . Well, what kind of problems? . . .

A   Oh, I really don't know what her problems are. I have heard a lot of hearsay and I don't like to quote hearsay. She has been involved with—it's my understanding from hearsay—the throwing out of a coach for what they claim to be teaching sexual things. . . . And she became pregnant, it's my understanding. . . .

Q   Did you go and talk to anyone at the high school to confirm whether or not this hearsay was true?

A   I did not want to involve myself in that hearsay.

Q   But you did conclude that Minda Brinkerhoff would not be a reliable witness because of this problem without checking it out?

A   Oh, I had enough people tell me as hearsay to give me adequate knowledge that it actually occurred. . . .

Q   When you use that phrase "questionable character," were you referring to this incident in high school?

A   No. I was referring to her conduct [during the interview] . . . things she did, the way she acted.

DEPOSITION OF JEAN ANDERSON HOWE
(Excerpts)

Q   (By LORETTA KEPLER)   Are you positive about how old you were?

A   No, I'm not. . . . I had to have been anywhere from eight to ten.

Q   . . . Would you describe from the beginning what happened?

A   Okay. I can remember being in the room and the nurse and the doctor talking. I can remember the nurse saying that she needed a shot—the doctor said I needed a shot. So they both went out of the room. He said that he would give me the shot. And then I can remember him coming back in and closing the door. He stood at the table and was preparing something. And I can remember him tugging and playing with his pants. And then he was still messing around with the shot at the table.

And then I remember him turning around. I can't remember if he had the shot in his hand or not. And then that's when his penis fell out of his pants. And that's when he asked me the question whether I was okay. . . . And then that's when he pushed his penis back up inside because I can remember seeing something brown. That's all I remember, was that it was something brown that fell out of his pants.

And I turned back—he turned back to the table and picked something off of the table and turned back around and he asked me another question that I can't remember, walked over to the table. He said that he had a kidney machine that he was going to put underneath me and that he wanted me to lift up the lower part of my body. And he slipped that underneath me. And I can remember it was nice and soft and warm.

And I can't remember how long that lasted. And he gave me the shot and then I guess I got my pants up and then we—he helped me sit up, and I can't remember anything after that. . . .

Q So what did [your mother] do?

A She took me home and I stayed with my dad. And then she went down to the police department and reported it. . . . And they said they couldn't do anything about it. . . . And she wrote a letter to the Medical Board. . . . She said they didn't do anything.

Four other witnesses were deposed. A Lovell housewife named Carol Beach testified that she'd been contacted by a relative and informed that a case was being made against Story at the Medical Board. She'd then written a letter about her own experience.

She testified that she'd told her husband on their wedding night, "This hurts just exactly like that pelvic Dr. Story gave me." She also charged that Story had manipulated her clitoris.

Her schoolteacher husband confirmed the wedding night conversation.

Kay Holm, housewife, substitute teacher, and wife of another Lovell Bible Church elder, deposed that Dr. Story had been her personal physician for seven years. She insisted that the charges were all gossip and lies—"Here goes Lovell again, another scam, another snowball, everybody jump on the bandwagon type thing. Lovell is pretty famous for that."

Peggy Rasmussen, a rural mail carrier and a Mormon, deposed that she'd been seeing Dr. Story for twenty-three years, that he'd given her frequent pelvic examinations, including one a week during a difficult pregnancy, and that she'd written a letter of support to the Medical Board. Her daughter Rhonda worked in Dr. Story's office as an aide.

33

Diana Harrison

Poor Diana. She's had a rough background. When you look at her, she wears that mask. Her hair's always perfect, and inside she's just a hurtin' lady. I would love to be able to set down and present Christ to her.

—The Reverend Kenneth Buttermore

DIANA MARIE BEAL HARRISON, five-two in her flats, was in a quandary. She'd worked for the man she called Doctor for six straight years, starting when she was nineteen, discontinued to follow her husband Bill to Cody and Cheyenne, then resumed part time in the last few years. She could honestly say that she idolized both him and Marilyn.

She could also honestly say that he'd violated at least two of his patients. One was her aunt, Emma Lu Meeks, a seventy-five-year-old widow, and another was one of Emma Lu's closest friends, Julia Bradbury. Aunt Emma was a Mormon pioneer, devout, lively, and as alert as most thirty-years-olds. Her husband Ted had served as town cop. If she said Doctor did it, Doctor did it.

But she'd told Diana in strictest confidence. Aunt Emma hadn't even told her bishop. She said she would die of shame if her secret got out, but she had to warn Diana so Story wouldn't do the same to her. "You trust that man too much," the old woman warned. "I trusted him and look what happened."

Diana's head weighed a ton these days. Her family's medical insurance came through the clinic, and her daughter's latest operation for a congenital urethral problem had cost $10,000. She and Bill would have lost everything if it hadn't been for that insurance. And the Storys had

179

always been so good to her, lent her money, given her days off when she needed them, treated her like family. She couldn't just dump them.

But she also had obligations to her aunt and the other victims. Some of the names ricocheting around town were friends, fellow Saints, former classmates at Lovell High School. She'd gone to Mutual with them, prayed with them, shared seats on temple excursions.

One evening when Bill came in from the malt barley that he raised for Coors and Budweiser on their six hundred rented acres, she told him, "I feel so bad about those poor women. Especially Minda. I'm the one who talked her into coming in. And then she was raped!"

Bill was a darkly handsome man, built like a cannon and just as soft and yielding. He was a studious scriptorian who looked with favor on the oldest teachings of his church, including polygamy. He instructed her to stay out of the controversy. It didn't concern her or the church. As far as men like Story were concerned, didn't the book of Nephi say, "Satan has great power over Gentiles"?

When an assistant attorney general arrived at the Harrison home to ask questions, Diana retreated into her standard defense of bubbly amiability. But in her nervousness, she let slip the basic information about the two unknown victims.

"Oh, Bill," she said afterward, "I'm so naïve. That woman let me go on and on and then she told me I could be subpoenaed and forced to tell the truth. I've never been in court. Honey, I'm scared to death."

Then Doctor's lawyers warned that sooner or later she would have to tell everything she knew or be held in contempt. Father in Heaven, she prayed, I'm getting it from both sides. I'll go to jail! What'll happen to my children?

She drove to Emma Lu's house. "They're pressuring me," she told her old aunt. "What's gonna happen if I have to say your name, and I can't, and they send me to jail?"

"I've had it with all those people!" Aunt Emma said. "Go ahead, Diana. Tell 'em I'll testify."

Two days before the formal Medical Board hearing, Diana answered the phone at home. "What's going on?" Doctor asked. "I just heard from my lawyer that Julia Bradbury and Emma Meeks are listed as witnesses against me. Diana, do you suppose you could come over?"

As she changed from her grubbies to head for the Storys', Diana felt like the rope in a tug of war. In the past, her allegiance had always been to her employer. Doctor had even delivered her children. She'd baby-sat Linda and Susan Story, exchanged holiday gifts, written poetic tributes to Doctor and delivered them tremblingly to his life-giving hands. The Storys always told her she was different from other Mormons.

When she'd returned to the clinic after several years away, she'd found a mess. Doctor's gross income was over $100,000 a year, but she saw ways to streamline the system and clean up unpaid bills. She even turned up a tax shelter where he could stash his profits at a good rate of interest. She had a secret laugh over that one; the administrators were LDS.

The very next year, the Storys took in so much money that they had to pay $25,000 in income taxes. Marilyn acted depressed, Doctor sulked, and they both made Diana feel guilty. She thought, They hate the government so much, they'd rather make less money than pay their fair share.

By then she'd begun to wonder about a few other things. One woman flat refused to pay her bill. "I'll never pay it and Dr. Story knows why," she confided.

Then Diana began to notice that Doctor was spending long periods in the examining room. She thought she detected a pattern: lengthy sessions with vulnerable women, single women, women whose marriages were troubled or whose husbands were sick or weak, and short workmanlike sessions with bright forceful women or well-married women or women whose husbands were important or powerful. His favorite patient was a married blonde whom everyone else in the office despised. He frequently dilated her for "headaches," sometimes even at night. The woman's arrival seemed to set Marilyn on edge. "Her again!" she would complain. "I don't like that woman. I don't know what's going on in there. I think she has designs on him." Marilyn would pace the hall outside the examining room.

Over the years, Diana had watched her dear friend change, beginning with Annette's death. Marilyn was no whiner, but a few complaints had worked to the surface. She said she couldn't relate to Lovell or its people. She'd wanted to leave from the first year, but Doctor had refused. They'd made few close friends. She'd always found physical closeness difficult, even with her daughters. More than once she made it plain that her sex life as a doctor's wife was mostly a memory.

As Diana drove toward the Storys' home, Aunt Emma's friend Julia Bradbury popped into mind. One day in the early eighties, Julia had stopped Diana on Jersey Avenue. "Diana," she said, "quit billing me, because I'm not paying for what Dr. Story did to me. Someday somebody's gonna clean that man's plow."

Diana had told Doctor, "We have a problem with Julia Bradbury. She doesn't want to pay. She is very unhappy about her exam."

"Give me her chart," he instructed. He brushed through it, snapped it closed, and said, "Well, forget it. We don't need patients like her anyway. We'll just write it off."

On an early morning not long afterward, she'd gone into Examining Room No. 2 to empty the wastebasket and found a wad of moist tissues with the strong smell of semen. She'd checked the appointment book and noticed that the blond femme fatale had been examined at 2 P.M. the day before. Diana had quietly resigned.

Dr. Story's latest words repeated in her ears as she pulled up in front of the house in response to his summons. *Diana, do you suppose you could come over?* It was so unlike him to plead.

When he ushered her in, she was already crying. She refused his offer of a tranquilizer. A red-eyed Marilyn sat on the sofa twisting her hands.

"Diane," Doctor said, "this is getting out of hand. Look at you. You're just too upset. Why don't you and Bill take some time off? We'll just send you to Hawaii. Then you won't have to go to that hearing."

"Please," she said. "No."

"All those women," he went on. "These two latest ones, Emma Lu Meeks and Julia Bradbury, they're good friends. They take walks together. They just worked up this story together."

Diana knew better. Julia had confided in Emma Lu, but not vice versa. Her aunt was still too ashamed.

After a while, Diana realized there was nothing she could say or do that would help. She didn't want to sit there and parrot polite falsehoods. She left as she'd come, in tears. She wondered if the long friendship was over.

34

Marilyn Story

MARILYN scanned the witness list and couldn't believe how many names there were. The hearing was set for the farm town of Worland, seventy miles south of Lovell, and was expected to last three or four days. John still treated it like Flag Day at the Ft. McPherson cemetery in his Nebraska childhood. He told Marilyn they would commute to the hearing, but Charles Kepler, Loretta's father and leader of the defense team, said, "I want you in Worland twenty-four hours a day. You need to be rested."

"I can't leave my patients," John insisted.

Kepler convinced him that he had to.

Reluctantly, they checked into a Worland motel. Marilyn couldn't shake the glooms. Some of these Wyoming places were so dry and bleak. Well, everything's in God's hands now, she told herself, but isn't it always? She turned to her journal for comfort. It was really a collection of entreaties and thank-you notes from her to the Lord. If she was too depressed, she didn't write for weeks. The last four entries showed her state of mind:

Jan. 12   Lord, forgive me. I have wavered and doubted and become depressed. I have fallen into the trap of looking at all this from a worldly perspective. Help me to be more stable and steadfast!

Feb. 22 There is still more than a month till the hearing. It seems like it will never end some days. Help us to be steadfast, Lord. Thank you for all the answered prayers.

Feb. 29 Another accuser has come forward. Satan wants us to "go under"—as long as Peter kept his eyes on the Lord, he didn't start to go under. . . .

Mar. 10 [A quote from] Oswald Chambers: "Have you been bolstering up that stupid soul of yours with the idea that your circumstances are too much for God?"

The hearings in the Washakie County courthouse were closed, even to family and press, and she spent her time walking in the crunchy crusts of leftover snow and reading Scripture in the motel room. Right in the middle of things, John had to rush to Lovell to treat his nurse's husband for severe stomach pains; it turned into an appendectomy.

On breaks from the hearing, John sometimes hurried back to the motel to see her, but he hardly mentioned the testimony. He still seemed bemused, and she was amazed at his tolerance. Even if he was completely cleared, those awful Mormon women had sullied his good name. That insult could never be forgiven.

35

The Record

The psychopath [or sociopath] makes a mockery not
only of the truth but also of all authority and institutions.
—Arnold Buss, M.D.,
Psychopathology

BEFORE THE WYOMING STATE BOARD
OF MEDICAL EXAMINERS
In the Matter of the License of JOHN H. STORY, M.D.
(Excerpts)

DEFENSE COUNSEL CHARLES G. KEPLER The thing that I find very
concerning, they are charging the doctor here with rape. You haven't heard that
term yet, but that's exactly what we're talking about. At some point they are
going to start talking about him using his penis to dilate a woman so that he
could conduct a pelvic examination. I can't conceive how that could be done
except by him placing his penis in her vagina. And I don't care whether you're
a doctor or a lawyer or somebody walking the streets, that's rape. The only
thing that I don't understand is why we are having it before this particular
board. It seems to me that rape is a criminal charge and it should go before a
criminal body rather than before a body of this kind. . . . I will try it as a
criminal charge just as if we were before a jury. . . .

ASSISTANT ATTORNEY GENERAL KATHY KARPAN Your Honor, I must
object. This is not a rape proceeding and I believe that your instructions to the
board and, I think, our statute will not be followed if Mr. Kepler is allowed to
transform this proceeding. . . .

HEARING OFFICER JOHN F. RAPER Well, the objection is sustained. . . .
This is a separate proceeding from a criminal proceeding. . . . If the prosecutors
of some county want to take an interest in it, that's fine. . . .

KEPLER I appreciate that. . . . I want to make clear also before I go on with evidence that I personally do not believe that the doctor is guilty of any of these charges. We are going to place him on the stand. And I think one of the things that is going to be beneficial to you is we're going to have his medical records which he kept meticulously. . . . I think it will give you an insight into not only Dr. Story and his very careful record keeping, but also as to the nature of the complaining witnesses. . . .

We're going to try to bring in evidence so that you understand the town of Lovell a little bit better than perhaps you do now. It is a small community. It is made up of many Mormon families. The Mormons are a very collusive group, closely related. You're going to find in the town of Lovell, half the Mormons are related to the other half or vice versa. They are close in their marriage. They are very clannish and they are certainly a rumormonger. . . . The Mormons in and of themselves and their clannishness will give you an explanation when this is all over with as to how these things came about, how these things got started.

You will find that two of your prime witnesses are sisters. The testimony will show that their mother had been an official and was an official not too long ago in the Mormon Church, and I think it will show that she used her official capacity to help at least orchestrate what you're going to hear in the next couple of days. . . .

TESTIMONY OF DEE COZZENS

Q . . . What year did you go to work in Lovell as the hospital administrator?

A August of 1968, I believe.

Q And how long were you there?

A Through November of 1974.

Q . . . What was the substance of the suggestion you made to Dr. Story?

A Just a suggestion that he have a nurse or someone in the examination room with him when he had a woman in there.

Q Did Dr. Story respond to your suggestion . . . ?

A No. He just kind of shook his head and that was about all. I don't recall he was upset at anything. We left it at that.

36

Diana Harrison

DIANA hoped she looked respectable. She'd spent hours deciding on her slack-pants ensemble and applying her makeup. She never left her house until she looked her best.

She'd been subpoenaed by both sides, and as she walked toward the witness stand, she felt torn. What did the state want from her? And Dr. Story's lawyers—did they expect her to deny what she'd seen in his office? Whatever happened, she was going to back up Aunt Emma Lu and her friend Julia Bradbury. Those dear old ladies wouldn't be going through this ordeal if it weren't for her.

The questioning went faster than she'd expected. The assistant attorney general drew her out about the day she'd talked Minda Brinkerhoff into coming into the clinic. Then she testified about her admiration for Doctor and Marilyn. "She's a very good person," Diana said.

She tried to keep her answers truthful, minimal, and inoffensive. She was just starting a sideline business in draperies and didn't need enemies on either side. She testified that she bore Doctor no ill will. From time to time she glanced his way, but he always seemed to be scribbling on his yellow scratch pad. He looked like an elf next to his three lawyers. The poor man, she thought. How did he ever get into a mess like this?

She was asked if she knew Minda Brinkerhoff, Meg Anderson, Arden McArthur, Irene Park, Carol Beach, Aletha Durtsche. Yes, she said. What about Jean Anderson Howe? Diana said she knew the name. She confirmed that they were all LDS.

The cross-examination was short but intense, much of it about office procedures. Diana testified that there were times when a nurse was present during pelvic exams and it didn't matter to her personally one way or the other. Her own exams had always been routine. Yes, it was possible to interrupt Doctor during pelvics; it happened on an average of once a day.

Q   (By LORETTA KEPLER)   What was his behavior toward women?
A   I always felt he was very polite. He liked a lady to be a lady. I should have wore a dress today. (Laughter.)
Q   Did he ever flirt with you?
A   No.
Q   Did he ever make obscene or lewd comments?
A   No.
Q   Does he ever compliment you?
A   Yes.
Q   Do these compliments have any sexual connotations?
A   No.
Q   What sort of compliments are they?
A   Very nice. He would always comment on how I looked. In fact, we had a little joke in the office. He wondered that particular day which airlines I had worked for.
Q   . . . Have you had an opportunity to determine the care which he takes in his medical practice?
A   . . . A lot. . . . His wife would also tell me many times that he had stayed up most of the night studying on that case. He's a very—I believe he's a dedicated doctor.
Q   What is Dr. Story's reputation for telling the truth?
A   I have never known him or caught him in a lie.
Q   I have no further questions.

Diana wondered, When am I going to be asked about Emma Lu and Julia? She was pleased when Kathy Karpan got up to ask more questions:

Q   . . . Were you allowed to turn the knob and walk into a room when the doctor was in the examining room with the patient?
A   No.
Q   Did you ever walk in that room?
A   No.

Q   Are you aware of any employees who did knock and then walk in the room?
A   No.

Then the defense attorney took over again:

Q   Was the door ever locked while Dr. Story was giving an examination to a patient?
A   I do not know.

That seemed to end the questioning by the lawyers. She was relieved that she hadn't been asked about the semen in the wastebasket and certain touchy matters like one woman's comment that she wouldn't pay her bill "and Dr. Story knows why," but she also wondered why no one had given her a chance to back up Emma Lu and Julia.

The four doctors on the Board began asking questions. How many patients did Dr. Story see each day ("Oh, probably fifteen"), and how many pelvics did he perform? ("Probably two or three").

Q   Did you ever notice women being upset when they came out of the examining room?
A   No, truthfully I haven't . . .
Q   Do you know whether or not there are locks on the doors to the examining rooms in Dr. Story's office?
A   I think there is.
Q   Are you still a patient of Dr. Story's?
A   Yes.

After a few more questions, the judge told her to step down. She thought, They still haven't asked about Emma Lu and Julia. Dear Lord, they'll bring them in here cold and cross-examine them and embarrass them to death. And there'll be nobody to confirm their stories or their integrity. She'd been asked about Doctor's own honesty and she'd given him a high recommendation. Why couldn't she do the same for her aunt and Julia? Was it because they were victims?

She stumbled across the courthouse lawn, crying. She just wanted to get away. "Diana!" someone called.

She turned. It was Kathy Karpan, running to catch up. "Diana, I'm sorry. I didn't have a chance to let you know. They won't let your aunt and the other lady testify."

Diana turned away. She was sure her makeup was dripping. "Why not?" she mumbled.

"The hearing officer said we turned in their names too late. I'm sorry."

She remembered how Bill had instructed her to butt out. She thought about the four stony-faced doctors sitting in judgment on one of their own and not being willing to listen to a couple of poor abused old ladies. She decided not to stick around.

37

Minda Brinkerhoff

LIVING in Gillette, Minda had begun to feel better, but for this morning inquisition some of her old symptoms came surging back. She had pain in her throat, her hips, her legs. She felt as though she were working the spotting rack at the Lovell Cleaners and getting stung every night at the Queen Bee Gardens. Maybe the problem was the long drive across the mountains from Gillette, or the sleepless nights worrying if she'd be a good witness, or her customary work load. Or just plain fright. Everything was so overpowering.

Before the 9 A.M. session on the second day of the hearing, Kathy Karpan showed her photocopies of her medical charts from Story's office. They were such obvious fakes that she almost forgot her discomfort in amazement. Who did the man think he was fooling? The penmanship varied, and dates were juggled around or omitted. Dozens of entries went all the way back to her childhood and consisted of a few scribbled lines each, but for the pivotal final date of their relationship he'd composed a minor essay:

4/21/83   1. Throat sore, and tongue hurts—3 days, cold 1 ½ weeks. 2. Nervous breakdown—rundown end '81. 3. Hips and back hurt all the time. Has been on Motrin 400—up to 10–12/d. Now on 6 daily. Hurts all over—esp. hips. 4. Stom-

ach (epigastric) pain couple months (one in hi-school). 5. Pelvic—lot discharge.
LMP—last week. Menses severe and bleeding excessive. Flow 62 days now (pre-
viously 3 days). Leg veins getting bad. EXM: Neck: Thyroid essentially neg.
Breasts: Neg. Heart: RSR good tonal no m. Lungs: clear A & P. Abdomen: ten-
der epigastric widely and RLW somewhat laterally. Pelvic: brief—didn't feel any-
thing right adnex (on half effort). Crux slightly diffuse erosion. No evidence infection
speculum. Extremities: No. Varicose veins (she mentioned). Back: Flexibility back
and hip motion. (Vitals next visit) Essentially full range of motion. Tender left hip
periarticularly. But no objective changes. Sugg. "Palindromic" syndrome. Fibro-
sitis reaction. Some is surely a "pushed-too-hard." Says sleepy all time now. Pres-
sure work, money, decisions vs folks, business problems. List—tongue, hips back
legs, etc. Epigastric burning etc. (with stress), Pelvic—mense pain (and tender right
lower quadrant). Given: Tagamet #8 1 each bedtime.

Minda thought, This is the man who never lies? She'd gone in that day
for a few minor ailments and ended up being abused. She perused the
entry again. It was puzzling. Where did he get so much biographical
information to lump under one date? Then she remembered her deposition three months earlier. She'd mentioned just about every point he'd
noted. Obviously he'd cribbed from the transcript and designed an
entry that made him look thorough and conscientious. How impressed
the Medical Board would be!

She noted the way he'd dragged in the phrase "nervous breakdown." That had been years ago and had amounted to nothing; she'd
seen a doctor once, then discarded the pills and healed herself. But the
simple notation "nervous breakdown" would make good reading for the
authorities. Who would believe the testimony of someone so unstable?

As she arranged her print dress down over her knees in the witness box,
she saw Dr. Story sitting to her right with his three lawyers, including
Senator Simpson's son. Four men in conservative suits sat in a row to
her left, along with the judge.

Story stared at her with a fixed smirk. As she started her testimony,
he went behind his hand to whisper to his lawyer, then resumed the
smirk. He took notes as though scoring her insufficiencies. She hated
his routine—it looked so rehearsed and manipulative—and avoided looking at him.

The lawyers went around and around, from the name and birth date
of each of her children to the name of every city she'd ever lived in and
every job she'd ever held. Construction crews outside the windows
forced her to yell her answers. The lawyers kept yapping at her to speak

louder or slow down or both. Gol, she thought, what time do they bring in the elephants and the twenty-one clowns in the Volkswagen?

Her direct testimony went on and on till her mouth turned dry. When Kathy Karpan finally said, "No further questions at this time," the court reporter slumped and the judge said, "Let me ask the reporter. Does your concentration need a rest?"

"Yes!"

Minda thought, How strange. The court reporter is saying a word and taking it down at the same time.

The judge commented that the testimony had been "most rapid" and called for a break. Kathy Karpan took Minda aside and told her she was doing fine.

Sixteen minutes later, the defense began taking her over the same ground. Her ulcer felt like a swallowed horse chestnut and the hard oaken chair aggravated her arthritic hips. She was sick of talking about Dr. Story. She'd told everything she knew in a long deposition; why couldn't they just use that? She knew that lawyers used various techniques, but she hadn't realized that the main one was repetition. There were times she could have sworn that Charles Kepler was deliberately trying to confuse her. It seemed unfair. Weren't things confusing enough already? He questioned her closely about visiting Story with Scott. Then:

Q I do note, just a matter of interest, you mention that three times doctor said he did not violate you, and then you say he said three times, Anything I can do to make things right.
A Right.
Q Did he have a tendency to repeat himself three times?
A He did that night, yes.
Q Rather unusual?
A Yes, it was.
Q Your given name is McArthur?
A Right.
Q That's what you were born with?
A That's my maiden name.
Q I see. But it's not your given name that you were born with. It's one that you have adopted since marriage?
A I think I'm lost.
Q I don't want to lose you. . . .

Oh, but you do, Minda said to herself. Anybody can see that. The object is to make me contradict myself. If I stick to the truth, I'll be fine.

She tried to concentrate. She wasn't going to allow herself to come across as a dimwit just because she talked fast and had trouble hearing him above the construction din outside. The interrogation about Story's p-e-n-i-s seemed endless. The word had always grated on her, made her feel crawly. She would have been happy to go to the Celestial Kingdom without ever hearing that word. The questions came fast:

Q And you had a sheet over you . . . and you raised up to see this penis?
A No, I didn't. I just turned my head off to the side.
Q And could see it from turning your head to the side?
A Uh-huh.
Q You did not raise up?
A No, I didn't.
Q Do you remember in your deposition saying that you raised up to look?
A No, I don't.
Q You don't remember that? When you—if I remember your testimony here correctly, you had to force his hands away?
A I pushed his hands up out of the way while I brought my hand up. He moved them out of the way.
Q So you touched him? This would be with your right hand?
A Right.
Q And you raised up this way?
A Uh-huh.
Q Did he say anything?
A No.
Q He said nothing about that when you were interfering with his examination?
A No.
Q Did he have [his lab] coat on that day?
A A white one.
Q And you could not see both ends of his penis?
A Right.
Q How much of the penis did you see? What dimension? What length?
A About the width of my hand.
Q So then some portion of it is in your upper leg?
A The end was pushed up against my leg.
Q And some portion of it is hidden behind his coat?
A Right.
Q The portion you saw is at least the width of your hand, and your hand is two or three inches, I suppose?
A Yes.
Q And you said nothing about it? You didn't say, "Doctor, that's your penis"?
A No, I didn't.

Q "Doctor, what are you doing?"
A No, I didn't.
Q "Doctor, please don't do that anymore?"
A No, I didn't.
Q Why didn't you say so?
A Because I really didn't think Dr. Story would do anything wrong. And in my mind I hoped that it was not a penis and I hoped that I was just seeing things.

She glanced at the members of the Medical Board. She hoped they understood why she hadn't made a scene. Their faces were pure Mount Rushmore. Kathy Karpan smiled from the counsel table. Dr. Story scribbled and smirked. She knew that Scott was waiting his turn in the witness room, and she had to defeat a claustrophobic urge to run to him for comfort.

Kepler got her to repeat that she'd once been near a nervous breakdown and that she'd been overdoing the Motrin, a prescription drug. She thought, He's making me sound like a lunatic and a drug addict. She wondered what these questions had to do with the case of Dr. Story.

The cross-examination finished in a volley of fast talk:

Q I hate to be logical at a time like this, but you have been worried for two and a half years and yet you only caught on and it has been going on for eight years. You know, there is a certain illogic here, Mrs. Brinkerhoff.
A No. He was doing the exams the exact same way from the time I went in.
Q And you don't remember in your examination of saying you raised up to see his penis?
A No, I don't. But it may be there. But I don't remember.
Q You don't remember that? Do you remember that you did raise up?
A I raised my hand up.
Q Oh, your *hand* up. Not your head?
A And I turned my head to the side to see.
Q I don't think I have any more questions. Thank you.

Kathy Karpan smoothed out a few points with some extra questions, and then asked if the incidents with Story had affected her marriage.

"Yeah, it has," the middle child answered. "It's terrible. Well, I would never tell Scott, but sometimes during intercourse, I think about—it feels exactly the same way it did in Dr. Story's office. And I think about it and it makes me not want to be around Scott." She swallowed hard.

"And I try to get over it. And I've never told Scott that. I would never. I'm sure he would be offended."

For once in her life, she was talked out. Kathy Karpan asked, "Mrs. Brinkerhoff, if you had it to do all over again, would you have written that letter to the Medical Board?"

"I would have done it sooner."

"No further questions."

She was just starting to leave the witness box when she saw Kepler rising to his feet. Criminy, she thought, not more!

He asked her a few mild questions, then held up a sheaf of papers. "On your deposition," he said, "you will be pleased to know that I have found, and you are correct—this is what you said. 'I laid there as this thing slipped through between my fingers. And then I decided it was time to look and see when he was pushing on my stomach. So I looked and he had his arms over my head and was pushing my stomach. And I turned my head and I pushed my hands out of the way and there was his penis lying on the table.' I apologize to you. I remember reading that, that you raised up. I just want you to know that I did find the passage and I'm in error."

Minda thought, Well, gol, I've just learned to hate this guy and he turns out to be a gentleman! "Okay," she said in her most forgiving voice. "I was really scatterbrained then."

Scott testified next, and Minda joined Meg in the witness room along with Aletha Durtsche, Irene Park and Carol Beach, all LDS sisters from different wards. While they waited, Minda helped Meg talk away some of her nervousness. Meg said a high school classmate had called and told about going to Story for acne and being ordered to strip for a pelvic. "She told him where to go," Meg said. "Don't you wish we did?" Meg said that a lot of the Lovell Mormons were still avoiding her, even in church. "It hurts, Minda," she said.

Minda said, "That's why we moved."

Scott finished at 11:57 A.M. He reported that they'd questioned him about the meeting at the hospital and Story's offer to wipe out their bill. He said Story had listened to the testimony with a smart-ass look on his face, "and I wanted to get up and knock him off that chair."

Minda said, "Shoot, why didn't you?"

38

The Record

BEFORE THE WYOMING STATE BOARD
OF MEDICAL EXAMINERS
In the Matter of the License of JOHN H. STORY, M.D.
(Excerpts)

TESTIMONY OF IRENE PARK

Q   (By Assistant Attorney General Margaret White)   When you were a child, Mrs. Park, did you go to Dr. Story . . . for a tonsillectomy?

A   When I was sixteen . . .

Q   And then, did you have a checkup?

A   . . . To have my throat checked so I could go back to school. . . . For some reason he did a pelvic on me.

Q   Did he ask your parents' consent before he did this?

A   No.

Q   Was there a nurse present?

A   Not that I remember.

Q   What was your reaction to this pelvic examination?

A   Well, I was a little startled. . . . I thought about it . . . and oh, four or five days, maybe a week later, this kept gnawing on me all the time and I thought that wasn't right, something is wrong. And so I finally told my folks what had happened and they were a little upset.

Q   Why is that?

A   Well, that's—tonsils and a pelvic is a long ways from one another. . . .

39

Meg Anderson

WHEN Meg's name was called for the afternoon session, her lips moved in prayer. She would have to tell the *whole* truth, and she was terrified that someone would ask about her years in Utah—the men, the "courts of love," the years of unworthiness and guilt. Kathy Karpan had promised that the proceedings would be secret, but that wasn't much consolation. Meg didn't want to be stripped to the bone in front of anybody, least of all a bunch of strangers in vests. *Ugh!* Only Danny knew the details—she'd never confided in another soul.

Kathy Karpan opened with a series of biographical questions and Meg tried to relax. She couldn't understand the deep emotion that welled up when she was asked to describe her feelings toward Story as a doctor. "I cherished the man very much," she said, and started to cry.

It was almost a relief when Kathy led her through the incidents in Examining Room No. 2—her "ugly black feelings," the cold sweat on her forehead, the sharp stabbing pain between her legs.

Q Now, Mrs. Anderson, you've testified that at this point you felt intercourse had occurred. Did you ever go back to Dr. Story's office after this?
A No.
Q Did you ever take your children back?
A Well, I took the children back, yes. I didn't go in for me.

Q Will you tell us how you came to take the children back?

A Well, Dr. Story is the only doctor I trusted with my baby. He's the only doctor I trusted, period. And I knew he was a good children's doctor. And I still didn't want to believe what was happening had happened. I, to this day, I don't want to believe that that's what happened. . . .

Meg kept hoping it would get easier, but it didn't. She stopped often to compose herself. She was relieved when Kathy Karpan said she had just one more question: "If you had it to do all over again, would you still write the letter to the Board of Medical Examiners?"

"I don't have any choice," she began, chewing on her lower lip. "I can't live with myself if I don't. I've lost enough self-respect, I couldn't lose any more. It just wasn't a matter of choice."

She took a deep breath. "After I heard that people had been offended for five years, I didn't have any choice. It was like the choice was then lifted from me and the burden was on my back. I just couldn't sit back." She stammered out the last few words and began to cry again.

The burly defense attorney named Kepler stood up. "I'm not sure I understood you, Mrs. Anderson," he said. "Did you say you taught public speaking, dramatics, or just took a course with it?"

The rest of his cross-examination went by in a blur. Kepler established that she was "rather ignorant of sexual matters," that intercourse had been painful till the birth of her second child, and that she'd had "an ugly feeling" in the examining room.

Q You're kind of in a dilemma. You hold Dr. Story in extremely high repute and you love to have your children see him and you feel that he is a good doctor for your purpose. Now, have I analyzed and stated correctly your feelings about this?

A Yes.

Q You cherish him for one reason, but you're willing to have his license removed for the other reason?

A I can't hate the man.

She admitted that she'd been shown Dr. Story's office records and found no entry for November 8, 1982, the date he'd violated her for the second time.

Kathy Karpan took her back for a brief redirect examination. "The important question, Mrs. Anderson, is are you sure you had a pelvic examination—"

"Oh, I'm positive," Meg interrupted.

"—By Dr. Story in November?"

"I'm positive I did."

Driving north toward Lovell across the badlands, Meg wondered if the Medical Board members could tell that some of the entries on her charts were faked. Or did doctors always take the word of other doctors? Story certainly fought dirty. How did that square with his religious beliefs? She was getting some new insights into the man she couldn't hate.

40

The Record

BEFORE THE WYOMING STATE BOARD
OF MEDICAL EXAMINERS
In the Matter of the License of JOHN H. STORY, M.D.
(Excerpts)

TESTIMONY OF CAROL BEACH

Q (By Assistant Attorney General Margaret White) Would you please tell the Board the circumstances under which you visited Dr. Story in 1961?

A Well, before you go on a mission, you have to have a physical . . . and then he gave me a pelvic examination.

Q How old were you . . . ?

A I was twenty-one.

Q Had you been sexually active at that time?

A No.

Q What happened during the examination, Mrs. Beach?

A Well, as he finished the pelvic and was turning away, he turned back and I think it was his left hand, as I remember the position, and he stimulated the clitoris. And he asked me if that was sensitive there. And I said, "Well, no." And he did it again and he said, "Are you sure?" And I said, "Well, no."

Q . . . Did you ever go to see Dr. Story professionally again?

A . . . [In 1976] I was getting married and needed a premarital examination. . . . And I had been going to Dr. Christensen in Powell at that time, and I believe that he was either ill—I don't remember if he was deceased at that time. . . .

Q   So in 1976 with no other doctors available, you went to see Dr. Story? What happened during this exam, Mrs. Beach?

A   He inserted an implement to begin the pelvic and then removed the implement and examined me with one finger. . . . And then he said, "Now I'm going to insert two fingers." And he held the fingers up for me to see, like this. And he repeated it again. He said, "Now two fingers, I'm going to insert two fingers." And then the examination started to become painful. . . . I finally said to him, "I don't know what you're doing down there, but you got to quit. That's hurting me too bad."

Q   What did he say?

A   He said something like, "Well, this will just take a few seconds more." And then when he got through, he said, "Oh, I didn't realize." I said, "Well, I haven't been promiscuous, if that's what you mean."

Q   . . . Had you been sexually active up to that point?

A   No, I hadn't.

Q   So when you went in, you were a virgin?

A   Yes.

Q   When it was painful, did you have any thoughts or feelings on what was happening?

A   No, not at that time. I don't think I probably realized what was happening until after I got married. . . . I told my husband, "That feels just exactly like that pelvic examination that Dr. Story gave me."

41

Aletha Durtsche

THE LETTER CARRIER hated waiting, but when her name was called late in the afternoon she wished she could just put the ordeal off for a day or two—or forever. She'd never been in court. It gave her goose bumps.

Every head in the room seemed to turn as she entered. She felt like Dorothy leaving Kansas for Oz. The only sound was her footsteps as she passed the doctors, the judge, then Dr. Story. She glanced at him and thought she saw a challenging look. *You'll never get me,* he seemed to be saying. *I'll get you first.* . . .

She liked the way Kathy Karpan opened the questioning by asking her to spell her name and then saying, "Thank you. I think I just won a bet with my cocounsel on how to spell your name. I feel pretty good about it." Aletha realized that the assistant attorney general was trying to defuse the tension.

The direct examination was easy, all about where she'd lived and worked and the incidents with Dr. Story. It helped that Kathy seemed sympathetic and the doctors leaned forward and seemed to be listening carefully. She wondered what she'd been so frightened about. She noticed Story and his lawyers whispering.

Then the one named Kepler stood up and began peppering her with questions. He got her to admit that her first suspicions had been in 1968 and yet she'd kept going back.

Q You were so convinced in 1967 and '68 that you did go to Dr. Story again in 1970 and '71, and you were convinced in 1970 and '71, but you still went to see Dr. Story numerous times including the Friday, February 12th examination of '83? I mean, you were convinced, but you still kept going back?
A I—yeah, I was convinced in 1968 and '71.
Q And kept going back?
A But I really didn't believe—I figured he had to have some instrument that was so similar to a penis, because I didn't think that he would ever do something like that, and I just wouldn't believe it so I never thought of it.
Q And you were convinced, but you didn't believe yourself even?
A Yes.
Q I see.
A I didn't want to believe it.
Q And all at once in 1983 you even convinced yourself, apparently?
A Yes. . . .
Q And yet you permit your children to go see Dr. Story after you became convinced?
A . . . I guess. We figured if we were in there, nothing could happen to them.

The questions turned more personal:

Q You've had problems with your husband off and on, have you not? Marital problems?
A Oh—
Q From time to time?
A Small ones. We had one big one a couple of years ago—three years ago.
Q Is that when you took an overdose of aspirin?
A Yes.
Q Were you attempting to take your life at that time, Mrs. Durtsche?
A I guess. Yeah. I thought that if I did that, he would be so sorry that he hurt me that it would—he would really—I just wanted to make him suffer. And then I realized that it was myself that I was doing wrong.
Q You went to the hospital?
A Yes, I did.
Q On your own volition?
A Yes.
Q And Dr. Story was called?
A Yes.
Q And you confided in Dr. Story then, too, didn't you?
A Yes, I did.

Q And your concerns with your husband at that time was his lack of fidelity?
A Yes.

When the questioning proceeded to Mike's prostate problems and a urinary infection and some unfounded fears about VD, Kathy Karpan interrupted: "Your Honor, I recognize that the scope of questioning in this hearing has been very broad, but I must question the materiality of asking Mrs. Durtsche to go into detail about her husband's problems."

Kepler said, "Your Honor, I have not questioned about her husband's problems. She has told us about them. I have been careful not to ask, and I really frankly don't care."

The lawyers squabbled for several minutes. A flushed Kathy Karpan argued that Dr. Story had had no business revealing confidential information about Mike's medical history and the defense lawyer shouldn't be permitted to bring up such privileged material now. There was a lot of jawing about "the rule of law." Story's lawyer said, "I think you'll find the rules of privilege do not apply when the patient is accusing the physician of a practice such as this."

The judge agreed, and the defense lawyer bore down:

Q Did you have a pelvic examination at that time because you were concerned [about VD]?
A Yes.
Q Yes. Fine. You have expressed concern to your working cohorts about men making advances to you on your mail route, have you not?
A I've had two men give me problems on the mail route.
Q In recent months?
A No. No.
Q But you have had two occasions?
A Yes.
Q And when you attended the Relief Society meeting and they were talking about incest and so forth, you did make the statement there, Well, you knew how that felt, that when you were young, I don't know whether it was a cousin or a relative or something, molested you? You did report that to the Relief Society?
A Yes.
Q I have no further questions.

Aletha vowed not to let anyone see her annoyance. What did these questions have to do with Story's guilt or innocence? Every young couple had marital problems. Did that justify raping the wife? Every female letter carrier had to repel advances. Her early fears about VD had been pure paranoia, based on ignorance. Was it okay to rape women who'd made half-hearted "suicide" attempts? As for the "incest"—a couple of her crazy cousins had fumbled at her breasts when they'd all been nine years old, and not one attempt had been reciprocated. Yet these silly points had been used to smear her in the eyes of the Board.

She shot a defiant glance at Story and his three lawyers. They'd fired their heaviest guns and hadn't shot her down. If they thought they were going to break her with their sleazy little questions, they were wrong.

She was excused at 5:20 P.M. As she was leaving she heard the lawyers agree to start the third day of hearings the next morning at eight. She told Mike that they'd tried to rape her legally, but this time she'd fought them off.

42

The Record

BEFORE THE WYOMING STATE BOARD
OF MEDICAL EXAMINERS
In the Matter of the License of JOHN H. STORY, M.D.
(Excerpts)

HEARING OFFICER RAPER Last evening as I was going into the Settler's Inn after yesterday afternoon's session, Mr. Kepler approached me and advised that he had an offer to make to the Board. . . . I think we should get it on the record. . . .

CHARLES KEPLER . . . At least two witnesses yesterday testified that they had seen Dr. Story's penis. Dr. Story is willing to submit to a physical examination by one or more members of the Board if the Board feels that knowing the size, characteristic, character of his penis would be beneficial in their deliberations. Our proposal would be that because of the embarrassment to Dr. Story, that Miss Karpan . . . not be present. . . .

RAPER . . . Well, the Board will take the proposal under advisement, and later today we'll come up with a ruling.

KEPLER Thank you. . . .

KATHY KARPAN Your Honor, at this time the State will call its last witness. . . .

TESTIMONY OF JOHN H. STORY, M.D.

Q Doctor, would you please state for the record your full name and your current address?

A I'm Dr. Story. Dr. John H. Story, 982 Nevada, Lovell, Wyoming.

Q Are you a licensed physician in the state of Wyoming?

A Yes. Yes, I am.

Q Doctor, could you tell the Board when and where you were born?

A In Nebraska, 1926.

Q And when and where did you graduate from high school?

A In Malcolm, Nebraska.

Q And when was it?

A 1944.

Q And where did you attend college?

A I attended two colleges. Wheaton College and the University of Nebraska.

Q And what year did you graduate from Nebraska?

A 1954. No, that's not right. 1950.

Q Where did you attend medical school?

A The University of Nebraska.

Q And what year did you graduate?

A 1955.

Q Did you complete an internship?

A Nebraska Methodist Hospital in Omaha.

Q For one year?

A Yes.

Q Could you summarize . . . what your professional career had been before you came to the state of Wyoming?

A You've outlined part of it. And then I was in Utah for some surgical residency. And then I came—then I came to Wyoming, and practiced one year in Nebraska before coming to Wyoming.

Q And where did you practice in Nebraska?

A Crawford, Nebraska.

Q What other states are you licensed to practice medicine in?

A Nebraska and Wyoming.

Q And do you remember what year you were licensed to practice in Wyoming?

A 1958.

Q Where do you practice medicine?

A Lovell, Wyoming.

Q And how long approximately have you done that?

A Twenty-five years.

Q Are you board-certified in any area?

A I have no board certification.

Q Doctor, how did you come to choose Lovell as the community in Wyoming that you wanted to practice in?

A Based on their need.

Q Could you describe in a general sense the nature of the practice that you had in Lovell?

A   It was a general practice, which includes general medicine, some surgery, orthopedics and obstetrics.

Q   At any time since you've been in Wyoming, Dr. Story, have you ever practiced medicine with another doctor in the same office?

A   Never. I never have.

Q   Doctor, as a general practice at this time, do you have as a rule in your office that when you conduct a pelvic examination a third person will be present with you in the examining room?

A   Currently?

Q   Yes, sir.

A   Yes.

Q   Has this always been your practice?

A   Since June of last year.

Q   Doctor, what is your understanding, based on your training and medical school and your experience over the years, as to what is the generally accepted standard governing whether or not a third person should be present during a pelvic examination?

A   I think because of legal implications it's come to be expected more than it used to be.

Q   Could you tell us what function you think that arrangement serves aside from legal protections?

A   It serves the function of a witness.

Q   Any other function?

A   I use her to dictate things to her that I would have done myself otherwise.

Q   Doctor, when you say that as of June you've had a nurse present, would that be as of June, 1983?

A   Yes.

Q   And would that have been one month prior to your informal interview with the Board of Medical Examiners?

A   Yes, it would be.

Q   . . . Do you recall . . . approximately 1972 or 1973 meeting with a gentleman named John Shotwell to discuss a complaint he had?

A   Yes. Yes, I met with him.

Q   Do you remember what year that was?

A   Approximately when you say. Approximately '72 or so.

Q   Dr. Story, as you can best remember, what was Mr. Shotwell's complaint to you?

A   He had no complaint. I asked him to meet with me. And I asked if I could talk to his wife and he said no.

Q   Why did you ask to meet with Mr. Shotwell?

A   Because I had heard that—I had heard that his wife was doing some talking that wasn't very advantageous to me.

HEARING OFFICER RAPER   Could you speak up a little more, Doctor?

A   Okay.

Q (By KATHLEEN KARPAN) Do you remember where you met with Mr. Shotwell?

A Yes. It was in the hospital.

Q Did you ask Mr. Shotwell if he could explain what the nature of these stories were, or did you understand it?

A No. I asked him if he would tell me about it, and he had nothing to explain.

Q What was the general nature of the comments that Mrs. Shotwell had been making?

A Oh, I believe—of course that's why I wanted to talk to her. I believe it was that I had mistreated her daughter. I never knew for sure.

Q Did Mr. Shotwell tell you at the meeting—

A No.

Q —Anything about his daughter?

A No.

Q Did he make any request of you?

A No.

Q Do you remember, Doctor, again in this same time period, 1972, 1973, a meeting with Mr. Dee Cozzens?

A No.

Q Did Dee Cozzens ever ask you to make it a practice to have a third person present?

A No, he didn't.

Q You have no recollection of that conversation?

A None.

Q Are you aware, aside from what you have heard in this hearing, of Dr. Welch contacting Mr. Dee Cozzens on this matter?

A I had heard unofficially that there was some association.

Q Dr. Story, at any time, and no restriction on years, at any time did Dr. Ray Christensen of Powell ever talk to you—

A No.

Q —On this subject?

A No.

Q Dr. Story, in the spring of this past year, 1983, did you have occasion to speak with Dr. John Welch on the subject of whether you ought to have a third person present during your pelvic exams?

A Not as a topic. I mean—

Q Did that subject come up, Dr. Story?

A I met with him twice. Yes, I think he did mention that, the second time I talked to him.

Q Was it your impression, Dr. Story, that Dr. Welch made any recommendation to you on this subject?

A The comment was that this is the only way—the only way to squelch this sort of thing is to have a witness.

Q Do you remember when that conversation was?

A My two conversations with him were in—I think in June. Both in June, I believe.

Q And have you changed your practice since June?

A Yes. Uh-huh.

Q Dr. Story, do you recall meeting with Mr. and Mrs. Scott Brinkerhoff in the hospital—

A Yes.

Q —To discuss complaints.

A Yes, I do.

Q As a matter of fact, Dr. Story, do you recall describing a part of that meeting to the Board of Medical Examiners during your informal interview?

A If I did, it was certainly a very small comment on it, I believe.

Q . . . Do you recall in the course of your conversation with Mr. and Mrs. Brinkerhoff if you made a comment to—and I may not be quoting exactly—of this having come up twelve years ago?

A I don't remember ever saying that.

Q Do you recall, Dr. Story, if during that meeting the subject came up of how you might change your practice of medicine in response to the complaints that were made by Mrs. Brinkerhoff?

A No. No, I don't.

Q Dr. Story, do you recall if during the meeting you indicated to Mr. Brinkerhoff that the current bill he had with you would be wiped out?

A No, I didn't make that comment. I didn't make it in the brief hearing.

Q Dr. Story, do you recall during the July 22nd informal interview with the Board that you did not know the identity of any of the complainants?

A Not officially.

Q Not officially. And, therefore, you didn't refer in the minutes to any individuals by name, I don't believe?

A I doubt that very much.

Q However, there is a reference in the minutes to your having—I believe the minutes say—lost your temper and told one of your patients that you would forget a bill of some thirteen hundred dollars, I believe it says in the minutes. Do you recall saying that to the Board of Medical Examiners?

A I remember not saying that.

Q The minutes are in error on that subject?

A The minutes are in error.

Q Dr. Story, do you recall being told by Mrs. Brinkerhoff at the meeting in the hospital that she intended to contact the Board of Medical Examiners?

A No, I don't remember that.

Q Accordingly, would you not recall—did you not say, "I can take care of them"?

A That I did not say. She may have commented on the Medical Board, but I did not say that.

Q Dr. Story, would you tell us what you believe and what you recall of that meeting with Mr. and Mrs. Brinkerhoff?

A   Yes. I asked them to meet with me, and after great difficulty I suc-
ceeded to meet with them. And due to this great difficulty, that conversation
was silence and lack of communication, and I had to finally tell them why they
were there. And, let's see, I finally told them why they were there because of
things I had heard from the mother and Joe Brown and through Dr. Welch.

Q   What had you heard, Dr. Story, in a general way?

A   That there were rumors about my abuse of those two girls, two daughters.

Q   That would be Minda Brinkerhoff and Meg Anderson?

A   And Meg Anderson, right.

Q   Dr. Story, do you recall what you said to Mr. and Mrs. Brinkerhoff that
night at the hospital regarding these accusations?

A   Yes. I told them they weren't true.

Q   Dr. Story, at the time of the informal interview of July 22nd, you recall
telling the Board that you had instituted the practice of having a third person
present for pelvic examinations?

A   Yes.

Q   Do you also recall, Doctor, telling the Board about a reduction in the
number of pelvic examinations you were conducting?

A   Yes.

Q   Do you recall what that reduction was?

A   No. I didn't give any numbers what the reduction was. I didn't—and it
wasn't quite that simple. It was a reduction in practice and reduction in pelvics.

Q   I believe the minutes state that your pelvics had been cut in half. Would
the minutes be in error?

A   Yes, the minutes—well, no, that could be almost true. That could be. It
could have been cut almost in half.

Q   Well, could you explain to us what the reduction in practice entailed
and why that came about?

A   Well, I interpreted it two ways: a recession that was evident at least
among all medical people in our area at that time and throughout the entire
year, and then the effect of rumors.

Q   Dr. Story, in estimating the reduction in the number of pelvics for
whatever reason, be it the recession or the dropping in practice, in coming up
with the figure of 50 percent, did you conduct a survey of the number of pelvic
examinations that had been performed in your office during any set period
of time?

A   Have I done this?

Q   Yes.

A   Yes, I have. Yes.

Q   You have. Could you tell us, Dr. Story, taking as a cutoff point June of
1983, approximately how many pelvic examinations you would have performed
in a month in your office?

A   Before the end of 1983?

Q   Before June of 1983. June will be the cutoff point because of the June
incident.

A   Yes. I can tell you pelvic exams for January of 1980, which I had access to, and it was thirty some, about thirty pelvic exams that month, January, 1980.

Q   And how many pelvic examinations did you conduct last month, Dr. Story? Do you recall?

A   I counted the pelvic examinations for the largest first fourteen days of January, February of this year, and that was about thirty-five pelvic exams.

Q   Dr. Story, you've mentioned the recession.

A   Wait! I think I have that reversed. I think it was thirty-five in 1980 and thirty for the fourteen days. And I also have percentages on that.

Q   Doctor, I may not be hearing you right. That doesn't seem like a reduction. You got thirty-five in one month in 1980 and thirty in fourteen days of this year. It sounds to me like you've done twice as many. . . .

A   . . . It surprised me that percentagewise I did more pelvics the first fourteen good days of this year than I did in 1980.

Q   Well, going back to your statement that was made to the Board of Medical Examiners in July that your pelvics would be cut in half, it would appear in practice that did not occur?

A   No, it didn't. . . .

HEARING OFFICER RAPER   Do you wish to examine at this time, Mr. Kepler?

CHARLES KEPLER   Just very briefly. . . . We will have the doctor in our case in chief. There's just no sense of doubling up, but only one or two points I wanted to clarify.

Q   In your informal meeting with representatives of the Board . . . was it your intention that you were representing to the Board that you would cut the number of pelvic exams?

A   No, I had no understanding of that sort.

Q   . . . The study to which you referred to this morning, when was that made?

A   Oh, three or four days ago.

Q   And it wasn't a very scientific study? It was just a sampling of fourteen comparative days?

A   Yes. Yes. . . .

KATHY KARPAN   Your Honor, having called Dr. John Story, the State would rest its case. . . .

CHARLES KEPLER   Our first witness, Your Honor. . . .

TESTIMONY OF IMOGENE HANSEN

Q   (By LORETTA KEPLER)   What is your occupation?

A   I'm a nurse, registered nurse . . . with thirty-seven years' experience. . . . I was employed as [Dr. Story's] office nurse for four and a half years. . . .

Q   Did anyone ever complain to you or tell you that Dr. Story had exposed his penis to anyone?

A   Well, not in that—those words, no. . . . Shortly after I went to work for

Dr. Story, I heard that there was some unprofessional conduct going on in the office. . . . Well, I was very indignant. I thought that that was just a vicious rumor that somebody had started. And that's what I told the person. . . .

Q Did you hear any rumors after that?

A No, I did not. . . .

Q (By KATHY KARPAN) How did you notify Dr. Story that he had received a telephone call?

A We knocked on the door and then he usually came to the door.

Q Did you ever walk in the door after you knocked, or would you wait for Dr. Story to come to the door?

A No. I waited for him to come to the door. . . .

Q (By BOARD MEMBER SAM T. SCALING, M.D.) . . . During the time that you worked for Dr. Story, was there ever a question in your mind about the validity of some of these rumors that you had heard?

A No. And this—you know, this hearing totally surprises me because I'm sure that subconsciously . . . I must have looked for some kind of something like that going on. There was never in any—all the time I worked there, ever anything that I could find or see that was out of line.

TESTIMONY OF NITA BRONKEMA

Q (By LORETTA KEPLER) . . . When did you work for him?

A From September 15, 1968, to . . . 1974, when he did surgery on me. . . . I was his office nurse.

Q . . . Now while you were working for Dr. Story, did you ever interrupt him while he was doing a pelvic examination?

A Many times. Many times.

Q And why did you interrupt him?

A Well, Dr. Story had very specific rules which I learned, and it's strange that I've never forgotten them. Number one is that if any member of his family [called], I would knock and wait until I heard his muffled voice usually saying "Nita," and then I would go in. However, if the hospital called and it was an emergency, I just knocked with one hand, had my hand on the doorknob, and was already in and say, "Hospital, Doctor," and he gets up and leaves and I take care of the lady. . . .

Q Did you ever have an opportunity to see whether . . . anything improper was going on?

A There was never anything improper going on that I ever saw, nor did I have any lady complain of any.

Q Now have you had the opportunity to observe Dr. Story's behavior toward women?

A Yes. He is very, very definitely one of the nicest gentlemen I have ever seen.

Q Does he ever flirt with women?

A No. . . . Dr. Story need not flirt. He has a gorgeous wife.

TESTIMONY OF JUDY GIFFORD

Q (By LORETTA KEPLER) What is your occupation?

A I'm an R.N.

Q . . . How long have you worked for Dr. Story?

A Two years and three months [part time].

Q . . . Did you ever observe Dr. Story doing anything inconsistent with proper pelvic examination?

A No. . . .

Q Now, would you have had occasion to learn how Dr. Story communicates to his patients?

A Uh-huh. . . . It's very poor. . . . I just feel that he's a very complicated man. I think he's exceptionally smart, and I think it's hard for him to relate to other people. . . . They will listen to what he says and take it just exactly the opposite, and then he becomes very frustrated. And I think sometimes he just kind of gives up trying to explain because it seems like everything gets mixed up.

Q (By KATHLEEN KARPEN) . . . Have you heard rumors about Dr. Story's pelvic examinations?

A . . . Yes, five and a half years ago . . . And my first reaction was, Boy, I'm not going to that doctor. And as time went on and the more I saw his work and got to know him, which probably took a year . . . I definitely decided that, yes, he was the doctor that I wanted to take care of me.

Q (By LORETTA KEPLER) . . . Does Lovell have a reputation for being the kind of town where there is a lot of gossip?

A It certainly does.

43

Arden McArthur

ARDEN strode toward the witness stand at 10:20 A.M. with her head held high. She was nervous, but she'd be danged if she'd show it.

She was glad to get away from Lovell for a day; the place was turning into a John Wayne movie set with the McArthurs wearing the black hats. Both the family stores were failing for lack of customers. She'd been snubbed in the streets by her own Mormon sisters and blood relatives. She'd received threatening phone calls and letters, including a neatly printed passage from Psalm 37: "The wicked plotteth against the just, and gnasheth upon him with his teeth. . . . Their sword shall enter into their own heart, and their bows shall be broken." One of the Saints had demanded her excommunication "for putting Dr. Story through hell." A mutual acquaintance had passed along what purported to be Dr. Story's latest comment: "I'll break Arden physically, emotionally, spiritually and financially. If she thinks she's poor, she doesn't know what poor is."

He'd telephoned several times, as sweet as sorghum, acting as though they shared the same problem. "What are *we* gonna do about this?" he would ask, and she would answer, "I don't know what *you* are gonna do about it."

His final call had been four days ago. "Arden," he'd said, "I guess whatever happens, somebody's gonna be hurt one way or the other."

As she took her seat in the witness box, it wasn't lost on her that she'd been subpoenaed by Story and not by the state. She knew the defense scenario by heart: the Mormons had plotted to destroy the kindly town doctor because he refused to convert; as Relief Society president, she'd brainwashed her daughters and then solicited and coached the other witnesses; she was a cheap gossipy laundrywoman who was just trying to beat the good doctor out of his bill.

A few days before the hearings began, she and Dean had paid their $2,125 medical account and another $213 for Meg and Danny, to spike one line of questioning. And she'd resigned as Relief Society president to spike another. As to the part about coaching the witnesses, it was just plain false and she could prove it by a dozen witnesses; from the beginning, she'd gone out of her way to avoid hearing their stories. She took no pleasure from hearing sexual details, least of all when rape was involved. She still didn't know exactly what Story had done to her own daughters except that it involved a "tube." Nor did she want to know, now or ever.

Under questioning, she insisted on telling the story her way, not just in bits and pieces. She started with Minda's first complaints four years back. Several times the defense attorney demanded that she stick to the point, but she thought she knew the point better than anyone in the courtroom and plowed the furrow straight. He questioned her for forty-five minutes and ended up on the subject of the bill:

Q (By CHARLES KEPLER) Over the period of years, you've had a substantial bill with Dr. Story, have you not?
A Yes, I have. But he's been paid well.
Q And when was he paid?
A You know when he was paid, Mr. Kepler.
Q I know when he was paid. The Board does not know when he was paid. You tell them, would you, please?
A Excuse me. He was paid last week. . . .
Q He's carried you for an extended period of time for a substantial sum of money and was paid in full last week?
A That's right.

On cross-examination, Kathy Karpan gave her a chance to unburden herself. "I can tell all of you in here today," Arden said, "that I know where Christ walked when he carried that cross, because I have fellow members of the church . . . that are saying, 'Crucify her. Crucify her!' And I've been there. I know what it is."

Q Are you satisfied that you've had an opportunity to tell your story?

A I don't think this Medical Board would know the story if they had a whole week to listen. But I feel that it's important that they do know it. I feel that Khrushchev said many years ago that he didn't have to worry about nuclear war in the United States because we are decaying from within. And I believe that's happening. . . . We have been accused of being an LDS community, but that's not true. Our hospital board is not run by LDS. Our school board is not run by LDS. Our town is not run by LDS. It's run by other organizations.

Q I've got one last question for you, Mrs. McArthur. All things considered, would you do this again?

A I would do it again if I lose every penny I had in this world.

She was standing on the courthouse steps wondering if anyone had believed her when Kathy Karpan tiptoed up and gave her a bear hug. "Oh, Arden," she said, "you're beautiful. You're *beautiful!* If you could've seen the look on Story's face . . ."

44

The Record

BEFORE THE WYOMING STATE BOARD
OF MEDICAL EXAMINERS
In the Matter of the License of JOHN H. STORY, M.D.
(Excerpts)

TESTIMONY OF DOUGLAS E. WRUNG, M.D.

Q (By CHARLES KEPLER) Have you formed an opinion on Dr. Story's qualification as a physician?

A I think he's a good, solid physician. I think he's competent and ethical from what I've observed. I think he's well read, particularly in orthopedic surgery, hand surgery. He is very introspective. He's not particularly pushy, but . . . he's usually pretty tactful. . . .

Q Have you had an opportunity to form an opinion as to his techniques in giving pelvic examinations?

A I would say it's standard from what I'm used to, at least what I've observed. . . .

Q Would you have any kind of feeling as to how much time he spent on a given pelvic exam . . . ?

A Maybe three to five minutes.

Q Is that an abnormally long, abnormally short, or normal period of time?

A I would say that's average time.

TESTIMONY OF MARILYN STORY

Q (By LORETTA KEPLER) How did you meet Dr. Story? Where? In Denver?

A No. I met him in Wheaton, Illinois. I was visiting or living with a cousin and my husband was going to school there and living in that same house and I met him there. . . .

Q Has the doctor asked you to cancel any bills?

A Oh, many. Yes.

Q It has been testified that the doctor offered to cancel Scott Brinkerhoff's bill. Does that surprise you? Is that untypical of Dr. Story?

A In that particular situation, he—he's the kind of person who says that if someone thinks they don't owe him anything, he doesn't want anything. . . . At times maybe I feel like he's too easy on people, but I'm very used to it. . . .

Q What do you recall about one of the last visits of Minda Brinkerhoff? Anything?

A Yes. . . . I do recall very specifically that she was in the room for a long time talking with doctor because you would hear her laughing a lot and talking a lot.

Q How could you hear her?

A Because she was loud, laughed loud, talked loud.

Q Could you hear what she was saying?

A No, we didn't try.

Q Did you interrupt any of her examinations?

A I don't recall specifically interrupting hers. I was very ready to, that day.

Q Why was that?

A Because it was taking so long. She was in there a long time and he was getting behind. . . .

Q What sort of husband is Dr. Story?

A A very good husband. Very affectionate. Very thoughtful. He's a gentleman. He's very respectful of me and our daughters. He treats them all—he treats us all very kindly and with a lot of consideration.

Q Have you ever suspected him of having an affair with another woman?

A Absolutely not.

Q Why not?

A I just know him. It's never entered my mind. Besides, he's always home if he isn't at the hospital. I always know where he is. . . .

Q Have you had an opportunity to observe your husband's behavior toward other women?

A Yes. . . . Very considerate, very respectful, very gentlemanly. He always opens car doors, helps them on with their coats. Every woman. Very kind. . . .

Q Is he protective?

A . . . He tries to protect me from anything that would be upsetting. . . . He never comes home with things like that. . . .

Q What sort of man do you think your husband is?

A Well, he's a procrastinator, but he's conservative, concerned, conscientious. He's protective. He's levelheaded. His moods never change. He's always happy, same always. He's affectionate. He's a very private person. He doesn't talk a lot. He's difficult to understand sometimes. I don't know. . . .

TESTIMONY OF JOSEPH BROWN

Q (By CHARLES KEPLER) Did [the McArthurs] relate to you that they had talked to their church people?

A . . . Minda had stated that she had gone to the bishop and that she had—he told her that perhaps she should get another doctor. And then she went to President Abraham of the Lovell . . . Stake, I guess it is, and he stated that he didn't quite understand how this could be. And he said would she get up on the desk and show him. And she said she did. . . .

Q What was your report . . . to your board?

A Basically that the witness was paradoxical in her behavior, her mother was contradictory in her statements but held to the fact that they wanted to go to the State Board of Medical Examiners. And since this was an occasion in the doctor's office, we had no—no other complaint in the hospital whatsoever. We had never had an off-color remark from Dr. Story's surgery or any part of the hospital. We've never had any of—my best-looking girls go to him and swear by him. . . .

Barbara Shumway, personnel director at the North Big Horn Hospital and the Storys' companion on their trip to Jamaica, testified that she'd sat in on the hospital meeting with Arden McArthur and Minda Brinkerhoff as a witness for her boss, Joe Brown. She described Minda's behavior: "Well, she was talking very fast. She cried. She would laugh. She would contradict herself on something that she just said before."

Verda Croft, a Mormon and director of nursing at the hospital, testified that Dr. Story was "picky," "professional," "very ethical," and never flirted. "We don't even dare tell a shady joke. . . . It's just not his personality. It's just not his character. He's very reserved. We just respect him that way. He just does not care for shady jokes or that kind of talk."

Jane Keil, a registered nurse for almost forty years, described Dr. Story as "very efficient," "very modest," and poor at communication.

Kay Holm, a pastor's daughter, wife of a Lovell High School teacher and active member of Story's church, reiterated most of her deposition testimony about his excellent character and Lovell's taste for gossip. "It's a little scary to us to have an innocent person attacked by a certain group, and then it snowballs and it happens over and over again." She described Lovell as "sort of like a Peyton Place, only worse."

Rural mail carrier Peggy Rasmussen testified that she hadn't thought twice about letting her daughter go to work for Dr. Story, because the charges against him were "totally ludicrous." She said that Minda Brinkerhoff had "a very bad mental problem, and I think her mother pushed it." Mrs. Rasmussen testified that her colleague Aletha Durtsche could talk herself into believing whatever she wanted to believe and "can't keep a secret."

After the last defense witness was excused, Dr. Story took the stand in his own behalf; his earlier appearance had been as a hostile witness for the state. This time Charles Kepler did the questioning, and the general content was a blanket denial of every charge or insinuation, sometimes reinforced by office records and charts.

Q   Do you ever say routinely, "I'm going to dilate you"?

A   Not routinely. I've heard that term more in the last three days than the rest of my life put together. . . .

Q   At any time, at any place, have you ever exposed your penis in [Meg] Anderson's presence?

A   No.

Q   . . . Insert your penis into her vagina?

A   No. . . .

Q   Have you ever had your penis out at any time under any conditions or place where Mrs. Brinkerhoff was present?

A   Or any examination, no.

Q   Did you ever insert your penis into her vagina at that examination or any other place or time?

A   No.

Q   What could she have seen that might look like a penis . . . ?

A   Well, actually, I haven't made a real effort to figure it out. . . . Maybe I should have. Other people have. I don't know. People wondered if I have taken my glove with me and had it on the table while I was examining her abdomen. But I don't really—I guess maybe I should strain my mind to figure some weird explanation out. . . .

Q   Do you think this is a Mormon conspiracy against you?

A   No. I have never said that. I've never thought it. I have put it a little bit differently—a small group of Mormons. And if anything, it's them using the church, not the church using them. . . . This is—they just have to be a small little clique of people.

It was 6:30 P.M. and dark outside when Kepler finished with the direct examination. Judge Raper announced that the final day of the hearings would begin the next morning at eight. It was already the longest such inquiry in Wyoming history.

In the morning, Kathy Karpan announced that the state had no immediate questions for Dr. Story and didn't intend to put on a rebuttal case. The members of the Board took over the interrogation. Most of their questions were medical and technical:

Q (By HAROLD D. THOMASON, M.D.) . . . And the electric table can be tipped up and down?
A Yes.
Q Forward and back and raise and lower itself?
A Yes. Right.
Q (By THOMAS V. TOFT, M.D.) Do you have any anatomic abnormalities of your genitalia?
A No, I don't think so. . . .
Q Do you ever find that doing pelvic examinations arouses you sexually?
A I don't think so. I'm interested in the anatomy, pathology, the finding, the recording, the knowledge I gain from it. . . .
Q (By DAVID VICK, D.O.) Do you see patients at night or on weekends without the benefit of a nurse or secretary in your office?
A Yes.
Q Would you ever do a pelvic under those circumstances?
A No. Last Wednesday I—a week ago last Wednesday I did a pelvic in the office on Wednesday afternoon, but that was with a cleaning lady and a husband there. . . .
Q (By SAM T. SCALING, M.D.) . . . What do you think [Arden McArthur's] feelings toward you have been over the years up to the point when this problem surfaced? Your honest opinion of what—how—what you think she feels toward you.
A Well, she wanted to, you might say, make points, per her testimony, and work on me. . . .
Q Do you do abortions, Dr. Story?
A No.
Q Are you a Christian?
A Yes.
Q Are you spirit-filled or born-again Christian?
A In a sense. Bible-believing at least.

Kathy Karpan went over a few final points:

Q Dr. Story, we've had a number of questions about religious zealots, and I noticed something interesting in looking at your medical charts. You put the religion of your patients on the charts, do you not?

A If they tell it . . .

Q Dr. Story, once you know the religion of a patient, does that affect your relationship with the patient?

A No. . . .

Q There is no significance, then, Doctor, to the fact that every complainant who has come into this room has been a Mormon? I'm suggesting that religious bias can run both ways, Dr. Story. . . .

A Some of them have convictions, and I have convictions. . . .

Q Is Arden McArthur a religious zealot in your judgment? You discussed a group of religious zealots, and I want to try to figure out who is in that group.

A You want to put names on them?

Q Oh, yes, sir. We have names in this hearing and they've testified, so we want to know. Is Arden McArthur a religious zealot?

A She is very committed to the group that she was born and raised in.

Q Is Minda Brinkerhoff a religious zealot?

A I don't know that I really want to put names on religious zealots.

Q But, Dr. Story, you've suggested to this Board that it's a group of religious zealots that are against you. Now if Arden McArthur is a religious zealot, why was she a patient for twenty-five years? Wasn't there a Mormon doctor in town at any time? . . . If religion is her basis for being a patient, why did she stay with you for a quarter of a century? . . .

A I can explain things. I don't know that I care to go further in a religious zealot conversation, though. . . .

At last the defense rested, and the hearing officer told Kepler, "It would appear that you probably already have the answer to your offer to have Dr. Story submit to a physical examination."

"I believe we have," Kepler responded.

Raper went on, "But let me state precisely that the Board rejects that offer unless there is some showing of anatomical abnormality that does not exist. So therefore the offer is rejected."

Closing arguments were completed by 10:30 A.M. of the fourth day, March 29, 1984. As expected, the Board took the matter under advisement.

45

Marilyn Story

ON THE TWO-HOUR DRIVE back to Lovell, John seemed confident. From the first day, his attitude hadn't changed. He felt that the hearing was typical bureaucratic overreach, and he would be cleared. He giggled when he recounted Arden's testimony about putting his name on the prayer roll. "She said she was levitated," he said. They'd often joked about the Mormons—their burnings in the bosom, their silly garments with the funny markings, their quaint ideas about baptizing the dead and holding "courts of love" for the living. Mormons held hands with Satan, but sometimes they were good for a laugh.

A week passed without word from Cheyenne. John went about his practice, but Marilyn was worried sick. What was taking the Board so long? What was there to deliberate about? A bunch of silly charges by a bunch of silly women? John kept telling her not to worry—the typical bureaucrat couldn't tie his shoes in less than three days.

Marilyn imagined the worst. An honorable career would end in disgrace in this seedy little burg that she despised. But at least she didn't have to worry alone. Friends kept knocking at the door with platters of fried chicken, cakes, plates of cookies. Fellow parishioners brought so much ice cream that she had to borrow space in a neighbor's freezer. After word spread that John's favorite meal was meat loaf, the

225

refrigerator sagged with its burden. Marilyn wrote in her journal: "Have received meals from Browns, Holms, Millers, Cheri and Janet. . . . What wonderful, thoughtful Christian friends we have."

But one close friend remained ominously silent. On May 11, six weeks after the hearing had adjourned, Marilyn wrote: "We have great concern over Diana. . . . We have had no contact with her since the hearing and keep getting word from others that she is *not* a friend. As an enemy she could do more harm to us than any other I could think of. I have been praying to see her, but feel no definite peace or leading—others have counseled me not to go. Lord, if only we could know Your will in certain things."

Another month went by. Then the Lovell *Chronicle* of June 7, 1984, broke the news under a headline an inch thick and six columns wide:

STATE BOARD REVOKES DOCTOR'S LICENSE

The article noted that the revocation would become effective June 30. Kathleen Karpan was quoted as saying that the reason was "unprofessional and dishonorable conduct likely to deceive, harm, or defraud the public."

"What a shock!" Marilyn wrote in her journal. ". . . Lord, how we need your wisdom to know what to do."

The next week's *Chronicle* was crammed with letters of support. An advertising column, "Cards of Thanks," rang with praise of John:

> Dr. Story has been our physician, our neighbor and our friend for twenty-five years. We believe and trust in him. Evy and Bob Richardson.

> Doc Story and Marilyn, you have been a lot of help to our family in time of need. Now let us help you. Wayman and Bernita Moody.

> . . .Thanks for being such a wonderful doctor! Hope to have you for another 25 years! Leola Mangus.

> We wish to thank Dr. Story and Marilyn for their love and patience with us as a family. . . . They are special people and we don't want to lose them. Calvin and Parthena.

> Doc and Marilyn, "The angel of the Lord encampeth round about them that fear Him and delivereth them." Psalm 34:7. J. C. Brown family.

> Doc and Marilyn, we love you and God shall turn your midnights into day. Psalms 30:5b. Ken and Janet.

We appreciate you, Dr. and Mrs. Story. Psalms 28. The Butch
Finks. . . .

For weeks the letters and ads appeared, many from prominent citizens.
Mayor Herman Fink and his wife wrote, "Dr. and Mrs. Story, we
thank you for your faithful service to our family and our town, you have
our support." Town clerk LaVera Hillman paid for a short ad: "Dr.
and Mrs. Story: our community is a better place because of you! My
love and support is with you!" The great old pioneer names of Lovell
were on some of the letters: Doerr, Bischoff, Thompson, Sorensen. . . .

Mrs. Ron Massine wrote in from Mesquite, Texas: "It amazes me
that anyone could take these charges against him seriously." Former
Lovell High School teacher and coach Dean Gerke, who'd been "pressured" to leave by the McArthurs and others, wrote from Columbus,
Montana: "What a loss Dr. John Story would be to your community."

In all the public support, Marilyn was glad to see so few sour grapes.
A predictable letter from Scott Brinkerhoff quoted Isaiah: "Woe unto
them that call evil good and good evil." One of Minda Brinkerhoff's old
girl friends, Rhonda Christensen, thanked the accusers for "having the
courage." But anti-Story notes were offset ten to one by letters like
the one signed by three Lovell women saying that the news had made
them "literally physically ill. . . . It is truly appalling to each of us that
such a wonderful doctor should be put to such a test," and the
letter from a young couple that was headlined, "Too much faith was
only fault."

At last John was beginning to take things more seriously. He enlisted
the aid of his most powerful patient, Cal Taggart, the heaviest-hitting
big-shot politico clear to the Montana border. Taggart owned half the
buildings on Main Street, flew his own plane, divided his time among a
big house in town, a cabin in the Big Horns and a home in Sun City,
Arizona. He'd built up his family insurance business and started his
own political career as mayor of Lovell. He was relaxed, approachable,
and as quick to do a favor as he'd been during his twelve years in the
state senate.

A smiling John returned from the meeting and confided that Taggart
had promised to use his pull with Governor Ed Herschler. Later Taggart
phoned Marilyn with a message: "I talked to the governor. Don't
worry. Doc'll be practicing real soon."

She wrote in her journal, "At noon a very beautiful brilliant rainbow appeared in the southern sky. It seemed a promise from God that 'there will be a brighter day.' "

A few hot days after the rainbow, on July 10, the Lord's promise was fulfilled. John's lawyers had a short but rewarding hearing before District Judge John Dixon in Cody, forty-six miles west of Lovell. Marilyn's scrawled report ran across a full page of her journal: "The judge gave John a stay on the revocation and a chance for appeal! Praise the Lord!" She thought how comforting it was to know that some people in Wyoming knew an innocent man when they saw one.

46

Arden McArthur

ARDEN rode her bike toward the dry cleaners and inhaled the sweet fumes from the sugar factory at the other end of town. The sugar campaign was just getting started. From now till the last truckload of gray-brown beets spilled onto the conveyor belt in February, the aroma of the refining process would be in every nose. At best the fumes smelled like hay after wet weather, at worst like bad feet. To Arden, the smell meant home and money.

She'd just pedaled past the Hyart Theater when Joe Brown pulled alongside in his car and called out, "Well, I hope you're proud of yourself." If it was for helping to put Story's tail feathers in a crack, she thought, he's right—I couldn't be prouder. She was glad when the hospital manager sped off.

After she opened the dry cleaners, she checked the latest edition of the Lovell *Chronicle* and wished she hadn't. An article quoted a judge named Dixon as ruling that Dr. Story could continue to practice while his appeal was pending, and the file on the case would remain sealed.

She called the attorney general's office and asked how long it would take the judge to rule on the appeal. "Months," the state lawyer told her. "And longer if he goes to the higher courts."

"How long could that take?"

"Oh, a year or two. If he files in the federal courts, maybe three or four."

Her voice skittered way up. "And he can practice the whole time?"

"That's Judge Dixon's ruling."

She asked why the state didn't just go ahead and file criminal charges; rape was still rape, and the simple lifting of a license didn't seem to fit the crime. "The criminal action's been dropped," the lawyer told her. "It's the Medical Board's baby now."

You mean it's their hot potato, she said to herself. Why are you folks trying to fob this off on someone else? She remembered other injustices that she'd read about: murderers sitting on Death Row for years, civil rights issues heard and reheard, courts reversing other courts, rulings overturned on technicalities and word games. She thought, Dr. Story is almost sixty. If he can keep the revocation on hold for another four or five years, he can retire and it'll be the same as if he'd never lost his license. Is that what Wyoming calls justice?

By fall, Dean was up and around, but he wasn't much use to himself or his family. Anyone could see that the stress was killing him. The pressure from Story backers was unrelenting. Each morning Arden had to lead a bicycle convoy to school. Inside the classroom, the McArthur children were taunted, teased and assaulted with Scripture, including passages from the Book of Mormon. When they sat together at athletic events, they were shunned. Now and then a brave friend would come over to show support, then slide away.

Arden and Dean decided to take Cal Taggart's long-standing advice to put up or shut up, and they went to see the new county attorney in his little office in Greybull, thirty miles south of Lovell. At first, Arden was unimpressed. His name was Terrill R. Tharp, "Terry" to his friends, and he certainly didn't make her feel like one. He had a farm-boy look that made him seem more like somebody's hired milker than the chief law enforcement officer of Big Horn County. He had long skinny limbs, thinning reddish-brown hair, a high pink forehead, and tightly drawn skin that showed the shape of his skull. He didn't look much older than thirty. She couldn't decide whether he took after Howdy Doody or Bozo the Clown. In his old parka, open shirt and battered boots, he looked as though he'd just ridden into town on a bad horse.

She wasn't surprised to learn that he'd barely heard of the case. Northern and southern Big Horn County were divided by twenty miles of mineral-rich badlands, and most public officials lived in the area around the county-seat community of Basin in the south. The only time the folks from the upper Big Horn Basin saw them was just before elections. She couldn't remember ever seeing this Tharp person.

He looked unhurried, so she gave him the full briefing, starting with her anger over the laudatory letters in the Lovell *Chronicle* and the phony twenty-fifth anniversary celebration. A few times she had to stop to compose herself, and when she talked about her family she couldn't hold back the tears.

Dean sat quietly while the county attorney blinked behind his rose-tinted glasses and didn't give her much encouragement. He had a funny little habit of repeating back your last few words in a kind of mumble:

"So I told Minda to go home and get some sleep."

"*. . . Get some sleep.*"

"We came down here as a last resort."

"*. . . A last resort.*"

When the echo of her final comment died away, he said, "If you and your daughters can round up twenty more victims, then maybe we can do something."

"Twenty?" Arden asked. The numbers game was getting tougher. "Why twenty?"

"Well, there's no magic in twenty," Tharp admitted in his lazy tenor drawl, "but if you have twenty, your chances with a jury are better than if you have two or three."

She said, "One should be plenty."

"One should be plenty," he repeated. After a long rumination while he stared at his pencil, he observed that it didn't make much sense to bring charges that wouldn't stick. A doctor with twenty-five years of service would have everything going for him. If he were brought to trial and cleared, he'd end up more powerful than ever. Was that what she had in mind? "Me neither," he said, without waiting for an answer. Then his face relaxed a little and he said, "Do you think some of the victims would visit with me? Mind you, I'm not guaranteeing a thing."

"They're sick of just talking," Arden said. "They already talked to their bishops and a bunch of lawyers and two state investigators. Six of 'em testified at the Medical Board hearing. I hate to even mention their names. I've got a daughter over in Gillette that's fed up with the whole thing. Plumb finished! Another one just sits and cries. And after all they've gone through, that dang Story is still up on the hill giving pelvics! And you want twenty names! These poor women, why should they talk to you at all?"

"Talk to you at all," Terrill Tharp said. He repeated that he'd be more than willing to listen to their stories. The McArthurs left, more upset than ever.

47

Aletha Durtsche

THINGS were getting sticky on the mail route. Formerly friendly shop-keepers, neighbor folks who'd sent flowers when she had babies, sisters and brothers who'd worked with her on church projects—all turned cold toward her. She would walk into a store with a fistful of mail, call out her usual "Good morning!" and conduct her business in a cold silence. She listened in church as the women stood up to give their testimony: "Dr. Story is being persecuted and we should all help him. . . ." "I can't believe that the man who saved my dad's life is being run out of town. . . ." "God bless Dr. Story. . . ." The grandmother of one of his victims announced in church that Dr. Story was "being crucified just liked Jesus Christ."

One day Aletha delivered mail to Ponderosa Floral on Main Street. "Good morning," she said to the proprietor, and laid the mail on the counter.

"Aletha?" Beverly Moody said. "Can I ask you something?"

"Sure."

"I just found out last night that you're one of the witnesses. We had a meeting at our church and Dr. Story gave us your names."

Aletha had heard that he was using the Lovell Bible Church for support and that he'd called for a boycott of the victims' business

233

establishments, but she was surprised to learn that Bev Moody was a church member. She'd always thought the chunky little florist was a Mormon from another ward.

"Yes," Aletha said nervously. "I testified."

"I can't believe you'd do that to Dr. Story."

"What do you mean?"

The woman emerged from behind the counter. "You Mormons!" she said. "You wicked *wicked* Mormons! Dr. Story's been preaching the word of God for over twenty-five years. He's been a good teacher for our children. He's a kind, loving, considerate human being. . . ."

Aletha backed toward the exit. Keep your cool, she told herself. Let her talk.

The woman's round face turned pink. "Are you claiming he raped you?" she demanded.

"Yes."

"Oh, you're gonna pay! You'll go straight to hell. You wicked people will pay dearly. . . ."

"Yes," Aletha said as she backed out the door. "The wicked people will pay."

She attended a family function at her Uncle LaMar Averett's house. The former police chief was a short barrel-chested man with white hair and glasses and the profile of an eagle. He was her mother's oldest brother and one of her favorite relatives. She'd hardly arrived before Uncle LaMar's daughter Carol began complaining about what "those women" were doing to Dr. Story. Another cousin noted that Arden McArthur was a liar.

"Well, he raped *me*," Aletha put in.

"Oh, Aletha!" one of the cousins said in the tone of an indulgent adult. The relatives sat in the kitchen and traded stories about Dr. Story and his skills. Aletha didn't take part, but she knew that most of the remarks were intended for her ears.

Not long afterward, Uncle LaMar cornered her at another gathering and said, "Aletha, we need to talk about all this shit that's going on."

"What shit is that, Uncle LaMar?" the plainspoken woman asked.

"Well, I hope you don't think I've ever called you a liar, but Doc Story's never done anything to my family. He's just been totally good to all of us."

"He was always good to my family, too, Uncle LaMar. That's why it hurt me so deeply when he did what he did. I couldn't understand why he'd do that to me—but he did."

"Well, honey," the old man said, "I just can't go along with that."

"Well, then, you're calling me a liar."

"That's not what I mean and you know it."

"Well, it *is* what you mean, Uncle LaMar! I'm saying he did it. If you don't believe me, then you're calling me a liar."

"I just don't want these bad feelings between us."

"Uncle LaMar, as long as you think I'm a liar, there'll always be bad feelings."

He shook his head and walked away. Aletha thought, He can't admit he was mistaken when he refused to take action. Why, he's one of the reasons this whole thing happened! What a shame; my favorite uncle would rather lose me than admit he was wrong.

Aletha dragged Mike to a postal workers' party and someone suggested a liars' game. A woman who'd testified for Story said, "I can't tell a lie. There's only one person in this room that's a liar." Aletha and Mike left quietly.

Mike had been supportive, but she knew he was being taunted daily at the bentonite plant. "I told you," he said one night after work. "Look what Arden McArthur got us into."

Aletha said, "Hey, nobody made me testify. I had to do it." But she let her voice drop off and wasn't sure he heard. They went to bed without speaking.

With Mike's support waning, her own spirits fell. She'd always shampooed her furniture every few months, kept her carpets spotless, dusted walls, spritzed bugs, ripped out garden weeds. For seven years she'd never failed to write in her journal daily. But now she let everything slide. She even stopped work on a sweater she'd been knitting for her daughter.

It didn't help that a few other women dropped hints that they'd been abused on the doctor's automatic table. When Aletha asked why they didn't come forward, they mumbled apologies. Once she wouldn't have understood, but she sure did now.

48

Arden McArthur

ARDEN hit on a way to meet Terrill Tharp's demand for twenty names.
If it worked, it would be the coup of a lifetime. She phoned the idea to
her childhood friend John Abraham. She suggested that his bishops
contact the victims who were known to them and urge them to get in
touch with Arden, anonymously if preferred. Object: justice. What
happened after that would be up to each woman's conscience.

Arden could tell by the stake president's tone that he didn't think
much of her suggestion. From the beginning he'd tried to keep from
involving the church. She knew his reasoning and had to admit he had a
point. Story was trying to make the Medical Board's action look like the
result of an LDS conspiracy. Arden decided she needed another plan.

She remembered hearing a rumor that Diana Harrison had tried to
bring two new victims to the Medical Board hearings. Maybe these
women would talk now. But who were they?

She drove to her old sewing companion's house and found her
working in the yard. At first, Diana didn't want to discuss the case.

"Diana," Arden said, "you've got to get off the fence."

"I'm not on the fence."

"Yes, you are!"

Diana sighed.

"What if this goes to court?" Arden persisted. "You're gonna have to decide, 'cause you know more about him than anybody. You tried to tell me about him the day I went up to pick up the laundry, and I just walked out crying."

The two Mormon women talked for an hour in the twilight. Diana finally admitted that her aunt, Emma Lu Meeks, was plenty annoyed about Story, and Emma Lu's elderly neighbor Julia Bradbury might have something to say, too. "Fine," Arden said. "I'll call the prosecutor. They can all get together in my home."

49

Terrill Tharp

HE'D LEARNED early in his short career as a rural county attorney that the more he acted like the shy farm boy he'd once been, the more cooperation he got. In the case of Dr. Story, it hadn't been hard to feign ignorance. Tharp had read a few newspaper items about the license revocation, but it seemed to be the Medical Board's show and he was just as happy to be on the sidelines.

A few weeks back, Lovell Police Chief Dave Wilcock had mentioned Story on the telephone and said that his victims were playing their hands so close that nobody even knew their names. "Well, what are we supposed to do about that?" Tharp had asked. "The damn Medical Board isn't about to release names. Doctors are more secretive than lawyers'll ever be."

Wilcock said he'd just wanted to bring him up to date.

"Well, I appreciate that," the county attorney had said. "Now, by God, all we can do is twiddle our thumbs and see if somebody comes forward." He knew this wasn't the perfect posture for a man sworn to uphold justice all the way from the Rockies to the Big Horns, but he didn't see where he had much choice.

He couldn't decide what to make of the McArthurs. The Mrs. had seemed articulate and respectable, if a little shrill and overprotective of her daughters and the other LDS women. She was certainly ultrarighteous, but that was the norm in Big Horn County, a land of stern and stubborn people. He'd been forced into jury trials for $16 traffic tickets, and he'd tried cases involving fanatics like the Posse Comitatus and the Minutemen and others who seemed to believe that their main right under the U.S. Constitution was—as he once put it—"to act like horses' asses in court."

Arden McArthur hadn't seemed quite that irrational. After she'd stopped snuffling and sniffling and waving the letters to the editor, she'd laid out her evidence pretty much like a good lawyer. He had to admit it was a hell of a case—if true. But why hadn't any of the victims made an official complaint in the twenty-five years this had been going on?

He summoned the police chief for a talk. Dave Wilcock was an odd duck for a cop—shy, reserved, soft of voice, with the command presence of a nervous deer. The joke on him was that when he yelled "freeze!" suspects had to ask him to repeat. But Lovell wasn't known for conventional lawmen. Most of Wilcock's predecessors had been farmers. Until recently, the Lovell P.D. had operated out of a storefront across the street from the Cactus Bar. Now it was squeezed into a two-room addition in the rear of the small Town Hall.

Wilcock was in his mid-thirties, an educated cop with a degree in police science. When he wasn't fighting crime, he was fighting weight. Tharp had seen him so big around the middle that he couldn't see his sox.

"Tell me what you know about Dr. Story," Tharp said as he poured a welcoming cup of orange pekoe. He avoided coffee; he didn't like doing business from his ceiling.

Wilcock was LDS, but the county attorney had seen enough of him to suspect that he was really a jack Mormon, one with the same casual air about his church as Tharp had about his own Lutheranism. He'd seen Dave Wilcock smoke and now watched him suck up his tea like a heathen.

"Story's a tin god in Lovell," the chief began in his quiet voice. "He's got his own church, his own clinic, his own fan club. He does almost all the surgery at the hospital. He's got a lot of funny ideas. When the migrant workers get hurt, we have a hell of a time getting him out of bed. It's always, 'Check 'em in the hospital and I'll see 'em in the morning.' Seems like he makes value judgments. He'll say, 'I've dealt with these people before.' That's his code for Mexicans: 'these people.' "

"Any evidence that he abuses women?" Tharp asked.

Wilcock drained his cup. "I heard a few rumors eight or ten years ago. Norm Doerr and some of the other policemen said it was hysterical bullshit. Then an old guy asked me in the café if I knew what Doc Story was doing to women, but he wouldn't go any further. He seemed upset, and I got the impression he might be talking about his own flesh and blood. I asked Chief Averett, and he said, 'I know Doc Story. It's gossip.' "

LaMar Averett's tenure had been before Terrill Tharp's time, but the county attorney had heard tales about the easygoing old Mormon. Other cops waded into barroom brawls; Averett negotiated. He was in the farmer-chief tradition of his predecessor, Solon Cozzens, who refused to carry a weapon on the grounds that guns were dangerous. Averett liked to take juvenile delinquents home for a good meal and "talk some sense into 'em."

The rumors about Story had resumed a year or so ago, Wilcock went on as Tharp leaned back to listen. "I asked Danny Anderson and he said it was just one of Arden's deals. Two weeks later Danny told me, 'The witnesses aren't supposed to talk about it and my wife's a witness.' Then Bud Owsley came through town for the State Division of Criminal Investigation and I asked him what was going on.

"He says, 'I can't tell ya.'

"I says, 'You can't tell *me*?'

"He says, 'Nope. This Medical Board stuff is secret. But you've gotta get into it later. There's a lot there.'

"I says, 'What are we talking about? Bad medical practices?'

"He says, 'We're talking about rape.'

"I says, 'Well, when you boys are finished, will you fill me in?' He promised he would. I'm still waiting."

The chief offered his cup for a refill. "A month ago I got a call from a woman in Colorado," he continued. "Said she'd heard that Story'd been cleared. I said the hearings were still going on. She said, 'Oh, that's good to know.' I says, 'Why?' She says, 'Because of what he did to me.' I tried to get her to talk, but she wouldn't give her name. I asked her to write me a letter."

Tharp wondered how he would ever get his teeth into such a twilight zone case. If he brought charges, who would testify for the state? An anonymous caller from Colorado? Burnt-out victims too nervous to talk?

And there was a more personal problem. Unlike many young prosecutors who viewed their jobs as stepping-stones to big-money careers as defense lawyers, Terrill Raymond Tharp intended to earn $45,000 a year as Big Horn County Attorney for the rest of his life. It was a perfect spot for someone who'd once raised bummer lambs for spending money. As all-state high school baritone saxophonist, he'd toyed with the idea of becoming another Gerry Mulligan, given up music for a journalism degree at the University of Wyoming, then abandoned journalism for law. In his first year of practice, he'd grossed $7,000 and lived on corn and beans. At last he'd found his niche in a county office that no one else seemed to want. He explained the charm of his job: "When it's dead here, you could sit all day and not have two phone calls. Then all of a sudden you're up to your ass in alligators." He enjoyed the peace and the alligators, and he also liked to catch rainbow trout and plunk rabbits and take his wife and baby daughter up to Devils Canyon in his new pickup truck.

His constituents were like members of his own family, tough old farmers and blue-collar folks who didn't like to waste their tax dollars. The whole Big Horn County government ran on nickels and dimes. If he lost a kamikaze action against the most prominent medical man in the northern half, two results were certain: (1) the evil doctor would come out of it stronger than ever, and (2) Terrill Raymond Tharp would be back on corn and beans after the next election, and so would his wife and daughter.

"There's a criminal case here, Terry," Dave Wilcock was saying. "I just wish I could figure out where to start."

"Where to start," Tharp echoed in his nervous way. But on the *other* hand, he advised himself, this thing can't be ignored. The allegations were enough to make a man sick—sexual molestation, child abuse, even rape.

He decided to move ahead, but not fast enough to attract too much attention. "Miz McArthur's gonna set me up with a woman named Emma Lu Meeks," he told Wilcock. "Why don't you sit down with some of the other victims? Develop it as far as you can."

The chief stood up, nodding. He seemed pleased.

"We got one shot at this, Dave," Tharp warned as they walked outside to the chief's car. "If we blow it, we're both finished. It's like that old saying, If you try to kill the king, by god you better succeed."

50

Emma Lu Meeks

THE OLD WOMAN had a clear memory of the pioneering days when her family first came into the country. She still lived on the plot where she'd been born in 1908, and yellowing pictures of her ancestors lined her walls so she could keep their memories fresh till they all joined hands in the Celestial Kingdom. She never tired of talking about the past. "My dad came here from southern Utah to work on the Lovell Canal. He brought cuttings from his favorite trees—cherries, oaks, apples, willows—and planted them in a little cove off the hill. Some of those other Mormons came up here to keep from being prosecuted for polygamy. One of my uncles had two wives, and he took good care of them. Each wife had a nice house.

"My dad burnt out thick patches of dead prickly pear that'd been here forever. He hitched a team of horses to a flat board called a slip and dragged it along the ground to clear his land. All of us kids rode on the slip. This was a rough country then: sagebrush and cactus, greasewood, mesquite, pretty little desert plants that would nip your hand. The river bottoms were full of wild roses and cottonwood and bullberry bushes. Most of the land wouldn't take up water. Mark my words, if you're ever gonna clear land, stay away from greasewood. It waterproofs the soil underneath, turns it hard and dry."

In her late seventies, Emma Lu Meeks had hazel green eyes, silver bangs, a pageboy haircut that swung from side to side as she walked, and a trim five-foot figure. She still tended her garden, took in sewing, painted in acrylics, and worked for her ward's Relief Society. As a young woman, she'd earned her teaching credential at a normal school in Laramie. "I taught over on Beaver Crick, fifty, sixty miles east of here. I had to board there 'cause we were snowed in all winter." She laughed. "One year cured me of teaching."

Emma Lu remembered how Lovell's first lots had been laid out with knotted ropes. She'd helped her late husband Ted, the town cop for fifteen years, to tear down her family's old log cabin and build their own two-story house in its place. "We used drystanding lodgepole pine from up on the Big Horns. We trucked it down, stained it with hot linseed oil, and chinked the walls with creosoted hemp. We traded our young milk cow for plastering. She died a month later." She giggled. "The plasterer was annoyed about that."

For years the couple had taken in troubled children as part of their LDS program of compassionate services. Ted would spot them walking down a road, wandering, lost, maybe drunk or drugged, and bring them home for a year or two. "I had a very tenderhearted husband," the old woman explained. "His temper concealed a soft heart." She still enjoyed helping people, calling on fellow Saints with their monthly religious lessons. She hoped it did them some good.

On the morning of her scheduled meeting with the county attorney, Emma Lu was walking home from a teaching session when a pit bull had to be pried off her leg. Up at the hospital, she took more stitches than she could count. She winced but didn't complain.

Her niece Diana Harrison drove her to the meeting in Arden McArthur's house at the east end of town. A child let them into the empty living room and disappeared in back. The county attorney was waiting next to the upright piano. He was a spindly young man who didn't look very glad to make her acquaintance.

She stammered as she told him that Dr. Story had raped her during a pelvic exam in the fall of 1977. "I was in shock when I left the examining room. His wife was there and I made out a check for eight dollars. I always paid my bills and I knew I wasn't going back.

"After it happened, I walked around town for an hour. I kept thinking, 'Why did he do that to me? What did I do that let him do that to me?' I took it on myself, as though I was responsible. But I didn't cry. I was mad.

"It was still light out when I got home. My husband was dying of colitis and circulatory problems. I looked at him and I thought, I can't tell you. I can't do that to you. He'd been hurt in his first marriage. He didn't trust women. It had taken me all these years to gain his trust. I thought, He'll get his gun and kill Story. It's not worth going to jail. And I had no proof anyway. So I didn't tell Ted. I didn't tell a soul.

"After he died in seventy-nine, Julia Bradbury came over one day and banged on my door. 'I've been raped!' she said. 'Dr. Story raped me!'

"We were old friends, and I thought, Oh, Julia, why didn't I tell you about Story? You'd've warned *me*.

"But all I said was, 'Oh, Julia!' I listened to her story, but I still didn't tell her mine. I felt sick that I'd let it happen to her. I felt responsible.

"She didn't cry either. She was just mad. I felt so bad about her, I could've crawled under the door."

Emma Lu was still upset by the pit bull's bite and didn't think she was making an impression on Mr. Tharp. She wished she could use all the words that it took to describe what Story had done to her, but some of them just weren't in the vocabulary of a Mormon lady. It hurt her feelings that the prosecutor hardly took notes.

Of course she couldn't tell him about seeing Story's thing. If she did, the nightmare would come back. It was a Technicolor dream about a tubular section of brown skin and some folds of clothes, exactly what she'd seen when she'd looked down the examining table seven years before. All these years she'd been waking up at night yelling, "You dirty son of a bitch!" Then she would have to read herself back to sleep.

The county attorney asked a few questions and left.

51

Marilyn Story

JOHN DECIDED to hire a new lawyer for the appeal, but in under-populated Wyoming it was hard to find the right one. Marilyn hadn't realized that attorneys sometimes refused clients. On July 20, she wrote in her journal, "Annette's birthday. Another shock today to read the letter [Atty.] Speight wrote . . . and his analysis of us. He misunderstood me—thought we had a poor demeanor. . . . He didn't believe John. Lord, you are closing all the doors in our faces!"

A few weeks later, after she received encouragement from a favorite source, she wrote: "It seems that all our prayer and efforts have been met with closed doors and deaf ears, but the Word met my need this morning with Heb. 12:1–4— . . . Jesus *endured* the cross—consider him who *endured* such hostility of sinners so you won't grow weary and lose heart. . . . You have not yet resisted to the point of shedding blood."

52

David Wilcock

POLICE CHIEF DAVID WELCH WILCOCK turned up the volume till his cubbyhole office resounded with the rich string passages of Tchaikovsky's Fifth Symphony. Ever since he'd blown sousaphone in his high school band, good music had helped him relax and think. When his men griped that the chief was playing "that classical shit" again, he was pleased; it propelled them to the street, where good cops belonged. Wilcock kept a cassette player in his office. The only local radio station was down in Greybull, and its programmers considered Elvis Presley a singer.

The chief was still trying to figure out how to investigate John Story and retain his job at the same time. He'd had coffee at the Rose Bowl Café with Mayor Herman Fink, just recovering from bypass surgery. His Honor asked, "What do you think about this Story business?"

"What do you mean?"

"I can't believe it," the elderly mayor said. "I *won't* believe it. I owe that man my life."

Wilcock swallowed and left. This case was tough enough without bucking his boss.

He called the State Department of Criminal Investigation in Cheyenne and asked if the agency was still providing help to smalltown police departments. A spokesman said that the DCI had already worked the Story case for the Board of Medical Examiners and its reports were under lock and key. "That's okay," Wilcock insisted. "We'll ignore everything you got for the Medical Board and start together from scratch."

An assistant attorney general named Kathy Karpan called Wilcock a few hours later and informed him that Story's license revocation was under appeal and no state agency could become involved in the case till a final ruling, which might be a year away. Wilcock realized that the Lovell P.D.'s detective bureau was on its own—all one of him.

In his first interview, with R. Dee Cozzens, the former North Big Horn Hospital administrator, the chief learned that Story's offenses might date further back than he'd imagined. Cozzens recalled that a bishop named Lyle Nicholls had reported confidentially that a teenaged girl in his ward complained about "improprieties" by the doctor. The girl, now an adult, hadn't filed a complaint; her parents were still in the dark, and the bishop was dead.

Wilcock filed the interview under "useless" and called Minda Brinkerhoff in Gillette. He wrote up their talk:

0956—Telephone Conversation   First Contact
  Minda Brinkerhoff expressed distrust and is unhappy with the way things are going. She feels that everything should be made public and has taken steps to try and achieve this. Minda stated she had written "60 Minutes" and the American Civil Liberties Union. She is also upset about the way Bishop Larry Sessions is trying to stop a petition against Dr. Story.
  Reporting Officer requested a more concise statement than that found in her letter to the Medical Board but was refused. R/O asked if Minda would be coming to Lovell in the future and was told no. . . .

Minda's sister Meg seemed equally reluctant at first, but after a little warm-up she let him turn on his cassette tape recorder. Meg proved touchingly eager for a friendly ear. It took Wilcock's schoolteacher wife Judy three days to type up the thirty-one pages of Q&A. But Meg's account had a glaring weakness. For all her certainty, she hadn't seen Story's penis.

Wilcock ran into more frustration when he called on a sixtyish woman named Julia Bradbury. She agreed to an interview, but soon began to fidget and fuss. Whenever she reached the scene in the examining room, she skipped ahead. The chief's own shyness was no help.

When he asked questions about the "tube" and "semen," he felt like Jack the Ripper.

An interview with Diana Harrison went better—nine pages after Judy finished typing it—but he came away convinced that Story's former receptionist had held back some of the less palatable details. Country people were like that.

He called the county attorney. "Terry," he said, "these interviews aren't going so well. I need some help, and I think it oughta be a woman."

"Maybe we should ask the DCI."

"I already did. The state won't touch it."

"What about a private detective?"

"I'd rather stick with law enforcement," Wilcock said.

Tharp gave the impression that he'd lost some of his inspiration since interviewing Emma Lu Meeks a few days back. The chief remembered what he'd said on the phone that night: "I can't charge a man with rape because of what some old woman imagines she felt seven years ago. By God, Dave, we gotta do better than that!"

Wilcock opened his office mail and a cassette fell from a wrinkled brown envelope postmarked Denver. He slid the tape into position and leaned back to listen. He hadn't heard five minutes of the forlorn, weepy voice before he was on his way to Tharp's office again.

Neither man spoke as they listened to the cassette. When the frail voice trailed off, the lawmen stared at each other and slowly shook their heads. Then Tharp said, "We're gonna get that sucker."

53

Terri Lee Timmons

"I WASN'T ABLE to sit myself down and write this all out, so I decided to send you a tape. I hope that your tape recorder will be able to pick up everything that I say. I've talked to people about what happened to me, after I grew up, but I've never talked to anybody about it in detail of exactly what happened, so this is going to be a little bit hard for me. I'll do the best I can.

"As I remember, it was the spring of 1968, and it seems that I had a doctor's appointment after school. I had been having pains in my right side for probably about a year since I had turned fourteen and my menstrual cycle had started.

"Just to preface this a little bit, when I was twenty-five and we had been married about six months I had my first miscarriage. At that time the records were found and gone through of my mother's pregnancy with me. It was found that she was given a drug called D.E.S. This drug affects the unborn fetus in that it makes the reproductive organs abnormal. I have a condition which is called D.E.S. exposure, so my insides are not formed correctly.

"Consequently, as I reached puberty and my hormones started working, I was in a lot of pain each month. At the time, they had no idea that this drug did this to the unborn babies, but this was what was wrong. We found this out about ten years later.

"Anyway, it seems like about three months in a row that I had gone in because I was just in so much pain. Each time he would examine me, Dr. Story would examine me through a pelvic exam, and he couldn't find anything wrong.

"The day in question, I went in and sat in the waiting room. Imogene Hansen, who was the nurse, took me back into one of the rooms and told me to undress. The doctor came in and did the preliminaries, asked me what was wrong and everything. I told him it was the same thing, I had a pain in my right side and had no idea why.

"He asked me to lay down and got out the metal instrument, put on his glove and got out the lubricant. He began examining me with his finger inside and pushing on top, like they always do, to see if he could feel anything around my ovary or uterus. He did this for a while. Of course, the door was shut, and it was just he and I. I was draped to where I could not even see him.

"Then all of a sudden he deviated from any other time that I had been in for an examination. All of a sudden, as I was laying on the table, my feet in the stirrups, I felt something start to push against my bottom in the area of my vagina that was very, very warm and fleshy and yet hard.

"I didn't know what to think. I had never been taught by my parents or anyone what intercourse was. I had no idea what a penis looked like, or anything like this. All of a sudden I felt it push inside of me. I started to cry, because it really hurt. It was much larger than his finger, and it was not a hand with a plastic glove on it. It was bare skin.

"At this point I couldn't imagine what he was doing, and yet I trusted him because he was my doctor. He kept pushing it in farther and I just cried really hard because it hurt very bad.

"He pulled it out and proceeded to rub it up and down in my crotch for a while. I could not even imagine what was going on. Then he would try it again, and each time he would try to push it in a little farther. Then he would take it out and rub it up and down on my crotch some more and push it in.

"By this time, I was just in tears, crying and crying. About the third time he pulled it out, all of a sudden I felt a warm fluid go all over my bottom on the outside and down on the table underneath me. I had no idea in the world what that was at that time.

"After this happened, he started to fuss around. He grabbed hold of the paper that covers the table that they always pull down for a new patient out from under me and he wadded it up and threw it away, and started wiping me off. After this happened he told me to sit up and to get dressed and he would be back in a few minutes, and so I did. Before he went out of the room and asked for me to sit up, he said to me, 'You did real good,' and then left.

"I got off the table and proceeded to clean myself up. The tissue which I used to clean my bottom was bloody and I was bleeding. I was very upset and in a lot of pain. I got my clothes on and sat there and a few minutes later he came back in and told me he could not find anything wrong with me, that he couldn't explain my pain. I left.

"I don't remember if my grandmother picked me up or if I walked home. It seems like I walked home, which was probably two miles, to where my grandmother lived. I remember saying to her, 'He hurt me. He hurt me.'

"She didn't know what I was talking about. I don't even know if she knew why I went to the doctor or what type of an examination it was. I was crying. She just gave me some ginger tea and put me to bed.

"I feel that by coming forth and turning this in to you, maybe I can help some other woman, some other young girl that, like me, might have happened to be a fifteen-year-old virgin and have to go through an experience like this. I have a little girl of my own. I would like to see Dr. Story get the help, the psychiatric help, that he needs.

"Just for your records, this is a statement from Terri Hansen Timmons. I live in Denver, Colorado. . . . We moved away from Lovell in May of 1970. It was over sixteen years ago that this incident happened to me."

Terri Lee Hansen Timmons, a thin-boned Mormon woman whose grandfather had been the first president of the Lovell bank, returned the borrowed tape recorder to her Denver neighbor a few days after she mailed off the cassette and wondered why she didn't feel better. How hard it had been to make that recording! She'd trembled for the whole twenty minutes. It was scary to say all those words, even in the privacy of her locked bedroom. It would have been impossible to say them face to face. But she knew that sooner or later she would have to give her testimony, either in this life or at the judgment bar.

Well, she told herself, at least I've quit bawling. Ever since her mother had called from Powell with the news about the Medical Board hearings, Terri had been crying. She was relieved that the Holy Spirit had given her the courage to make the first move. For days, the Spirit had told her, "Call the Lovell police," but she'd held off because she didn't want the cops to think she was crazy. Chief Wilcock turned out real nice. If he'd said one wrong word, she'd have hung up.

At thirty-two, Terri had reason to be leery of men. Her truckdriver father had been difficult—"ornery," as she put it in her journal. A pack of young Lovell Mormons had raped someone very close to her. Dr. Story had done his evil, not only to Terri but to one of her aunts. And she'd wasted three years—from fifteen to eighteen—on a handsome schoolmate who went off and married another woman.

She hated to think of the years she'd spent trying to block out the Story incident. She'd had nightmares and daymares, flashes of horror, attacks of anxiety and panic. At Brigham Young University, there'd been times when the memories ruined dates. At home, she would be doing the dishes or washing her hair when she imagined herself back on the examining table. For a few years she improved, but when she returned to Lovell to see her dying grandmother, she spotted Story standing at the nurse's station in a black turtleneck and dark trousers. Black suits him, she said to herself. The memories surged back.

Every day she thanked her Father in Heaven for her husband. Loyd "Red" Timmons was the miracle in her life. When she'd met him in Powell, she'd felt an immediate burning in the bosom. He was a halfhearted Protestant with red hair to his shoulders, but 369 days later he'd turned himself into a neatly cropped Mormon who talked to the Lord and knew the Scriptures. They were married in the temple at Salt Lake City.

Terri had hoped that her life would turn around, but at first the events of her wedding night only deepened her depression. She was almost twenty-three, and she'd never been positive what Story had done to her, only that she'd bled and hurt. But after her wedding night, she knew. For a long time she couldn't explain to Red why she flinched at his touch. She sat around brooding.

One day she started to tell him, "A long time ago, this doctor did something to me. . . ."

After a few sentences, Red said, "No! That didn't happen. Don't tell me that!" He'd been born and raised in Big Horn County. He knew what family doctors did and what they didn't do.

They'd left their hometown of Powell to start a new life in Colorado.

Red landed a good job as a manufacturing engineer for Robotics & Co., but he still didn't seem to comprehend what she was going through and neither did the leaders of her Denver ward.

In 1981 she planned to kill herself, then changed her mind when she remembered that Mormon doctrine equated suicide with murder and held that it brought an eternal curse. She went to her bishop for counseling. "Terri," he told her, "there are people on this earth that we call tender spirits. They're more vulnerable to the pain and suffering that go with the wickedness of the world. You're one of them."

For three more years she'd lived in limbo, and then came the nice talk with Chief Wilcock. A few days later, the Lord informed Red that it was time to quit his Denver job and return to the Big Horn Basin with his family. If someone at home needed her testimony, Terri would be available.

54

David Wilcock

HE WORKED quietly, tiptoeing around the mayor and other Story supporters. He asked each interviewee to keep their talk confidential, and to his amazement each seemed to be comply. He suspected that Lovell's reputation for gossipmongering was just another lazy cliché about small towns. He regarded such generalities as a substitute for original thought, and tried to avoid them.

It bothered him that he still wasn't getting the job done, at least to the county attorney's satisfaction. As Tharp reminded him almost daily, it was one thing to lift a doctor's license and another to send him to the penitentiary. Wilcock and the victims were still having problems relating to each other, and some had been so affronted by Story's easy return to practice that they'd refused to cooperate with anyone in law enforcement. Minda Brinkerhoff wouldn't even return his phone calls to Gillette in Campbell County.

One wasted day followed another as the cottonwoods turned deeper shades of gold and the wind from the Rockies sharpened and chilled. He had a long interview with his next-door neighbor, Aletha Durtsche, but she couldn't swear that she'd seen the doctor's penis. A Medical Board witness named Irene Park swore that the only beef she'd ever had against Dr. Story was that she'd gone to him for a tonsil check and was given a pelvic. Any other complaints? "None." How had the doctor treated her? "Fine."

Arden McArthur tipped him to the victimized Mae Fischer and suggested that he approach the family through the father, a former bishop. John Shotwell admitted that he'd had a showdown with Dr. Story, but said the doctor had explained everything. Wilcock asked if the Shotwells' daughter could be interviewed and was told that she was still skittish on the subject. It seemed that Mae hadn't told her bad-tempered husband Bill, and probably never would.

Tired and frustrated, the chief cued up some Shostakovich just before dark on a Saturday evening in October. Across the room, his wife Judy pounded on the typewriter, transcribing his latest futile interview. He looked out the window of their rental house on Carmon Avenue and saw a parked car with a 17 prefix on its license plate. Wyoming licenses were numbered according to county population, and his cop's memory told him that 17 was the designation for Campbell County.

It was a long shot, but he phoned next door to Aletha Durtsche and scored a hit. Minda Brinkerhoff was visiting. Two months had passed since he'd first talked to Minda on the telephone, and she sounded as reluctant as ever. "I just don't want to go through this again," she insisted over the phone. "Criminy, chief, try to understand."

"Look, Mrs. Brinkerhoff," Wilcock said, "all I need is five minutes of your time." He'd heard that Minda was a talker, so he didn't want to tell her too much about his investigation.

"If you guys are onto him, how come he's still doing pelvics?" she asked.

"The judge gave him a stay," the chief explained.

Minda asked how he could expect decent folks to take part in such a phony baloney operation for land's sakes; they were all just spinning their wheels, and why waste everybody's time, and oh shoot maybe she could see him Monday morning at her mother's house on Quebec Avenue. By the time he got off the phone, his ears rang.

On Monday, Minda put up some token resistance, but once the words started rolling off her tongue he knew he had a better chance of stopping the afternoon train to Casper.

He called Tharp. "This is solid," he burbled into the phone. "Story abused her for years, and she's not just going on some dark ugly feeling like her sister. Minda felt it, saw it, and—"

"That's great," Tharp interrupted. "Now get me a dozen more."

Wilcock's hopes rose when a woman from the little oil town of Deaver, fifteen miles north on the road to Billings, walked into the cramped police headquarters and told about a pelvic examination back in 1970, when she'd been seventeen. He dutifully reported:

She states her vagina was first penetrated by a cold instrument, described as metal, round at the top, flat at the bottom, and hinged. This instrument was withdrawn. Her vagina was then penetrated by a warm object. She recalls thinking, "It's about time something was warmed up around here." Dr. Story soon withdrew the object and stated, "I'm having trouble inserting you. Can you help me?" Dr. Story then asked for her hand. She placed her hand under the sheet between her legs, near her vagina, and grasped Dr. Story's penis. She said it felt like he had a rubber on. Wilcock asked if she could have mistaken any other object, such as a gloved finger, for Dr. Story's penis. She replied firmly, "No. I couldn't get my hand completely around it. It was round, warm and firm. . . . It gave off its own heat. . . ." When she grasped Dr. Story's penis, she can't recall if she said or just thought, "Whoa, I'm not going to do this." She let go of Dr. Story . . . and [he] did not persist. . . .

When she got home, she did tell her husband. She states he became very upset and wanted to kill Dr. Story. Late that evening, they called Bishop Lyle Nicholls, who went to their home. . . . She states both she and her husband talked to Bishop Nicholls about filing a complaint, but the bishop advised against it.

The woman had a crippling liability as a complaining witness. Her husband had a police record for entering women's homes and stealing their underwear. Terry Tharp said he couldn't use her as a complainant. A competent defense lawyer would destroy her credibility on the witness stand.

Wilcock was afraid he'd made all the progress he could make without assistance. He was thinking about shelving his investigation when the county attorney called from Basin and said he was scouting around for an outside investigator. A few days later, Tharp reported that help was on the way. Right now, he said, she was about halfway up the Wind River Gorge, driving a bright red Pontiac Fierro. He said Wilcock would know her by her hair color. It was a little lighter than her car.

55

Judi Cashel

SHE HADN'T WANTED to say good-bye to her kids and her husband to work an out-of-town case, but the challenge was irresistible. How many chances would a female cop get to investigate a doctor charged with sexually abusing his patients? There was a modish new name for that contemptible crime—"doctor rape"—and she'd read a few reports on the subject. It seemed about on a par with mugging nuns.

Her name was Judith Ann Gilmore Cashel. She stood five-two after a shampoo and five-six after she'd fluffed out her wedge-cut red hair. She combined an innocent face, a command voice that rattled windows, and an understated figure featuring 112 pounds of femininity and three pounds of .38. She liked to dance, didn't smoke, seldom drank, spent weekends biking on her Kawasaki 440, and sometimes shocked her friends by wearing Dolly Parton wigs. She'd been baptized Presbyterian, raised Methodist, and now attended the Assembly of God. At thirty-four, she'd been a housewife, mother, cosmetologist, firefighter, meter maid, street cop, and now a Casper police sergeant. As an undercover agent for WYCAP, the Wyoming crime-attack team, she'd worked a string of dope cases, but almost no sex crimes. Once she'd joined in a raid on a brothel, but only as a witness. The men had all the fun.

When Chief Edward Kenyon told her he was lending her to Lovell for an undercover job, she had only one question:

Where's Lovell?

The local chief of police had promised to meet her at the first restaurant on the left as she entered town. She parked her red Fierro in the rear lot and took a look inside. No one resembled a police officer. A roly-poly man in an ill-fitting gas station uniform took up two seats in a booth and blinked at her tentatively. She took a closer look and realized that he was the chief. She put on a smile and walked over and thought, Oh, my god, how can I work with *this*?

They talked for an hour. David Wilcock turned out to be bright, articulate, and deeply concerned about the case. She couldn't remember when her mere presence had so disarmed a fellow officer. It usually took a long time to break through masculine doubts and distrust. Wilcock sat there beaming, refilling her coffee cup, already treating her as his peer.

He handed over a thin file of interview reports. She halfway expected to read a bunch of vague complaints about improper comments during Pap smears—sexual innuendoes, maybe even a few lewd suggestions, nothing prosecutable—but she was startled to see that this case involved full penetration and went back years, maybe even decades. She thought, This is the 1980s. How can this be possible?

By the third cup of coffee the two officers had discarded the idea of sending her up the hill for an undercover pelvic. That was a little more gung ho than she'd had in mind, although she'd certainly taken bigger risks. Wilcock told her about an out-of-state woman who'd been driving through Lovell with her husband, stopped at the Story clinic for a back spasm, and ended up being raped. But that had been a long time ago. The rape doctor figured to be much more cautious now.

Wilcock kept stressing the county attorney's stance about credible witnesses. "I doubt you'll be needing your gun," he said.

She pulled out a microcassette tape recorder. "I brought something more lethal," she said.

She checked into the new Super 8 motel next door and an hour later hit the street. Her first interview was with a woman named Meg Anderson, whose shoulder-length hair looked spun from silver. Her figure was full and her voice had a mellow, professional quality, as though she'd been trained.

The two women talked in a small room in the Town Hall, and in a few minutes Judi turned off the recorder and dropped it into her purse. The woman was obviously inhibited by the machine and was retreating into giggles and tears and silliness.

It proved to be an attack of nerves, and when Meg settled down she told a horrifying story. Judi thought, How could this happen? How could an educated lady just lie there and let him do his sick thing? She had a lot more investigating to do.

56

Jan Hillman

The double standard is the basis of the [Mormon]
patriarchal order: men have privileges that women do not
have. . . . Patriarchy is a sham. . . . Justice is never bestowed, but that it is always wrested by intelligence and
courage out of the hands of fate. . . . [The Mormon Church]
poses by far the greatest threat to equal rights for women
in this country of any New Right group.
——Passages highlighted by
Jan Hillman in her copy
of Sonia Johnson's
From Housewife to Heretic

SHE'D NEVER BEEN ABLE to sit idly by while others were being mistreated, and now it was happening in her own hometown. She heard
from her mother LaVera at the Town Hall that a female police sergeant
was already interviewing the so-called victims. The police office was a
cramped brick afterthought tacked onto the furnace room of the Town
Hall, and her mother was in position to see the comings and goings. Jan
thought, It's those damned McArthurs again. Dr. Story is just their
latest victim.

She remembered how Arden and Minda and a bunch of other prudes
had run a good teacher out of town despite several letters of support to
the editor, including a personal one from Jan herself. And Jan's disk
jockey sister swore upside down that Arden phoned KMNZ to complain
that the station's hard rock music helped make Minda pregnant (and
Arden swore upside down that the story was false). Another McArthur
woman was always griping that men made passes at her.

Jan thought, What a bunch of flakes. She'd met Arden at a recent
social gathering and found her to be a typical Mormon. Her inflections,
her voice, her manner, her righteous air—she was LDS from her
galoshes up.

Janice Hillman knew exactly what ailed the Mormons. Their problem was that they had a monopoly on the truth. Women like Arden McArthur seemed to say, I'm perfect and my children are perfect and my church is perfect; join us and we'll make you perfect, too, you poor slobs. It took a hell of a lot of gall to be perfect. And some ignorance, too.

Jan had grown up as a Lutheran surrounded by Mormons, and she prided herself that her four closest schoolmates had been LDS and they'd never exchanged a harsh word. Of course when you made friends with Mormons you had to accept certain conditions, such as the fact that they went to Mutual on Wednesday nights and you couldn't, and they were always making weird "temple excursions" and missionary trips where they did off-the-wall things like baptizing the dead. Jan didn't profess to understand and didn't want to understand. It was Mormon mumbo jumbo.

She was a large, robust woman, given to jeans and loose-fitting athletic sweatshirts. Her neatly coiffed curly brown hair framed a handsome oval face behind big glasses. Her voice was husky, almost a whiskey alto, oddly befitting a woman who'd tended bar for years, now owned one, but seldom took a drink. Back at the old Cactus Bar, when she was twenty-one, she'd heard too many drunks shout, "Hey, nurse, bring the medicine!" She knew exactly how therapeutic those bourbons and gins were. But she and Jack Bischoff weren't ashamed of owning and operating the new Diamond J Bar together. The Mormons frowned on the place, but who could keep up with all the LDS prohibitions and restrictions? Those folks who wore funny underwear also disdained hot or cold drinks of any kind. Jan thought, Imagine a religion that would damn you for sipping ice water.

"The bishops think I must be a prostitute if I run a bar," she explained, "but that rubs right off me. I'm an arrogant person. That's my defense. When I think people look down on me, I hold my head that much higher." In a town full of churches and piety, she'd lived with Jack Bischoff for fifteen years and had no plans for marriage. The prigs chattered about that, too. Jack was a cattleman and fencemaker, descended from pioneers who'd faced down the Hole-in-the-Wall gang. The Bischoffs weren't famous for kissing backsides.

Jan seldom had need of her personal physician, nor had she undergone his pelvic examinations, but she knew Dr. Story and his methods. One black midnight in 1981 she'd rushed Jack to the hospital with a fever of 105 and an abdomen that made him look as though he'd swallowed a slot machine. There was no time to fly him to Billings, and there were no other surgeons on hand to assist. As the nurses wheeled him into the operating room, Jan was aghast to spot her family doctor sitting at the nurse's station reading a book on problems of the bowel. An aide explained that he studied up before every operation, even tonsillectomies.

At 3 A.M. Dr. Story stepped from the operating room in a blood-spattered surgical smock and told her that Jack was unblocked and doing fine. She could have kissed the little man, but before she had a chance to offer thanks he sat her down, impaled her on his owlish brown eyes, and asked her why a fine woman like her persisted in living in sin. "You weren't raised like that," he admonished her.

"That's the way I want it," Jan assured him.

"I know your mother," Dr. Story went on. "I know your family." He'd treated her asthmatic mother and paraplegic father for years. "I'm not condemning you. I just want you to explain why."

"I *am* explaining why," she insisted. "That's the way I want it. And despite what you think, Dr. Story, it's *my* choice. Okay?"

She would never forget his conciliatory smile. It said, Okay, *okay*, don't be annoyed. You can't blame me for trying, can you? She'd admired him all the more after that.

Her first word of his trouble had come on a wintry day in 1983 when her old friend, McKay "Muck" Welling, the best blade operator in the whole Big Horn Basin, had suggested that she stop going to the clinic up on the hill. "He's going to lose his license," Muck said. "Some women are talking about improprieties in his office."

Jan was shocked. "What?" she said.

"Oh, yes," Muck said. "It's a fact."

"No it isn't! And if you repeat it, then you're no better than those gossipy women."

"Would you believe it if I told you Arden McArthur said it?" Muck was LDS. Evidently he believed that women like Arden McArthur were reliable.

"Now I *definitely* won't believe it," Jan said.

"Would you believe it if I said Caroline Shotwell?"

"Nope. She's another one. How'd you find out?"

"Arden came to my wife for more dirt."

Jan blew up. "You're just adding fuel to the fire! If we're gonna be friends, Muck, you'd better stop spreading this gossip. That's a horrible thing to be saying about Dr. Story."

A few months later she'd run into Diana Harrison in the IGA market. "What in heaven's name's going on with Dr. Story?" she asked.

"Oh, Jan, you would *not* believe what they're trying to do to him. It's the McArthurs, and you know *them*."

"Is there anything I can do?"

"You can write letters to the Medical Board about what a great doctor he is."

Jan's mother had been even more upset than Jan when she heard about the charges. LaVera Hillman was from Morton, Mississippi, and after thirty-six years in Lovell she still said "Y'all." She was a Baptist who'd converted to Lutheranism for her husband, a farm implement dealer who later sold guns and fishing tackle, but she also enjoyed Reverend Ken Buttermore's colorful sermons up at the Lovell Bible Church. In 1982 her husband had died of cancer under Dr. Story's care; LaVera herself suffered from emphysema, bronchitis and asthma and twice had been operated on by the family doctor. Sometimes he gave her cortisone so she could breathe. LaVera was dependent on the family doctor and praised his name.

One night just before the Medical Board hearing, Jan had called Dr. Story on impulse and asked what she could do to help. He advised her to pass on anything she heard about him. After the license revocation, she went to his office and renewed her pledge of support.

She'd learned about causes from her father. After a 1952 automobile accident had put him in a wheelchair for life, he became cantankerous about everything from local politics to veterans' rights. Jan remembered his fight for ramps at the courthouse, for special parking places in Billings, for recognition of the needs of the disabled.

Father and daughter proved to be a matched pair. At Augustana College and the University of Wyoming, Jan took double majors in sociology and psychology, protested Vietnam, and wore an MIA bracelet. She spoke out for racial equality, the ERA and the women's movement, and against capital punishment. In 1968 she wore a black armband to the Wyoming-BYU football game because the Mormon university wouldn't allow blacks on its team. "Mormons," she told her Laramie friends, "are the worst racists and sexists." She wrote letters of protest and signed petitions. Like her father, she felt unfulfilled without a cause.

When her mother mentioned the Lovell P.D.'s new investigation, Jan asked her to take notes on the cops' activities. As a clerk in the Town Hall, LaVera handled travel vouchers and phone slips.

"Oh, I couldn't do that," her mother said.

"You don't have to *do* anything, Mother," Jan explained, a little impatiently. "Just get me the information. I'll do the rest."

LaVera had to admit that the cause was just.

Jan had worked as a skip tracer in a collection agency and knew the techniques. As fast as her mother brought in the police department's phone slips, Jan dialed the numbers. In a brisk voice, she pretended to be selling siding, or announced in an upbeat manner that the party was a finalist in a contest, or said disconsolately that she was searching for a missing relative. It wasn't hard to convert raw phone numbers into basic information.

She hand-delivered her findings to Dr. Story, and together they discovered ominous patterns. The Lovell police were contacting ex-residents, mostly women, in places as far removed as Maine and California. The names meant nothing to Jan but seemed significant to the doctor. One number turned out to be the bank in Salt Lake City where the accuser Jean Anderson Howe worked as a vault teller. Another was listed to a nursing home managed by Tom West, an early administrator of the Lovell hospital. When one call was traced to "Dean Price" in Salt Lake City, Marilyn Story explained that only Diana Harrison knew about their tax-sheltered account with the Price firm. Another call was traced to the U.S. Passport Agency in Seattle; apparently the gumshoes were worried that Dr. Story might be planning to skip.

The inside information seemed pretty much of a mishmash to Jan, but Dr. Story acted grateful and told her to thank her mother. LaVera was pleased.

57

Marilyn Story

> . . . The astonishing power that nearly all psychopaths
> and part-psychopaths have to bind forever the devotion of
> women.
> —Hervey Cleckley, M.D.,
> *The Mask of Sanity*

IN MID-OCTOBER, Marilyn wrote in her journal: "We are hearing rumors this week about our enemies pressing criminal charges. Investigators are in town—one a young woman. . . . May we get our armor on and STAND!"

And what a relief it was to stand shoulder to shoulder with Christians! Every edition of the *Chronicle* was filled with ads wishing John well. He'd taken the pulpit at the Lovell Bible Church and explained the whole mess—the vulnerability of doctors, the unreliability of his accusers, the pervasiveness of Satan, the trials to which God subjects his followers. If there'd been any doubts about his innocence, they were dispelled by his talk. Prayer vigils were scheduled, and the energetic Reverend Buttermore drummed up support at every service.

Marilyn was glad to see that John's legions of admirers only grew. One by one, Lovell women showed their faith by making appointments for Pap smears and pelvics. John fitted them all in. He figured later that he did more pelvics in the three months after his license revocation than in any three months before.

So many Lovellites offered their help that it was almost embarrassing. Bob Negro, the Lutheran owner of the Big Horn IGA market, contributed box after box of food. One night eighteen or twenty supporters formed up on the front lawn, singing "We Shall Overcome" and waving banners saying WE'RE BEHIND YOU 100% and DON'T GIVE UP, DR. STORY! Marilyn was thrilled to see Mormons among them. The gifts filled the big living room: frozen chops and steaks, glazed hams, pungent casseroles, pies bursting with fruit, gallons of milk and ice cream. Marilyn was afraid she'd have to borrow more space in Iva Lee Meeker's freezer. Her eyes filled. How could she waver when others stood so strong?

The new lawyer, Wayne Aarestad, didn't seem quite as optimistic about the outcome as the Keplers had been, but he was bursting with ideas and energy. He wasn't quite forty; he practiced in Fargo, N.D.; he was a member of the Christian Legal Society, and his fee for handling the appeal would be $50,000—if they managed to talk him into taking the case. "I don't want a Wyoming lawyer," John had explained. "I want somebody who isn't tied into the local politics. And, most of all, I want a Christian."

Aarestad's first requirement was that John pass a lie detector test, which was quickly done. Then he was ordered to submit to extensive testing by Denver psychologist James R. Dolby, author of many professional papers including "I Too Am Man: A Psychologist's Reflections on Christian Experience," and "Jesus—As Seen by a 20th Century Follower."

Marilyn enjoyed the trip to Colorado. At last they were doing something in their own behalf, not waiting around for another Judas to appear. The trip gave her a chance to see her folks. Marilyn loved to talk Bible with her father. Except for John, no one knew the good book better.

On the long drive back to Lovell, John said he felt good about the tests. "Dolby and I talk the same language," he told her. She knew what that meant; the two men of science had spent half their time talking religion.

While awaiting the results, they made friends with the new lawyer. Wayne was a bulky six footer whose suits always looked a size too small. He had alert blue eyes, flaring nostrils, and sandy hair that drifted in wisps over his face. He spoke in the accents of the northern border: "accoracy," "North Dakawta," "mawst" for "most." His ancestry was half Norwegian and half Swedish. He'd been a hippie and a Peace Corpsman before taking off on his own and winding up in Katmandu.

Marilyn admired his refreshing, uplifting spirituality. Some Christians stressed the negative—believers would suffer, be cast out, set upon, even killed. Aarestad's approach was more like a happy evangelist's: God will provide, God performs miracles, God wants you healthy and wealthy. If you will love God and honor his teachings, He'll do the rest. . . .

Marilyn realized that both points of view could be substantiated by the Scriptures—it was all a matter of emphasis—but at the moment the concept of a benevolent God was welcome. Not that John needed reassurance. He was his same confident self, secure in his twin strengths of faith and innocence.

She couldn't bear to tell him that although she shared the passion of his beliefs, there were nights when she worried more hours than she slept.

58

David Wilcock

IN THE BEGINNING the chief had entertained a flicker of doubt about Casper Police Sgt. Judi Cashel, mostly along the lines that no one who looked so comfortable in a red Fierro could possibly be a complete cop, but he'd learned to recognize male chauvinism even in himself and withheld judgment. A good thing, too, he soon realized. He could hardly keep up with the woman. Together they began a blitz of sixteen-hour days and seven-day weeks. They knew they could be shut down any minute, if not by the mayor, then by the mayor's nephew, who was the councilman in charge of the P.D., or by several other power figures.

Both investigators smelled a leak early but couldn't pin it down. Judi began working out of her motel room to avoid a telephone tap. Wilcock used pay phones whenever possible. The leaks seemed to diminish.

Soon he began hearing gossip that a sexy little carrot-top was running hookers out of her room at the Super 8. The madam's full figure, it was said, had already earned her the nickname "Boom Boom" among the hot-eyed young men from the mineral plants and the sugar factory. One night she'd been seen in the Medicine Wheel Bar on Main Street. Now was this a whorehouse madam or what?

Wilcock told Cashel, and the two cops enjoyed a rare laugh.

Another investigator limped onstage, a young half-Indian from California named Dan Flores. He explained that he'd damaged his leg in a car crash while working a free-lance case for the Wyoming public defender's office out of Cheyenne. As Wilcock listened deadpan, Flores claimed that he'd been hired by a lawyer who was developing information on behalf of Minda Brinkerhoff and Meg Anderson. The sisters were planning a civil suit against Dr. Story. Flores said that Minda had contacted "60 Minutes" in New York and expected a crew to arrive any day.

Wilcock thought, Why the hell didn't Minda and Meg tell *me*? "Look, Dan," he said, "you couldn't've picked a worse time. Work someplace else or you'll screw things up. I hear there's some victims over in Powell."

Flores agreed to cooperate. Soon afterward, Wilcock heard that he'd started hanging around the Lamplighter Inn in Powell. He didn't seem to be opening his mouth, except for drinks.

While Judi Cashel beat the bushes for victims, Wilcock searched out others who might be helpful. From former mayor Jim Wagner he learned about Dixie King Marchant, a divorcee who'd suffered serious brain damage in an auto accident. Wagner said the epileptic woman had come to him in 1976 with a complaint that Dr. Story tried to take liberties with her, but Police Chief LaMar Averett had refused to listen.

Averett's name came up again in a Cashel report on a gypsum worker named Nelson St. Thomas, who claimed that his wife Annella had been abused by Story in 1972. Wilcock read:

Mr. St. Thomas spoke with LaMar Averett, Lovell chief of police (now retired). Mr. St. Thomas was told that it would be his word against Dr. Story's. Mr. St. Thomas was advised [by Averett] to forget this situation. . . .

Mrs. St. Thomas wrote a letter of complaint, which Mr. St. Thomas distinctly remembers was sent to the State Board of Medical Examiners in Cheyenne, WY. Mr. St. Thomas recalls receiving a reply from the Board of Medical Examiners stating that they would need more corroborative evidence before they could proceed.

At some time after this, Mr. St. Thomas received a letter from the office of Dr. J. H. Story and signed by Dr. Story. This letter was in reference to the St. Thomas family's outstanding bill to Dr. Story. Mr. St. Thomas recalls that the letter stated that if the bill was too high, he, Dr. Story, would adjust it down. Mr. St. Thomas was angered by the letter and he immediately destroyed it.

Nelson St. Thomas didn't mind discussing the case further. He was a Catholic, an easygoing cowboy type who'd drifted down from Montana, married a Lovell Mormon and joined the regiment of hardworking men wrenching a living from the badlands. When he wasn't clogging his lungs with bentonite or gypsum dust, St. Thomas photographed birds and butterflies, smoked his big pipe, and drove his pickup a little too fast on the desert road. He had flyaway black hair flecked with white gypsum dust, heavy pork-chop sideburns and a handlebar mustache. His labored breathing could be heard across the room as he spoke about the incident twelve years back:

"The night 'Nella told me what Story did to her, I racked my twelve-gauge in my old Chevy pickup and drove to town. I parked down the street from Story's house. Then I took and walked up to the front door. I was gonna waste him and get away without being seen.

"It seemed like forever till I reached that door. I was so mad I was shakin'. My finger was inside the trigger guard. I thought, I'll give him one barrel for waving that thing in front of my wife and the other for poking it in her side.

"Just before I pushed the doorbell, I thought, What if his wife answers? Then I'm in trouble. That hesitation saved me. I said to myself, Why go to prison for killing that stupid son of a bitch—excuse my French. For what? It's not worth it.

"I got back in the truck and drove to the police. I pointed my finger at Chief Averett and I said, 'You better arrest Dr. Story for rape.'

"He sat back and stared.

"I said, 'You better find that son of a bitch before I do, or he's dead meat.'

"He said, 'Mister, if you don't put that shotgun down, I might just throw you in jail.'

"I'd clean forgot I was carrying my gun. I says, 'He raped my wife. You better find him.'

"The chief told me I was wasting my time."

Wilcock drove to the Averett home to check out the story. As soon as he was ushered inside, he felt the antagonism. He asked his questions in a low key and gave no hint of his concern about Averett's behavior. The former chief's face reddened as he admitted talking to Nelson St. Thomas. "I told him he would have to get him a lawyer and get a complaint made up," the old man recalled. He insisted that he would do the same again "because anybody that thinks Doc Story would do them things has gotta be plumb loco to begin with."

After the short interview, Wilcock returned to the little police office behind the Town Hall and a few minutes later looked up to see Averett bursting through the door. "Look," the former chief said, "if you try to use anything I said in court, just remember one thing. An old man has an awful convenient memory."

Wilcock started to speak but ended up saying it to himself. *For god's sake, LaMar, you're supposed to be a cop. . . .*

Sgt. Cashel uncovered a victim who was distantly related to Mayor Herman Fink. There were even more Finks than Asays in the Lovell phone book, some thirty in all. They were Lutherans descended from a colony of Germans who'd been lured to Russia by Catherine the Great and thence to the Big Horn Basin, duped both times by promises of gold.

"We've got a new name to check out," Judi told Wilcock. " 'Hayla Farwell.' Story did it to her in 1968."

"Did what?"

"I don't know the details yet."

The name was familiar. "Say, who's Hayla Farwell?" Wilcock asked police dispatcher John Fink.

Fink looked up from his wheelchair. Years before, he'd fallen from a tree in the snowy Big Horns and snapped his spine. Dr. Story had been in the rescue party. "She's my sister," he said.

"Oh, I'm sorry, John," Wilcock said. "How long have you known about her and Story?"

"A month or so."

"God, John, why didn't you say something?"

The details made the chief sick. Hayla Fink Farwell, a round busty woman with a pretty face, had suffered slight loss of brain function after inhaling butane from a defective burner. The German-hating family doctor began giving her pelvic exams. Hayla hadn't realized what was going on till she saw his penis, and then she kept the information to herself out of fear and shame.

Wilcock had worked closely with Hayla's paraplegic brother and knew that reticence was a deep family tradition. John had told him about an ancestor who said of her own pregnancy, *"Um dis spricht man nicht.* No one speaks about this." Another family expression dated to the nineteenth century on the Volga: "When little men try to act big, they usually use their pecker."

59

Judi Cashel

THERE WERE nights when she fell into bed at the Super 8 with the unwholesome feeling that she was making a sick situation sicker. Lovell women were naive, shy creatures, hugely different from their counterparts in cities as close as Casper and Cheyenne. She admired them, respected their principles and ideals, but also felt that some of them must have been living in caves while the twentieth century passed unnoticed. They squirmed at the merest mention of sex and cried at the simplest questions. The mere mention of her birthday made Aletha Durtsche break into sobs; she'd been raped on that day.

Sometimes Judi had to break off interviews and reschedule them. Most of the women referred to "my bottom," "down there," "my sex." Breasts were "boobs"; one woman called her breasts "my flowers." Every victim had to be asked if she'd seen Story's erect penis, and several answered that they knew how erections felt but not how they looked. Apparently sex was performed exclusively in the dark in Lovell. The women seemed to think that it was unworthy of them to discuss the subject.

After a while, Judi found herself opening each interview with an explanation that there was nothing to be ashamed of, that women didn't need to accept victimization, that they had basic rights. "I want you to talk to me," she would plead, "and we'll see this through together." She called it her "I am woman, hear me roar speech." Dave Wilcock, working hard on his own contacts, kept threatening to bring in the Helen Reddy song on a cassette.

Aletha had turned in Mae Fischer's name as a possible victim, and it proved to be one of Judi's hardest interviews. Caroline Shotwell's daughter gave a full statement but begged that it not be used. "My husband doesn't know and he'd kill Story." A few days later she phoned to say that she'd told Bill and he was in a rage.

Not long afterward, Bill Fischer made a hostile remark to Dave Wilcock in the Rose Bowl Café. The next day he strode into the police office and warned, "You got exactly two months and then I'll handle this myself."

"We're working on it," Judi told him.

"You got two months!" He had a strange look in his eyes.

Judi called on Caroline Shotwell to corroborate daughter Mae's story and ended up finding another sobbing victim. The wife of the former bishop lamented that she'd been violated by Story and failed to warn her daughter. The Shotwell woman still hadn't told anyone in her family about her own involvement. She thought she would get around to it soon, if she could only stop crying.

Plump little Wanda Hammond was another vale of tears, but behind the hysteria the grocery checker had almost perfect recall of the day she'd been raped fifteen years before. Judi made a note that she would be a superior witness.

Dorothy Brinkerhoff admitted that she hadn't made an official complaint, and she refused to make one now. Minda Brinkerhoff's mother-in-law seemed to feel that the police had voodoo techniques for learning victims' names and she'd better come in before she was found out. Otherwise, Judi was convinced, they wouldn't have heard from her at all. She cried throughout the interview and acted thoroughly ashamed. She'd only told her husband a month before.

Judi began to get a line on the victims' thought processes. To her, they seemed like docile, subservient creatures, raised to serve males and continually reminded of their low station. Most of them seemed to consider themselves property, not much more important than a bell cow or a blue-ribbon hog. When the realization had hit them that they were being "dilated" with a penis, their minds simply shut down in a combination of shock and denial. Some thanked the doctor and left. Some politely asked how much they owed and wrote checks. Some scheduled new appointments. They reminded Judi of accident victims she'd seen sitting on the curb applying lipstick. In the face of unexpected horror, the mind held itself together by reverting to the familiar.

She discovered that the reason most of them had kept quiet was not the oft-mentioned rationalization that their husbands might kill Story and go to jail, but the fear of personal embarrassment and ridicule. Each wondered if she'd done something to bring on the attack and therefore deserved it, at least partially. Alone in her shame, almost every victim was sure that she'd committed adultery, or, at the least, fornication, and that she could be excommunicated. In a godly town like Lovell, that amounted to social death.

After a few weeks, Judi felt the strain herself. She'd never become so personally involved with crime victims. The constant emotional scenes, the handholding, the midnight phone conversations—it was so *draining*. There were nights when she'd almost have dumped the case for a spin on the Kawasaki with her husband.

In the daytime she couldn't relax; she had to go about her work while maintaining a low profile. She and Dave Wilcock knew that someone was keeping watch. Five or six times she picked up the police office phone and heard breathing. Her personal behavior had to be impeccable. She warned herself, Nothing will sabotage this case faster than some sort of confrontation where I can be made to look bad or the facts can be twisted against me.

So she didn't take her usual daily jog or her long walks at night; her red hair and her petite figure were too conspicuous. She ate every meal in the Big Horn Restaurant next to the motel. She always sat in the corner booth with Dave Wilcock or Patricia Wiseman, the town's new Family Violence/Sexual Assault coordinator, who was counseling some of the victims. Rather than study the long menu, she always ordered nachos. Once in a while the three of them would share a carafe of wine, make jokes and act silly. It was their only recreation.

She drove thirty miles to Powell to interview Terri Lee Timmons and found the woman to be an emotional wreck. After mailing the microcassette tape from Denver, Terri had returned silently to her hometown and tried to forget. Dave Wilcock had located her only after a frantic hunt.

The Timmons woman was small, pale, feminine, slightly prissy, and totally credible. Judi called their session a two-Kleenex interview—two packages. At the end, Terri mentioned that an aunt had been violated by Story twenty years before; she now lived in another state. It might be difficult interviewing her; she'd always been "a little . . . different."

Judi confirmed the information with another family member and sought interagency help. Back came a report from a detective:

Basically Betty claimed that when she was approx 15 she went to the doctor's office and Dr. Story told her to lay on the table and he was going to put an instrument in her mouth, that he wanted her to suck on it like a baby bottle. She was to close her eyes and not open them. She did and he placed the instrument in her mouth. She sucked for several min. before gagging. As she opened her eyes the doctor turned around quickly. He told her that she was not finished, to close her eyes again. She did and the doctor continued by placing the instrument back in her mouth. He did push it in and out as she recalls. He did have an erection according to the victim. He did not ejaculate that she recalls.

Other juvenile victims turned up. Jean Anderson Howe had been a deathly ill ten-year-old when Story violated her. Another woman told how she'd watched him stick his finger into her three-year-old daughter, then explain, "She might as well get used to it."

Carol Beach, a Lovell schoolteacher's wife, proved to be another prim and proper victim, the type who would make a good witness. She brought some of her information in writing so she wouldn't have to say certain words. Judi relaxed her with the "I am woman" speech and the interview went smoothly. At the end, Mrs. Beach asked, "How do you think it feels to be thirty-six years old and find out on your marriage bed that your doctor raped you?" Judi said she couldn't imagine.

60

Marilyn Story

ONE MORNING when the silvery-chrome sun was so bright that it hurt her eyes, Marilyn tore open the long-awaited envelope from the psychologist in Denver. What did an experienced behaviorist think of her husband? John had felt good about the interview and the man; Dr. Dolby seemed to know his Scripture and his psychology. But how far would he be willing to go in a sworn affidavit?

Marilyn settled into a chair in the atrium in back of the house. "Dr. Story is a small, 58 year old, Caucasion male," she read. "He is average in build, wears glasses, and his face has some lines in it." Well, she said to herself, whose face wouldn't?

The report noted that John seemed almost fatalistic about the charges, as though the matter were in God's hands and out of his own. The psychologist had found John cautious and thorough, a strong conservative who believed in hard work, moral values, self-denial, obedience, and "a minimum of governmental intervention in one's work or private life."

"It appears that his father was his key model," Dr. Dolby observed. "E.g., neither he nor his father are very socially gregarious, but they both have/had many good friends."

Marilyn wasn't surprised to learn that the MMPI (Minnesota Multiphasic Personality Inventory) and other tests had shown "no evidence of psychopathology." She read that her husband had a "need to suppress unacceptable impulses," and that he was especially angry about the recent intrusions into his life, "but even here his anger is blunted and expressed obliquely, e.g., cutting remarks on the side. He tends to approach his life and work compulsively."

Marilyn paused to imagine the results of the same scientific tests if they'd been administered to women like Arden McArthur, Meg, Minda, Aletha, some of the others. Would they show "no evidence of psychopathology"? And yet the Medical Board had acted as though John was the weird one! How would the Board have ruled if they'd read this report? Dr. Dolby was a licensed psychologist, a graduate of Baylor University, a former teacher at Wheaton College, John's own alma mater. His findings were hard evidence, not malicious gossip.

Marilyn agreed with the doctor's evaluation of John as a "private person who has spent an adult lifetime serving people as a physician" and a deep believer in religion and ethics. His sexual fantasies, according to the psychological tests, were "normal and unimaginative," and he lived a normal, "provincial" sex life with neither sadistic nor aggressive fantasies. Above all, he was emotionally stable and mentally healthy, and the charges against him were "inconsistent with the results of this diagnostic examination."

As part of his fee, the Denver expert had agreed to study the case and distill his findings into an affidavit. Marilyn felt relieved as she read his sworn observation that female patients frequently indulged in sexual fantasies about their physicians, and that this "could be a powerful dynamic which might be the core fantasy around which a myth is built." Dolby likened the case to the Salem witchcraft trials. The accusers, he noted, seemed to "have a difficult time thinking and functioning as independent units."

A covering letter ended with a ringing statement that if John were convicted, it would "indeed be a travesty of justice."

Marilyn felt like dancing around the sunstruck room. Dr. Dolby had never seen or heard of John before they'd met in Denver. Who could disregard impartial testimony like this?

After Wayne Aarestad read the Dolby report, he formally agreed to take the case. In the first strategy session, he insisted that John take the attack. "You've got to speak up," he said. "Look at you, Doctor.

You're an intelligent, likable, honorable man. You represent the highest principles of medicine. Why can't you get that across?"

"I can't brag about myself," John insisted. "And I don't like to bad-mouth my patients." Marilyn thought, John would rather drink formaldehyde than violate the rule of doctor-patient confidentiality.

"If you can't talk about yourself," the beefy lawyer said, "we'll have to find someone who can."

Marilyn suggested Dr. Douglas Wrung, John's colleague at the hospital and a fellow member of the Lovell Bible Church. John had helped to bring Doug to town and they'd become social friends, at least to the extent that the homebody Storys were social with anyone.

Marilyn stayed up past midnight, running off a fresh set of depositions and transcripts on the clinic's clunky old copying machine in the back of the storage room. The next morning a sympathetic Doug Wrung promised to study the two thousand pages and respond with his own honest interpretation.

As far as Marilyn was concerned, the result was a masterpiece of logic. "Frankly," Doug wrote, "Meg Anderson's testimony reveals *no direct visible witness* of anything improper or irregular in her examinations by Dr. Story." Doug stressed how "bizarre" it was for Minda and Meg to bring their children back to the clinic after claiming that John had molested them.

As she read, Marilyn found her head bobbing in agreement. She was sure the courts would be equally impressed. Doug suggested that Minda suffered from emotional instability and other disorders, including a tendency to be incoherent, agitated, talkative, disoriented about time, overly dependent on her mother, and highly insecure. According to Doug, she was just after attention.

Marilyn blushed when she came to an especially frank passage. John's fellow physician noted that he'd conducted tests in his own examining room and concluded that Minda's allegations made no sense unless John's flaccid penis measured at least ten inches. Poking her in the side with such a huge instrument, Doug wrote, "would seem an anatomical feat that only a *rare* individual might possess. . . ." On the other hand, he went on, Minda might well have imagined it.

Wayne Aarestad seemed pleased with the Wrung report but insisted that more letters and affidavits were needed—"all we can lay our hands on." What better way to expose the Medical Board's error and reverse the revocation?

Marilyn thought of a psychologist who'd briefly rented space at the Story clinic and attended the Bible Church before moving to Grand Forks, North Dakota. John and Dr. Russell Blomdahl hadn't always seen eye to eye, but Russ was a good Christian and he'd recently expressed an interest in the case. Marilyn made another photocopy of the massive Medical Board material and mailed it off for comment.

The reply came fast. Russ Blomdahl modestly discounted his comments as "not intended to be a comprehensive, complete diagnosis," then produced a penetrating analysis of the McArthur girls and their motivations. He noted that Minda hadn't received enough love and attention from her parents, especially her father, and that she'd engaged in rebellious acting-out, including premarital sex and a subsequent marriage at seventeen. This was her way of punishing her parents, Russ wrote, "as well as forcing them to take notice of her."

The groove in Minda's tongue appeared to be a conversion reaction or hysterical reaction, Russ explained, and was common among sexually disturbed women. He called Minda's relationship with Arden "significant," as shown in remarks that she would climb into her mother's bed and "get cuddled," "Mother would climb into my bed," and "I always listen to my mother."

The psychologist discerned a love-hate-jealousy triangle among Arden, Meg and Minda, with poor John in the middle. He observed that Minda had a strong need for a real or imaginary relationship, and when John treated her in a friendly, caring manner, she became infatuated. The report went on:

Without doubt, she very much enjoyed, subconsciously, the pelvic exams and had fantasies of intercourse with mixed feelings of guilt and anger—guilt relating to her husband, mother, and the Church; anger that the exam was uncomfortable during the instrumentation and bimanual manipulation. She expected that the fantasies of intercourse with this otherwise pleasant, gentle man should not be painful but it always was. . . .

Russ suggested that Minda suffered from "pseudoneurotic schizophrenia" and "erotomania." He described her accusations about John as "explicit examples of psychotic illusions."

As for sister Meg, the Blomdahl report noted "numerous emotional and personal problems including her marriage, relationship with her mother, and sexual functioning." Russ likened Meg's childhood experiences to Minda's and noted that "indept psychological evaluation would undoubtedly reveal significant distorted perceptions and emotional functioning."

Marilyn was jubilant when she read his conclusion: the McArthur girls shared a mentally disturbed relationship known as "Folie A deux . . . a communicated emotional illness between two persons."

In other words, Marilyn whispered to herself in glee, they're crazy. She could have hugged the two behavioral scientists and Doug Wrung. Together the three professionals had answered a question that had troubled her sleep for months. *Why would so many women make so many insane charges against an innocent man?*

The dogged Aarestad warned against complacency. He agreed that there'd been a conspiracy against John, and the best defense against a conspiracy was exposure. He hired a husband-and-wife detective agency in Red Lodge, Montana, and a female investigator from Casper. LaVera and Jan Hillman were still providing confidential information, but it wouldn't hurt to bring in a few seasoned gumshoes. From now on, the conspirators would be watched at every step.

61

Judi Cashel

It is estimated that for each rape that is reported, there are anywhere from 3 to 10 others that are not reported.
—Coleman, Butcher, and Carson, *Abnormal Psychology and Modern Life*

IN THE BEGINNING she'd thought, How will we ever get this case into court? But after Judi had interviewed nine or ten victims, clear patterns began to emerge: the repeated use of Examining Room No. 2; the automatic table, so out of place in a smalltown general practice; the frequency with which Story conducted pelvic exams (sometimes ten a day) and the length (up to forty-five minutes); the repeated instructions to slide a little bit past the end and contract the vaginal muscles; the pelvic exams for sprained limbs, colds, sore throats, infected earlobes; the peculiar requests ("Do you want to help guide it in?") and the inappropriate comments ("You have lovely breasts"); the instructions to strip and jump in place; the little touches and feels. . . .

Now if the victims would just cooperate, Judi said to herself, we might just be able to bring some charges. But there were still big problems. Minda McArthur Brinkerhoff, one of the most important witnesses, was acting reluctant. When Judi suggested that they meet in Gillette, Minda said, "Shoot, you won't do anything. How do I know you're not working to get him off?"

Judi felt a flush of anger. There was the suggestion of corruption in that remark—payoffs, malfeasance, the standard slanders about cops. But she kept a smile in her voice till she extracted a grudging okay.

She drove seventy miles in her Fierro and was welcomed inside the Brinkerhoff home. Her first thought was, Oh, God, another Mormon family with wall-to-wall kids! How am I supposed to do an interview? Two towheads with gleaming faces and plastered-down hair squealed at one another while a third banged a piano with a wooden hammer and a fourth sucked on a bottle of pop. The floor was deep in toys. At a word from their mother the kids quieted down.

"I hear you're planning a lawsuit," Judi began.

"You bet."

"Why?"

Minda looked disgusted. "Well, gol, it's been eighteen months since we wrote the Medical Board, and he's still practicing."

"How much are you suing him for?"

"Mooga-bucks, that's all I know. The lawyers are handling it. We're giving the money to charity. We don't want his dirty money."

It didn't take long for Judi to realize that she was dealing with a severe case of disillusionment. You poor kid, she thought, you placed your trust in all those LDS absolutes about chastity and worthiness and then you learned that there's more to real life than the Book of Mormon.

When Minda got started on her story, it was almost impossible to take notes. She sounded like a schoolgirl trying to recite the history of the world in three minutes. Judi remembered that Meg had also seemed kind of fluttery for a while, but that first impression had proved wrong. What made these McArthurs put their worst foot forward?

Minda giggled even more than her sister; it seemed to be the family's all-purpose nervous reaction. Judi reminded herself that giggling rape victims make bad witnesses. You want a woman who wrings her hands and sobs, like Terri Timmons, Caroline Shotwell, Wanda Hammond. Minda might be the Joan of Arc of this case, the first one to take on the male establishment, but that's no reason to let her blow it.

Even when the rape story came gushing out, Judi didn't feel that she'd gained the young mother's trust. Minda seemed as fed up with the justice system as she was with Story. She seemed to be saying, Look, I'll go along with you and give you this information, but you're not fooling me for a second. . . .

The sugar factory's white smokestack looked good as it came into sight on the return trip. Judi drove straight to the police office and learned that while she'd been gone, Wilcock had turned up more victims. The investigation was snowballing. Even the out-of-state leads were paying off. At Judi's request, a Pennsylvania state trooper had interviewed a woman named Susan Moldowney who claimed that Story had locked the examining room door, pulled on a condom, and "dilated" her so cruelly that she begged him to stop. "The doctor continued for a few minutes," the report noted, "telling her that he had to do this."

A detective in Mesa, Arizona, had located a Mexican-American woman who said that Story had dilated her three or four times and finally revealed his erect penis. She acknowledged that her twenty-year-old son might be his but refused to take the matter any further.

At Judi's request, a policeman in Maine interviewed another Mexican-American, Emma Briseno McNeil, who said that Story had dilated her and then turned to the sink and washed his penis in full view.

On October 16, two more Hispanic victims made it clear that there was a Mexican connection. Juana Garcia told how Story had probed her for fifteen minutes with something that felt like a finger, "only it was bigger." She could feel his clothing rubbing against her inner thighs.

Bettina Diaz said that Story accompanied his assault with advice: "Never let a man touch you. They only want one thing," and "Your body is too beautiful to ruin by having children." Toward the end of a pelvic exam, he began sweating and making "funny noises—panting, heavy breathing, grunting."

Over nachos at the Big Horn restaurant, Judi talked demographics with Dave Wilcock and the area's new rape counselor, Patricia Wiseman. By now they'd interviewed two dozen victims and had the names of more. Of the total, four were Hispanic Catholics, one a Lutheran of German descent, and the rest Mormons. "Does that make sense?" Dave asked. "No Methodists, no Presbyterians, no Baptists? Not one member of the Bible Church? This town's only half-Mormon, you know."

Pat Wiseman said the numbers made sense if you understood that rape was a crime of hatred and rage, not passion. Dr. Story had abused ethnics, whom he'd always referred to as "those people," and Mormons, whose "satanic" doctrines enraged him, and poor Hayla Fink Farwell, who seemed to qualify for rape because of her German ancestry. He'd made a move on another woman of German descent, the motelkeeper Eloise Benson, but she'd stalked out of his office in anger. Minutes later, he'd told a nurse, "Those damn Germans!"

Judi picked up a nacho and put it back down. "He's pretty consistent," she observed. "Don't you wish we had stats on all his rapes? I wonder what they'd show."

Pat Wiseman said that only about one rape in five was reported to police, and most went unsolved or unprosecuted. Reliable figures were hard to come by, but it was doubtful that more than one rape in every thirty or forty resulted in hard jail time. Judi wondered how much more shocking those estimates would be in a back-eddy town where women were afraid to say "vagina."

In the office, the investigators set about bringing their files up to date for the demanding county attorney, Terry Tharp. Under the heading "real good," they listed the victims who'd seen Story's penis or been asked to guide it in. Under "pretty good," they listed the women who hadn't seen or touched it but were positive they'd been violated. Under "not-courtroom," they listed the ones who were "pretty sure" or merely had patterns of unusually frequent pelvics. In trial, these weaker cases would diminish the impact of the others.

Then there were the "ah-hahs!"—the fondled children, the women who were asked to do naked gymnastics, the victims who went in for sore throats, the ones like Dorothy Brinkerhoff whose intimate parts had been stroked. Wilcock and the two women agreed that the "ah-hahs" constituted sexual abuse, but not the kind that would sway a jury.

Pat Wiseman explained, "That kind of abuse is a power and authority thing. 'I can make you do something, bitch. You can cry and blush and be embarrassed, but by God you'll do it.' It's the classic woman-hating syndrome."

"It may not be courtroom material," Judi put in, "but it sure makes the pie whole."

Toward the end of October, the investigators had a thick sheaf of statements and more leads than they could check out. Wilcock was working two shifts a day and losing some of his rotundity. His pretty wife's fingers were sore from typing reports gratis. And Judi was having nightmares.

"Let's set a deadline," she suggested wearily, "and then let the prosecutor take it from there." They agreed on Halloween night.

A week before the deadline, she drove her red Fierro two hundred miles over the Rockies to Evanston, in the far southwest corner of the state, and interviewed a former Lovell physician, Henry Eskens. She typed up the report herself:

Dr. Eskens said that he was aware, through conversations with some of his patients and friends, that Dr. John Story raped women in his office during examinations. Dr. Eskens recalled that the first day he entered the North Big Horn County Hospital in Lovell, WY, a man walked up to him, asked him if he was the new doctor, and what he could do to keep Dr. Story from what he did to his (this man's) wife. . . .

Dr. Eskens said that there were two major reasons for his leaving Lovell. . . . One reason was a disagreement with the hospital board. The other reason was that Dr. Story's unethical conduct concerned Dr. Eskens, and he felt that if he remained in Lovell, his reputation would be tainted. Dr. Eskens said he did not want to be known as one of those dirty little doctors from Lovell. Dr. Eskens said that Dr. Story was a very strange man, that when you talked to him, you couldn't get in touch with his emotions.

Dr. Eskens said that at least twenty women told him about being assaulted by Dr. Story. Dr. Eskens said that his wife, Esther, had headed the legislative committee which rewrote the sexual assault statute. The subsection which specifically refers to doctors, Dr. Eskens referred to as Dr. Story's own law.

When I spoke to Esther Eskens, she confirmed that she, too, had conversations with women about their being assaulted by Dr. Story, and that because of Dr. Story, a special subsection referring to doctors had been included in the sexual assault statute. Dr. Eskens said that what Dr. Story did to women while examining them was certainly not a matter of malpractice, but was felonious misconduct. . . .

Dr. Eskens said "that a properly done pelvic examination would take about twenty seconds," "pelvic examinations are not done on pregnant women except occasionally on an early first visit and then near delivery to check the cervix, unless there was a special problem," that when he gives pelvic examinations, he never is closer to the patient's body than about 14 inches, and that there is no examination tool used to give pelvic exams which could be mistaken for a penis.

Judi showed her report to Wilcock and asked, "Enough?"

"Enough," he said.

62

Arrest

I wake and feel the fell of dark, not day.
What hours, O what black hours we have spent
This night.

— Gerard Manley Hopkins

DAVE WILCOCK knew their cover was blown and the arrest had to be quick and dirty; otherwise there might be more trouble than a seven-man police department could handle. He was firmly convinced that Story's supporters were capable of violence.

It was noon on Halloween, Wednesday, October 31, 1984. The justice of the peace didn't seem to understand the urgency. He read the warrants with aggravating slowness, then read them again. He kept wringing his hands and saying, "This is so sad. Oh, this is so terrible."

He asked Judi if she realized what she was doing to Dr. Story. Judi said "Yes, sir" and kept smiling. At last he signed the warrants and handed them over.

The arrest plans had been carefully laid, but Wilcock had spent ten years learning that nothing was predictable in the Rose Town. The program called for officers to serve a search warrant on the clinic while Judi, Dave, and Deputy Sheriff Bill Dobbs carried out a quiet arrest. Before Story's hot-eyed supporters knew he was in custody, he would be pressing his fingertips to an ink pad in the Big Horn County Jail.

Mrs. Story answered the front door of the house on Nevada and Judi asked, "Is the doctor here?"

"No," the small woman answered. Her wide brown eyes told them that she knew why they were here. Lately the Storys had seemed to know everything before it happened. "He went downtown on an errand," Mrs. Story explained. "He'll probably be right back."

Judi Cashel said, "Thank you, ma'am." Wilcock thought she sounded like a waitress who'd just accepted a nice tip.

As they walked back down the driveway to the two police cars, the chief blew on his hands. When he'd finished his day's work at 3 A.M. the night before, the temperature had registered 14. He guessed it was now in the forties. But he still felt cold and apprehensive. Any minute now, he could be out of a job.

They were driving downhill toward the Town Hall, Deputy Dobbs in one car and Judi and Dave in the other, when Wilcock spotted a short, slight man in front of the Coast to Coast store at Main and Nevada. It was the only intersection in Lovell with a stoplight and the last spot in town he would have chosen for the arrest.

Story was walking toward his parked car with a large package under his arm. Wilcock jumped out and said, "Dr. Story, we have a warrant for your arrest. The charge is second-degree assault. You'll have to come with us."

Story blinked through his heavy-rimmed glasses. "Oh, you're kidding," he said in his thin voice.

"No, sir," Wilcock said. "Will you come with us?"

Story stepped toward the curb and the chief grabbed his arm. It felt like a child's. Story looked annoyed and said, "I just want to put my package in the car."

Wilcock let him unload the package and guided him into the backseat of the patrol car between himself and Judi. Normal arrest procedure called for handcuffs, but they'd decided to waive their own rule.

"Doctor," Wilcock said, "this is Sergeant Cashel." Story offered no handshake or acknowledgment.

On the half-block ride to the Town Hall, he said, "This is utterly ridiculous."

Wilcock read him his rights and handed over a written Miranda waiver. He refused to sign. The chief said, "Dr. Story, this paper just confirms that we've given you your rights."

"I'm not signing," he mumbled.

———

Judi had been rehearsing the interrogation in her mind. She didn't expect to get much—a minor admission, a slip of the tongue. That was about the most you could expect from a fox like Story. She was glad that the plan called for her to conduct the interview. This was the county attorney's case and technically she was his investigator.

She wasn't surprised when Story immediately demanded to know who'd sent her from Cheyenne to get him. The old sexist power game was on. It fit his profile perfectly. The unstated message was that a female couldn't exercise authority on her own. "Was it the Medical Board?" he asked. "The governor's office?" Judi thought, What a grandiose little egoist you are!

She'd already arranged the furniture in the front room of the police office. There was a "hot seat" for Story and a large chair for Wilcock. Judi would sit behind the desk, slightly elevated. It was basic interrogation technique, rooted in upmanship psychology and taught in every police academy.

Story made a beeline for Wilcock's chair. "No, sir," Judi said firmly. "You'll have to sit here." The hot seat was the lowest chair in the room.

From her position behind the desk, she opened her notebook, penciled in the time—1442—and said, "Your name is John H. Story. Is that correct?"

"Yes." He seemed bemused.

"What's the 'h' stand for?"

"Is that important?"

"It's just for our records."

"My middle name is not important," he said, peering through his glasses. She had to strain to hear.

"Date of birth?"

His eyes narrowed as he asked, "Why do you need that?"

Judi knew exactly what he was doing. He was trying to trivialize the interview and put her on the defensive, a standard technique of miscreants from speeders to mass murderers. *Who, me? You've made a serious mistake, officer.* . . . If Story only knew how banal his performance was. He peered at her as though she'd just crawled from a swamp.

Dave Wilcock had already done a 10-27 through the sheriff's office and collected Story's driver's license vitals, but she repeated her request for his date of birth. He waved his hand as though chasing gnats. Such biographical minutiae were plainly beneath his notice.

She wrote in large block letters JOHN HUNTINGTON STORY and added his D.O.B. She angled her notebook to make sure he could see it. He looked at the printing and nodded. He almost seemed to be enjoying the game.

She showed him a copy of the arrest warrant and asked, "Doctor, do you know the women on this list?"

"Yes," he said.

"Do you have any idea why they would want to bring charges against you?"

He sniffed and said, "I have *every* idea."

"Well, would you tell me?"

"Tell *you?*" he said. "No." Once again she caught the subtle put-down. "You'll find out at the proper time. I might be filing suit." She thought, When is he gonna say, *I'm the doctor here?*

He confirmed that he'd given pelvic examinations to some of the women on the list. He denied ever discussing sexual complaints with any hospital official; he said he'd never been advised to have a nurse in the examining room, but one could come in if she wanted to; he'd never given pelvics to patients with broken wrists or sore throats, and he'd never abused a woman.

For a while they talked about the paraphernalia of pelvic exams—speculums, swabs, stains. She asked if it might be possible for a woman to mistake a doctor's fingers for an erect penis.

"Not unless she was strange," he answered.

She asked if he'd offered to void the bill of Minda and Scott Brinkerhoff. "That's correct," he said. "That young man was using profanity and I didn't want a nickel of his money with those profane thoughts."

"Why'd you stop billing Julia Bradbury?"

"I didn't. She just refused to pay."

"But why?"

"I never tried to find out. Some of those women on your list, they're quite hyper ladies—I mean women."

Judi smiled and said, "Why'd you change your wording, Doctor?"

"My . . . wording?"

"You called them 'ladies' and then 'women.' "

He frowned. "If they were ladies, they wouldn't be accusing me."

"I see." Judi stared at the desktop as though she were reading confidential files. "Doctor," she asked, "why did you move to Lovell?"

He paused, then looked from her to Wilcock and back again. "Because I was needed here," he said.

She shuffled some papers as the silence congealed. She noticed that his hands were in constant motion, smoothing his pants, brushing back his hair, one finger tapping another.

"Come on now," he said confidentially. "Who paid you to do this to me?"

She began reading off the charges and asking his reaction to each. He denied two or three and then said he'd talked enough. "That's your right," she said, and slapped her notebook closed.

Marilyn sat in the darkness, feeling sick and cold. Hours had passed since John left to buy the plastic trash can. She'd tried to call him at the Coast to Coast, but the line had been busy.

At last her phone rang. "Marilyn," John said, "you're not gonna believe this."

"I know," she said.

They talked for a few minutes. In the background, she heard someone warning him that his time was up.

John said, "They're taking me to Basin."

"I'll call Aarestad," she said.

"Okay." She could tell that he was trying to sound calm. That was always his way. He hated to see her worry.

She drove the two blocks to the clinic. A big deputy sheriff blocked the door.

"I'm Mrs. Story," she said. "I need to look up my attorney's number."

"Sorry, ma'am. Nobody gets in till they finish searching. And that won't be till late."

She refused to cry. As she drove home to try North Dakota information for the lawyer's phone number, the streets seemed unusually dark. Someone had turned off her porch light. Then she realized that every house was black. A power failure! She thought, John's leaving the city limits right about now. It's a sign.

She couldn't reach Aarestad. Her fingers scratched and fumbled at the phone as she dialed Ken Buttermore's number for help. When the preacher answered, she was crying so hard she could hardly speak.

The Reverend Kenneth Buttermore, an energetic young man who usually prepared his sermons three or four days early, had been polishing up his remarks for the Wednesday night prayer meeting when Marilyn telephoned the disastrous news in wrenching, gasping gulps.

The preacher loved every member of his flock, and none more than the Storys. He'd been pastor of an old church in Maxwell, Nebraska, when the doctor had come back home on a visit, heard one of his spellbinding sermons, and convinced him to take over the Lovell Bible Church. It proved to be the perfect marriage of leader and flock. "I try not to preach the negatives," the handsome minister with the thick brown wavy hair liked to say. "I preach love." Personally, he found it a challenge to love some of the Mormons, but he kept those negative feelings to himself. Too many pastors had tilted against the Saints and been run out of town.

After he finished consoling Marilyn, Buttermore phoned a lawyer friend and was informed that Elder Story would have to remain in jail till a judge set bail in the morning. The preacher refused to believe that God would allow such an injustice to one of His most faithful children, but the lawyer sounded positive.

Buttermore began dialing other officials of the Bible Church. Joe Brown's advice made the most sense. "Tom Holm and I'll drive to Basin," the hospital manager said. "You get on your knees with the congregation and pray."

By 7 P.M., the little wooden church resounded with prayer. The pastor led his parishioners with elegiac fervor and tried to maintain a positive note.

Marilyn prayed by the phone. An autumn squall roared down the hill like a tornado. She thought, Another sign! She looked out the atrium window and saw leaves and trash and other debris flying by. Willow branches lashed the air like horsewhips. The storm moved off toward the Big Horns, leaving behind a charged silence. No more trick-or-treaters knocked. She couldn't help hoping that the Lord had driven Satan out. Now if only John would walk through the door. . . .

Friends set up a front-room vigil. Apparently the news of John's arrest had spread. A reporter from the *Chronicle* called for details. Marilyn's sister Marge arrived on an impromptu visit from Colorado and started to cry.

Just after 9 P.M., the phone rang. John said he was passing through Greybull, thirty miles south, on his way back home.

At ten o'clock, lights flickered against the living room walls and a car pulled into the driveway. Marilyn ran across the lawn and hugged him. He was grinning, but he looked tired. She'd seen eyes like that on cowboys just coming in from riding night herd.

He seemed calm enough as he told the story. She thought, John, where's your anger? Where's your outrage? But that just wasn't his way. On the way south, he told her, the police car had stopped at the South Big Horn Hospital and a technician had drawn a sample of his blood. When he'd protested, they'd shown a court order.

John said that Joe Brown had yelled at the jailer, "You can't keep this man! He performed surgery this morning. If anything happens to his patients, you'll be responsible." After ninety minutes, John had been freed.

Marilyn told him that the police were still searching the clinic. Someone had called and said they'd seen two deputies carrying out the Ritter table. "I hope they got a hernia," Marilyn said. John seemed too tired to care.

Ken Buttermore phoned. "Marilyn," he said in his hearty voice, "the Lord opened the jailhouse door. The Lord pulled the string on the judge's heart and stopped the mouth of the oppressors. I don't know how he did it, but this has to be the work of the Lord."

Marilyn agreed.

"At first I was really surprised," the preacher went on, "but then I thought, God shouldn't surprise me anymore."

The final call of the night came from their friends the Nebels, Rex and Cheryl, fellow Bible Church members. Rex had been an undersheriff and knew the law. Cheri was quick and bright. Both were deeply religious. "Almighty God takes care of his children," Cheri told Marilyn enthusiastically. "Rex tried to say that the blackout and the storm were coincidence, but I believe in a realm of darkness that battles against the true men of God. This time the men of God won."

She said that she'd talked to people who'd driven by the clinic. Police cars were lined up outside, and neighbors were standing around gawking. The storm had caused broken windows and roof damage on the hill, but the clinic was untouched. "Let's call it the Passover Wind," Cheri told Marilyn, "like when the angel of death came and killed everybody and passed over the Jews."

For once, John was first in bed. Marilyn hadn't seen him so exhausted since med school. What a blow it must have been to be thrown into a cell! The most decent, the most law-abiding, the most pious, gentle, *useful* man in Big Horn County! She wrote in her journal:

10 31 84 Halloween. This afternoon the police—local, sheriff's department, and a Casper policewoman—arrested John downtown like a common criminal. . . .

Caroline Shotwell heard about the arrest by jungle drum and almost cried with relief. For the first time in ten years, she slept through the night.

At eight the next morning, she gave a prayer of thanks. Then the phone rang and she learned that Story was back at work at his clinic.

Chief Wilcock's home phone rang in the middle of breakfast. "You're hurting the town, Dave," Herman Fink said in his quavery voice. "These witnesses might be talking to you now, but when they have to testify under oath, they'll all be gone."

"I hope not," Wilcock said. He waited for the mayor to tell him he was fired, but all he heard was a click.

Aletha Durtsche's morning mailbag overflowed with copies of the weekly Lovell *Chronicle*. This November 1 edition carried a three-paragraph story under the headline:

COUNTY MAN
CHARGED WITH
SEXUAL ASSAULT

She laid a copy on the counter of Ponderosa Floral. Every delivery day since her last confrontation with owner Beverly Moody, she'd called out a cheerful "Good morning!" It was intended as a mild irritant and obviously accepted in the same spirit.

This time the florist looked up from some roses and said, "Oh, you're still struttin' around, huh?"

"Yep," Aletha said.

As she was walking out the door, she heard, "You women are really sick!"

———

That same post-Halloween evening, Marilyn Story wrote in her journal:

We were called before the judge for a bond setting ($10,000). John is required to check in every day to the police department. Can't leave state without telling the judge or getting permission. Harassment! Ps 3 "O Lord, how my adversaries have increased!" Ps 5 "For it is thou who dost blest the righteous man, O Lord. Thou dost surround him with favor as with a shield." A civil suit has been filed by McArthur girls, 1.5 million.

BOOK THREE

Justice and
Denial

63

Terrill Tharp

I'll tell you why Story has so many backers. He used to counsel his patients. He asked questions like, "What positions do you and your husband use when you make love?" He knows a lot of personal secrets. People are scared to death he'll tell if they come out against him.

—Arden McArthur

THE PROSECUTOR felt as though he'd broken open a hornets' nest. Angry letters appeared in the Lovell *Chronicle*:

It's bad enough that some venomous women accuse Dr. Story of rape, but to have him convicted in your Policia station is showing complete disdain for the U.S. Constitution.

The way in which he was arrested showed he had already been convicted. Three squad cars surround his car on Main Street in Lovell when a phone call or one police officer would have been sufficient.

Is there a difference between a rifle butt search warrant served on a Jew's door in the dead of night or a pistol butt search warrant on a doctor's office. . . . I would recommend each of your officers be decorated with a yellow swastika.

In Tharp's small office in Greybull, eight miles up the road from the county seat town of Basin and thirty miles south of Lovell, the telephone clanged all day. Newsmen demanded interviews. Anonymous callers suggested that he resign before they booted him out. Bible Church members informed him that prayers for the rehabilitation of his soul were being said daily.

Cal Taggart, Lovell's most prominent citizen, made the situation worse by charging publicly that Dr. Story's accusers were "emotional" and "given to hearsay." The former state senator predicted from his carpeted office in the Taggart Building that "some of these women will find it difficult to get on the witness stand." To Tharp, the statement had the ring of an attempt at a self-fulfilling prophecy.

Intimidated witnesses phoned for reassurance. The victims had always been fearful about telling their stories in a courtroom, but now they also feared for their lives. One said her husband was pressuring her to drop out, and another called to say that she was no longer sure she'd been violated.

Tharp dictated a letter to the witnesses, suggesting that they avoid talking about the case, especially to the press and outside investigators. "If you are harassed or there is any overreaching on the part of anyone," he wrote, "please call this office. . . ."

No local judge would agree to handle the preliminary hearing. The Lovell justice of the peace declined because Story was his physician, and the Basin J.P. declined on the grounds that his mother had nothing but good to say about Story and "I thought it better to withdraw."

A justice from adjoining Washakie County finally agreed to preside in Basin on Tuesday, November 13, two weeks after the arrest. For the occasion, Story's lawyer subpoenaed every listed complainant. The women sat on stiff-backed wooden benches outside the courtroom, waiting to testify. They'd never been together as a group, and the place resounded with sobs and shrieks of surprise: "Not you, Wanda!" "Oh, gol, Mary, you too!" Sgt. Judi Cashel ran errands and tried to maintain morale.

As the day wore on, a few victims who'd been frightened by the latest uproar recovered their courage out of sheer annoyance at the six-hour wait. Mae Fischer advised her high school classmate Terri Timmons: "When we go in that courtroom, I want you to remember: we've got to do this because we're gonna be facing Satan himself." Aletha Durtsche knitted with red, raw hands; she'd come down with nervous eczema. Minda Brinkerhoff laughed and giggled and chattered about everything under the sun. Her sister Meg looked serene with her long straight silvery-white hair: the Madonna of the abused. The two oldest victims sat quietly by themselves. Julia Bradbury had been under the weather but refused special attention. Her friend, Emma Lu Meeks patted her hand.

As Terrill Tharp surveyed the group, he felt annoyed that they'd been subpoenaed at all. None of them took the stand. Most of the hearing was spent in the judge's chambers, discussing three newspapers' demands that the proceedings be open. Story's new lawyer, Wayne Aarestad, argued, "In weighing the balance between the defendant's right to a fair trial and the public's right to know, I believe caution must be exercised in favor of the defendant." The visiting J.P. agreed and kept the hearing closed.

At 7 P.M., Story was bound over on seventeen counts of sexual assault: three involving Minda Brinkerhoff and one each involving Meg Anderson, Juana Garcia, Aletha Durtsche, Julia Bradbury, Susan Moldowney, Hayla Farwell, Emma Lu Meeks, Dorothy Brinkerhoff, Wanda Hammond, Annella St. Thomas, Terri Timmons, Caroline Shotwell and her daughter Mae Fischer, and Emma Briseno McNeil. The offenses dated from 1967 to 1983 and the victims' ages ranged from fifteen to sixty-eight. If convicted on all counts, the defendant could be sentenced to life.

After Story pleaded innocent eight days later, his supporters turned up the heat. Dave Wilcock swore he was being followed, sometimes by a man, sometimes by a woman. Kenneth Buttermore suggested from the Bible Church pulpit that the victims were doing the devil's work. Two of Story's former nurses recanted information against him that they'd given police in earlier interviews; then one turned up on the defense witness list. Story backers like Jan Hillman, Beverly Moody, and Rex and Cheryl Nebel made a point of refusing to go through Wanda Hammond's checkout line at the Rose City Food Farm. Others sat outside in their cars and glared at her through the glass.

On November 21, three weeks after the arrest, the latest pro-Story endorsement created still more problems for the besieged prosecution forces. Lovell's former Methodist minister, Mark E. Christian, penned a Thanksgiving Eve epistle calling Story "a man of conviction about medicine and morality . . . a man of deep commitment to his family, his profession and his faith."

Christian wrote, "Although these types of things do not seem to impress many people these days let it be said that anyone who commits and invests a lifetime to build his family and medical practice in a small Wyoming community will never throw it all away by practicing cheap and disgusting behavior behind closed doors."

The young pastor's letter stressed common sense and fairness:

> I know that most of those ladies that have stepped forward believe that something wrong took place in Dr. Story's clinic. However, the only "wrong" thing which happened was that there was no third party present who might now substantiate Dr. Story's innocence. . . . Any man who could do the things of which Dr. Story is accused would be broken and long gone from the community by now were he guilty. . . .
>
> I am no fool for I would not come forth on such a delicate issue if I were not absolutely convinced of Dr. Story's innocence. I am not calling any of the ladies involved liars. What I am saying is that they are confused between fact and fiction and also are being used by some who know how to manipulate and mold fiction into supposed fact. . . .
>
> He is innocent no matter what the final verdict is.

One sentence caused Tharp more trouble than all the other pro-Story diatribes put together. "Already certain ladies are backing down with their testimonies," the pastor had written from his observation point in Billings, Montana, "upon realizing that they will have to tell those stories to objective, impartial audiences."

When the Lovell *Chronicle* gave the letter special play under the headline DEVASTATION OF LIVES MUST STOP, the prosecutor began receiving anguished calls from witnesses who were convinced they were being abandoned. At best, Tharp thought, the minister's statement demonstrated ignorance of the facts. At worst, it was an attempt to intimidate rape victims who'd already been intimidated enough. Once again he dashed off an advisory to the complainants:

> . . . Some letters to the editor appeared in the Lovell *Chronicle* which contained a great deal of misinformation. One letter states some victims are beginning to recant their stories. This is *not* true and I don't know where the writer of the letter obtained such information.

He reminded the women to make use of the psychological assistance available from Patricia Wiseman at the Big Horn Behavioral Health office in Lovell. "She is trained in counseling in family violence and sexual assault and may be able to help you put a perspective on these events." He added, "Once again, we are all in this together. The case against the defendant is a good one and will continue to be as long as everyone is resolved to see it through."

A few weeks later, another letter to the *Chronicle* lifted the county attorney's spirits, at least for the moment. Mrs. Bryce Wrigley of Delta Junction, Arkansas, wrote, "Mr. Christian says, I quote, 'I am no fool,' but from where I sit I would differ. Mr. Christian goes on to say he wants justice, yet says he really doesn't want justice because no matter what the verdict he won't accept it unless it goes his way. Now is that justice?"

Of course it's not justice, Tharp said to himself. But he'd long since realized that justice wasn't the issue for most Story supporters. The issue was denial—denial that a respected member of their community could commit such offenses, denial that the city fathers would allow his outrages to go on for twenty years, denial that so few victims had had the courage to come forward. Tharp saw that the issue wasn't only Story's guilt, but Lovell's.

It was clear enough that the doctor had a thorough knowledge of psychology and was bending the phenomenon of denial to his advantage. He'd focused his supporters' outrage with his own denial to the Bible Church congregation. From the beginning he'd refused to admit that he had a problem, nor would he volunteer to change his practices or seek treatment. Tharp knew from unhappy experience that such offenders were the hardest to convict. A guilty defendant who trumpeted his innocence could sway jurors by the eloquence of his denial—it happened all the time. A guilty defendant who lacked conscience or a sense of shame could pass lie-detector tests. Psychologists called such types sociopaths, psychopaths, antisocial personalities; the terms were synonymous. Tharp was fascinated to learn that Story was so impressed by Dr. Hervey Cleckley's *The Mask of Sanity,* the classical study of sociopathy, that he'd insisted that Marilyn and his two daughters read it.

Judi Cashel said she felt sorry for Story's supporters. She told the county attorney, "He's manipulating them the same way he manipulated the victims."

Tharp had to confess that his Lutheran compassion didn't extend quite that far.

64

David Wilcock

THE CHIEF was glad to see that Terry Tharp was throwing himself into the case, even to the point of conducting lengthy reinterviews. Most lawmen felt that prosecutors should stick to prosecuting, but this was no ordinary case. Together the chief and the county attorney reinterviewed Julia Bradbury, Wanda Hammond, Hayla Farwell and five or six others. Tharp said he didn't intend to put anyone on the stand who didn't know her story backward. "I hate surprises," he explained.

Additional complainants kept surfacing. "Write 'em up," Tharp told Wilcock. "If we lose on the first seventeen counts, we'll hit him with seventeen more." The number of bona fide victims soon passed fifty.

Some of the complainants spoke of strange phone calls and being followed. Confidential information was still being leaked. Wilcock wished he had the time and resources to mount a counterintelligence effort and throw some misguided supersleuth in jail, but he was already working twenty-hour days.

The lame private investigator named Dan Flores returned to Lovell, and the chief set about mining him for information. Flores said he was still nosing around on behalf of Meg and Minda. "I've done everything but go door to door," he claimed. He seemed tired, dispirited; Wilcock had heard that he was drinking heavily.

All during their talk in the P.I.'s room at the Super 8, Flores played loud guitar music by Villa Lobos and Albeniz on his cassette machine. Go ahead and distrust me, Wilcock said to himself. My pocket tape recorder's off, and I love music.

The two men fenced and parried but exchanged little solid information. Flores hinted that he'd accumulated the names of a hundred victims. The chief thought it seemed unlikely but not impossible.

When he reported the conversation, the county attorney showed his redheaded temper. He called the civil suit "stupid" and said it endangered the case. By suing for $1.5 million each, the McArthur daughters were opening themselves to charges of moneygrubbing. They'd sworn that any award would go to charity, but that wouldn't keep Wayne Aarestad from painting them as opportunists. As a defense lawyer, he would be remiss if he didn't.

Wilcock noticed that in all the reinterviewing, Tharp didn't question Meg or Minda. It was odd. It seemed as though they should be his key witnesses.

December blew in with icicle air that numbed the chief's nose and turned his forehead purple. He asked a gas station attendant to install the police cruiser's snow tires for a business trip to Utah. The trip, to poke into Story's past and interview a few potential witnesses, had been Terry Tharp's idea. "We can't afford to miss a bet," he'd told Wilcock.

Lately the county attorney had seemed pessimistic about the case. Wilcock remembered his warning that both their jobs were on the line. It no longer mattered much to the chief. He wasn't sure he wanted to stay in a part of the world where a man like John Story could abuse women for twenty-five years and you couldn't get Tchaikovsky on the radio.

He made the long cross-country drive to Ogden, where Story had spent his surgical residency, and encountered a medical cone of silence. Not one hospital staffer would discuss the Lovell doctor or make any records available. He was told to return with a subpoena.

He looked up the retired Dr. Thomas Croft and asked if he'd noticed anything special about Story before leaving Lovell in 1962. "Yes," the old Mormon said, "I noticed that he was very slow and thorough." Further questioning adduced a memory that Thelma Walker, one of Story's earliest nurses, had once complained about smelling semen in Story's office and found a used condom in the trash. "After that," Dr. Croft said with a nervous titter, "I was suspicious of Story. I expected somebody to shoot him."

Wilcock traced the Walker woman to Salt Lake City and phoned for an appointment. She became upset when he told her his mission, and he attached his pocket tape recorder to the phone:

Q   Did you ever smell semen in an examining room?
A   Yes. Well, I thought I did.
Q   Did you find a prophylactic containing semen in a garbage can in the examining room?
A   Yes, but he could have used it by himself, for his own gratification. Some men do those things, you know.
Q   Did you save the prophylactic?
A   I'm not going to talk to you any more.
Q   Thelma, you obviously know quite a bit. Why won't you help us?
A   I don't see why you want to drag all this up. Dr. Story never hurt anyone I know.
Q   What about the one-time patients, people who were just passing through?
A   I could tell you a lot about that, but I'm not going to.
Q   Thelma, I know you saved that prophylactic. What did you do with it?
A   I threw it away.
Q   How long did you keep it?
A   Not very long.
Q   Why did you talk to Dr. Croft? Weren't your suspicions bothering you?
A   I've said too much already. I'm not going to say any more. I've got to go.

When Wilcock returned to Lovell on December 5, he learned that the service station attendant who'd put on the snow tires had tipped off Mayor Fink about the trip. The chief wasn't surprised when he was summoned to the mayor's home and informed that Story wanted him fired. "Why are we involved?" Fink asked. "This isn't our case."

"Well, Herman, yes it is," Wilcock said. "If it isn't ours, whose is it?"

"The county attorney's."

"Yes, but it happened in Lovell and it's a Lovell case."

"Why'd you bring that Casper policewoman up here?"

"Because it happened here, Herman."

"Look at the money you're wasting on this!"

"Herman, so far the county's picked up almost all the tab. You paid for some travel expenses. Before this is over, the town of Lovell is gonna want to say that it paid some of the expenses."

The mayor glared. Wilcock thought, Here comes the ax. He's just been reelected and he's got to reappoint me or name a new chief.

Fink asked, "Do you know what this is doing to the town?"

Wilcock parried, "Do you know what it'll do to the town if we don't take action?"

The mayor looked tired. It hadn't been long since he'd undergone bypass surgery. He mumbled, "Dr. Story didn't do these things, Dave. It's plumb impossible. You don't know him like I do."

"Herman, I'm sorry," Wilcock said softly, "but I think I know him better."

He stood up to leave. "Wait a minute, Dave," the old man said. "Will you—will you be my police chief again?"

Wilcock felt ashamed that he'd talked so sharply. "Thanks," he said. "Let me think about it."

By mid-January the leaks had become serious. Before Wilcock reached for his handkerchief, the Story forces knew he would blow his nose. His suspicions focused on the town treasurer's office. For security reasons he'd held back the receipts from his Utah trip, but now he needed the reimbursement.

Fifteen minutes after he turned in the papers, he watched as the clerk LaVera Hillman headed up the hill toward Story's home. He admonished himself for not catching on earlier. His good friend LaVera and her daughter Jan had been outspoken Story supporters from the beginning. He thought of calling Terry Tharp and discussing a felony charge of obstruction of justice, but he couldn't bring himself to such drastic action against the sweet southern lady who still said "y'all." He would just have to be more careful.

He drove up to Billings and within an hour had to shake a persistent green Cadillac. Later he spotted the same car in a parking lot and checked it out with the Billings P.D.

"That sounds like Zack Belcher," a detective told him. Zack and Mary Belcher operated Silver Run Productions, a detective agency in Red Lodge, Montana. They were highly regarded and didn't come cheap.

Wilcock reported the incident to Terry Tharp. When the prosecutor complained to Wayne Aarestad, the defense lawyer explained that Story was considering a conspiracy defense and therefore the surveillances were proper.

"They think you're a conspirator, Dave," Tharp warned on the phone.

Wilcock thought, In eleven years of police work, that's one name I haven't been called.

65

Marilyn Story

WHAT she would have given for John's strength of character! Watching him treat the loyal patients who came in for pelvics, she realized again what an uncommon man she'd married. He was a marvel of consistency in what he did, how he felt, how he acted and reacted. He didn't sulk or brood, and he wasted no time on worry. Emotionally, the two of them were almost opposites. Around Thanksgiving, her doubting soul had convinced her that he was going to prison. "Have been filled with horrible fears . . ." she'd written in her journal. "Can't seem to control my thoughts or emotions. Can't pray—don't know what to ask. . . ."

Both Storys remained high on the ex-hippie Wayne Aarestad, even though his asking fee had risen with the filing of criminal charges. When the lawyer came to dinner, he talked about the power of the Holy Spirit. He explained that he'd been raised as a member of the Two by Twos, a sect that derived its name from its practice of sending out evangelical teams in twos, after Matthew 11:2. The "Two by Twos" were such hardheaded fundamentalists that the fifteen-year-old North Dakota boy had quit in disgust. "I didn't hand my life back over to the Lord till three or four years ago," he confessed to the Storys. "Christ is everything to me now." He urged John to find a prayer partner and meet with him on a regular basis—"starting *tomorrow!*" as Marilyn noted in her journal.

She wasn't surprised when John refused. He honored God in his own way. Once or twice he reminded the lawyer that God loved them all, and God's will would prevail. To Marilyn, it sounded like his old Christian fatalism again. The most dire prospects left him unperturbed. God is in charge, he would say. God knows exactly what He's doing.

One morning at five she answered the phone to a soft male voice saying "You are going to die." Twenty minutes later John took the same message, mumbled something, and went back to sleep, cloaked and protected by God.

She couldn't keep up with the legalities—postponements, pretrial motions couched in Latin phrases, tedious depositions. One gloomy day she wrote, "Lord . . . help us to be braced for this new shock wave." A few days later, her mood improved and she wrote, "We have been having some wonderful times of fellowship with Wayne. Have gone on several mountain outings with him. He is confident about the outcome. . . ."

When the McArthur girls had filed their $3-million civil suit, both John and Wayne had surprised her by seeming pleased. "That's the biggest mistake they could have made," the lawyer said at the time.

R. Scott Kath of Powell had been retained to hit Meg and Minda with a $10-million countersuit and also to assist in the criminal trial. The Wyoming newspapers were full of news about the legal maneuvering, and soon a new batch of pro-Story letters and ads began to appear. A woman from Vashon Island, Washington, wrote to the *Chronicle*: "Why are these people doing this sick, unspeakable horror to a man like Dr. Story? This week my question has been answered. We get down to the nitty gritty . . . the almighty dollar."

Wayne Aarestad pointed out another benefit of the poorly timed lawsuit. In criminal proceedings, there were strict limits on how deeply he could delve into the complainants' personal lives, but by bringing a civil suit, Meg and Minda had made their lives fair game. They could be questioned till their teeth rattled.

The day Meg was deposed John and Wayne returned from the downtown session wearing grins, and when Marilyn read the transcript, she saw why. Meg had been forced to admit that a relative had made her feel his penis—and not just once. Wayne had made her recite a shameful inventory: five incidents of fornication during a two-year relationship with a man in Logan, Utah, three more in a three-month relationship that followed, three more in a third relationship that lasted a year, and a whole year of premarital intimacy with Dan Anderson. This was the paragon who claimed that John made a "dark ugly feeling" come over her!

Soon another accuser was stripped to the bone, this time in the latest psychological profile by John's old friend Dr. Russ Blomdahl. Marilyn thought, How fascinating to read the truth about Aletha at last! She'd never understood why the mail carrier had been willing to air so much of her own dirty linen just to ruin a fine man. But Russ's analysis made it all so simple—she'd been in love with John!

Of course Russ hadn't been able to interview the Durtsche woman in person, but he'd studied the transcript of an earlier deposition plus additional records that Marilyn had mailed from the clinic. His report noted that Aletha had been devastated by sexual guilt since childhood and felt "expressions of infatuation for Dr. Story [as] described in her recollections of baking bread and taking it to him; painting a picture for him; and bringing the mail into his office. . . ."

In his analysis, Russ considered the question of whether Aletha might have gone to John's office on that fateful February day "to relieve the unconscious desire to engage in sexual fantasy again." When John didn't give her the comfort she sought, Russ explained, Aletha became angry.

The report concluded that Aletha had been caught up in the mass hysteria and "collective obsessions" of certain Lovell women and allowed her fantasies about Dr. Story to become real in her own mind. Nothing that she said could be considered "in accordance with reality or creditable."

Marilyn saw the hand of God in the timing of Russ's report, as she'd seen it in the fortuitous exposure of Meg Anderson's sex life. Just a few weeks before the Durtsche analysis arrived, the Reverend Buttermore had suggested that each parishioner select one of the accusers as a personal special project, pray for her and fast for her, and ask God to keep her from hurting John. Marilyn had selected Aletha.

Two weeks before the trial, there was more good news for her journal: ". . . We found out (via the news media!) that six women accusers have been dropped from the case! The prosecuting attorney seemed to state that they would be damaging to his case. We are praising God, for his hand is beginning to move."

66

Terrill Tharp

"WE HAVE TO GO to trial with as clean a profile as possible," the county attorney explained in his monastic, undersized office. "The McArthurs were just too damn big a problem."

"Where'd we be without the McArthurs?" a baffled-looking Dave Wilcock asked.

"Nowhere. But that's not the point."

In the pretrial maneuvering, the defense strategy had come all too clear to the young prosecutor. Story's private detectives were putting the finishing touches on a highly effective smear campaign. The McArthurs would be depicted as architects of a conspiracy to destroy an elder of a rival church. Studies by a friendly psychologist would show that Meg and Minda had lusted for their family doctor. Meg's modest sex life would be picked over. Minda would be characterized as an immoral flake, and both sisters would be forced to admit they'd been censured by their church. Arden, matriarchal leader of her ward as president of the Relief Society, would be painted as a fanatical schemer who dreamed up the conspiracy after her idol refused to convert.

"I could've handled all that bullshit," Tharp told the police chief, waving his long saxophonist's fingers, "but then Meg and Minda had to

309

go off the reservation and file their damn three-million-dollar suit. So we had no choice, Dave."

The prosecutor had also dropped three or four other counts because the complaints lacked essential elements. "The weaker cases drag down the strong," he explained to Wilcock. "Defense attorneys club you to death with the weak ones. I did it myself when I was a public defender."

The chief seemed to understand.

"Dave, I'll tell ya one thing," Tharp reassured him. "We're not gonna let the bastard walk."

He was surprised when Wilcock said he intended to quit his job, no matter how the case came out. "Judy and I are moving over near Seattle," he said.

Tharp said to himself, You poor guy, you look stressed out. No wonder. He'd worked this case night and day for three months.

"You'll hang in till trial, won't you, Dave?" Tharp asked.

"Try and get rid of me."

Tharp said he hated to see Dave go, and meant it. Back-of-beyond towns like Lovell didn't often see his like.

The county attorney felt bad when he read that Minda had called the dismissals "a slap in the face." She was quoted in the Casper *Star-Tribune,* "I don't know where the justice is. . . . I thought it was the people's case. I felt like I have been led on. It took me a long time to decide to go through with this and now he treats it like what happened to me is nothing."

He wished he could call her and explain the dynamics of criminal prosecutions, but that would have to wait. The McArthur women were the real heroines; people would find out soon enough. His spirits improved when he read a few inches deeper in the same article:

> Aarestad has been reluctant to discuss Story's case prior to this week. But Thursday he blasted Tharp, the alleged victims, the investigation of the case, and what he perceives as a lack of communication between his office and the prosecution. . . .
>
> The Story case is "Wyoming's version" of the widely publicized Jordan, Minn., child abuse and sexual assault case, Aarestad said.
>
> In Minnesota, he noted, "the prosecution jumped the gun and through a complete and total investigative failure, began premature prosecutions of innocent people."
>
> In Story's case, "the decision to prosecute was made and then the

real investigation began," the lawyer said. "If this case had been properly investigated . . . then none of this would have occurred."

The allegations against his client "are unsupported by any evidence," Aarestad said.

"All you have is the unsworn, bold assertions of the ladies . . . who,
in many respects, pulled the wool over the eyes of the prosecutor and
the investigators. They are now beginning to realize they don't have a
case."

Tharp was pleased to see that he'd struck a raw nerve.

As the April, 1985, trial date approached, he got word of the new
prayer schedule at Story's Bible Church. Vigils were being held from 6
P.M. till dawn. Sometimes Reverend Buttermore presided, sometimes
elders like Tom Holm and Joe Brown. They prayed for Dr. Story, for
his wife, for the judge and jurors. They even prayed for the county
attorney. Tharp told his wife, "I'll take all the help I can get."

The victims kept phoning for reassurance. He had no choice but to
hear them out. Now that he'd narrowed the list, every witness was
crucial.

Aletha Durtsche told him, "I delivered to Reverend Buttermore's
house, and his wife said, 'Aletha, I want you to know that in spite of
everything, we still love you. I want you to know that you're welcome in
our home at any time.' I said, 'Well, thank you. I appreciate that.' But
good heck, she's never welcomed me in her home before! Why now,
Terry? It makes me feel so guilty, like I'm doing some terrible thing to
Dr. Story and his wife."

"You're not guilty, Aletha," Tharp reminded her. "That's how
they'd like you to feel. Story did this to himself."

Aletha thanked him and said she would try to feel better.

The reclusive Hayla Farwell phoned. As a lifelong Lutheran, she
was a key witness, along with the Presbyterian Julia Bradbury and the
Catholic Emma Briseno McNeil. All the other complainants were Mormons and could be used by the defense to further the claim of religious
conspiracy.

"I'm afraid to go downtown," the Farwell woman complained.
"People glare at me. I'm the type that likes people to like me." She had
a childlike voice, and Tharp remembered hearing something to the
effect that she'd been gassed and suffered mild brain damage years ago.

"Don't worry, Miz Farwell," he assured her in his farm-boy drawl.
"Everyone'll like you after the trial."

Wanda Hammond came to his office for a pretrial interview and referred to Story's "thing."

"You mean 'penis'?" Tharp asked.

"Uh . . . yes." She said she wouldn't be able to use that word in court. "I didn't know what it was called till this case came up."

Tharp suggested that the round little woman intensify her counseling at the behavioral clinic in Lovell. Patricia Wiseman and Judi Cashel had been trying to raise the consciousness of the victims, but some seemed as backward as ever. A few still hadn't told their husbands.

After several counseling sessions, seventy-six-year-old Emma Lu Meeks confessed to Tharp and Dave Wilcock that she'd been holding back vital information. "I saw Dr. Story's, uh—his *penis*," she said. "I couldn't say that word before." When the chief started to leave the room, the pioneer woman said, "You sit back down and listen, David Wilcock! I've got to practice saying it. . . ."

Terri Lee Timmons called from Powell, so upset that Tharp could hardly understand her. He urged her to talk to a counselor. He thought, She was fifteen when Story raped her and he damn near ruined her life; I've got to get her before the jury. But Terri had sounded ready to quit.

67

Terri Lee Timmons

SHE'D HAD fits of despair since she was seven, but never like this. She couldn't stop crying. Antidepressants only aggravated her ulcer. For three months she'd walked around in a daze, an icy pain in her throat from holding back tears. Her cat ate more than she did. Terri was thirty-two, but her gaunt body made her look like an anorexic child in a gypsy-shag wig.

Loyd had been out of work for almost a year now, ever since the Lord had moved him to give up his job in Denver and take his family back to Powell. They were crammed into her parents' one-story house and rubbing one another raw. Wyoming winters were so depressing. She picked her way around the snowbanks and skidded on dirty ice. Chinook winds roared down from the Rockies, pruned the old trees and made the branches clack against the house like skeleton bones. The kids went from virus to virus. Sometimes little Trevor couldn't catch his breath; his chronic bronchitis seemed to be deepening into asthma. She rocked him for hours, their tears mingling. She seldom slept past 2 or 3 A.M. She ached all over, and no doctor could help.

Her Celestial Father and her earthly husband were all that kept her from killing herself. "You're worried about that trial," Loyd told her. "Why don't you think of it as the end of eighteen bad years? This'll settle things once and for all."

Loyd's priesthood blessings were such a comfort that it was hard to imagine he was a convert. An elder by now, he kept his own sacred oil in the refrigerator. She would kneel in front of him while he anointed the crown of her head. "Terri Lee Timmons," he would say in his tender voice, "by the power of the Holy Melchizedek Priesthood and in the name of Jesus Christ, I lay my hands upon your head and anoint you with this oil that has been consecrated and dedicated for the healing of the sick in the household of faith. In the name of Jesus Christ, Amen."

He would lift his hands, then return them to her head and say, "Terri Lee Timmons . . . I seal this anointing upon you and give you a blessing." At the end he would say, "And this blessing you will know comes from your Heavenly Father."

After her tearful telephone conversation with the county attorney, she rushed to her bishop for counseling. A few nights later she summoned the strength to drive the icy road into Lovell for a group therapy session with some of the other witnesses. A speaker from the State Rape Crisis Center reminded them of their rights as women. They were urged to stop turning John Story's crimes in against themselves; they were *his* filthy acts and his alone. The women were no more responsible than the victims of a rattlesnake or a tornado.

It felt good to visit with the other women and learn that the same questions were tormenting them, but it was painful to see how easily they lost control, to watch their hands tremble as they spoke, to get a preview of how dumbstruck they would be on the witness stand . . . herself included.

It took her three weeks to write about the meeting. Her journal had always read like latter-day Dickens: sick children, family problems, her dyslectic brother's death in a car crash, personal guilts, unpaid bills, unemployment payments running out, aches, pains, depressions, tears. Now she added another chapter:

It was a good evening. I expressed the fear that Story's followers might hurt me and my family, and I am afraid that they will take one of my kids. This really bothered me, so I talked to Taya's teacher at school about it. She talked to the principal—they decided not to tell the other teachers and that I should talk to Taya about what she needed to do to stay safe. So I did, and it upset her.

Wed and thurs nights the 30th and 31st she did not sleep a wink. Scared me to death. She had been complaining of headaches and stomachaches for weeks. . . . I took her to the doctor. He checked her over, and said she is a victim of "stress." I rubbed her back and neck the next few nights and made sure she was asleep before I went to bed. . . .

Counseling brought more insights. She discovered that behind her depression lay a blind rage against men, especially the handsome genius who'd dumped her for another woman after a three-year courtship. A few weeks before the trial, she wrote rapidly and with her usual disregard for spelling:

> *Loyd took me to dinner at the church for Prime Rib. That night and for two more nights I had terrible nightmares again. I was sick for three days. The trial will probably affect me worse than that. . . .*
>
> *I found I was full of very bad feelings for ——— again. I found them from very deep inside of me and they were very strong feelings. I have been in agony for days now again. Why can't this end. I want all these bad feelings against him resolved. I found I wasn't angry with him because he married someone else, but because of the dishonest decietful munipulative way he treated me and used me throughout our whole relationship. The pain from all these feelings was very hard to bear.*
>
> *The Lord blessed me by helping me understand that there wasn't anything wrong with me, it was ——— that had the problem and probably still does. I have felt a lot better about it since then.*
>
> *I am basicly dealing with my nerves on this Story trial in two weeks. I feel like I want to throw up a lot of the time. The stress and headaches are difficult to get through sometimes. Then other times I feel like I want to stand on a chair and shout, "By damn Satan, your not going to beat me!" The strenght will come, I know it will. . . .*

She kept telling herself, "I'm sick and tired of men taking advantage of me." She set about improving her self-image. The mirror was no help. At ninety-nine pounds, she looked slack-skinned, half alive. The last time she'd gone to Story, she'd been a healthy, chunky fifteen-year-old with well-defined muscles and curves.

Spring came and her counseling continued. She learned how to say words like "intercourse" without turning red, and how to breathe on the witness stand, and how to listen carefully to each question before answering. Over and over she was reminded that she was as good as any man in the courtroom, including the judge, and there was no need to tremble in their august presence.

She enrolled in a weight-lifting course to build herself up for the ordeal. By the time the last patch of snowmelt disappeared, she felt as though Heavenly Father was making her into a different woman.

68

The Trial

THE SQUARISH FORM of the Big Horn County Building bulked large among Basin's billowing trees and frame houses and the small shops and stores that ran for less than a mile along a widened stretch of the two-lane Wyoming Highway 16. The town had been called Basin City back in the days when the word "deadline" alluded to the fate of any local sheepman who crossed into cow country. Basin hadn't grown much through the years. Its population was still barely 1,400.

The County Building was the tallest structure in sight. Its walls were of light brown brick and its roof of terra cotta. The architect had created his own version of a Potemkin front: four handsome Ionic pillars tinted in the faintest pink repeating a shade found on cliffs to the east. Heavy white doors opened on a vestibule housing a 35-cent pop machine. A small lobby served several public offices staffed by women in skirts and white blouses and men in Pendleton shirts and lariat ties with pointed metal tips. A broad staircase led up to a movie-set courtroom carved in rich dark woods. A narrower staircase led to rabbit-warren offices on the top floor.

The comfortable old building was set back from the street by a broad reach of lawn and shaded by a forty-foot weeping birch and two thick spruces in deepest blue-green. An angled parking area in front accommodated five or six cars and was seldom full. Across C Street, Bernadine's fabric shop and Odds 'n' Ends Recycle flanked a fading sign, BASIN REPUBLICAN-RUSTLER. Big Horn County still had its share of rustlers and more than its share of Republicans, but the newspaper had long since gone to its rest.

The trial of John Huntington Story, M.D., opened on the first day of Holy Week, a coincidence which wasn't lost on the eighty-five members of the Lovell Bible Church. District Judge Gary Hartman, a quiet man with a reputation for toughness, had cleared his calendar for the month.

In one of many pretrial rulings, the white-haired judge had banned any mention of the Medical Board hearings and placed strict limits on testimony of the law officers involved, since almost everything they knew was hearsay. The preliminary rulings were victories for Story and Wayne Aarestad; they meant that the verdict would turn almost entirely on the testimony of the complainants.

Prosecutor Terry Tharp took his preliminary losses and waited. Except for Aletha Durtsche, none of the listed victims had ever appeared against Story. He hoped that their testimony would be fresh and convincing. And if it wasn't—well, he still had his sax and his law degree. He could start over. Somewhere.

In the tedium of jury selection, the defense looked for impressionable females and the prosecution for hard-nosed married men. Unacceptable candidates were sent home by the carload. The first reject, John Gams, turned out to be a Story patient. So did several others. All were excused, as were several of Story's fellow churchmen. Some members of the venire were dropped after confessing to fixed opinions. Mona Lee Averett admitted that she was convinced of Story's guilt. A dubious Nancy Moore said, "I don't know how this could happen to any woman and not know." Mrs. John Pru said she lived across the street from the accused and believed that he was innocent "because of his lifestyle." Mrs. Burke, a nursing home volunteer, admitted that "we maintain loyalty to the doctors." A rancher named Hyatt said, "Well, to be right truthful . . . anytime a doctor steps into a room with a patient without an accompanying nurse he is asking for trouble." Mrs. Preis was excused when she explained that she was hard of hearing. A farmer explained that he was in the middle of planting; another was calving, a third lambing. One woman was eight months pregnant and another was "against men right now." Prospective juror No. 93 nodded off during the proceedings. No. 98 didn't seem to understand the questions. All were excused. Eleven women and three men survived. Two would serve as alternates.

Both sides made spare opening statements. Tharp told the jurors that Story was charged with six counts of forcible rape and three of sexual assault spanning the years 1967 to 1983. He listed his witnesses, synopsized what each would say, and was back in his seat in twenty minutes.

Aarestad spoke for half as long and came off as warm and friendly, his deep growly voice somehow easier on the ear than the intense young prosecutor's stressed treble. "I suppose you have figured out by now that I am Wayne Aarestad, one of Dr. Story's attorneys in this case," he opened. "And I don't know if congratulations are in order for being selected to this case."

He reminded the attentive jurors that twenty-seven years back, Lovell had lost its physician and Dr. Story "responded to that call."

"The evidence will show that he is a dedicated physician," Aarestad continued in his pleasing North Dakota drawl, "and we will further show that in some respects he was a little bit out of time sequence in that he almost practiced nineteenth-century form of medicine in the twentieth century. . . . He was extremely caring and considerate and kind to his patients. He did devote a lot of time to them. . . . Oftentimes he acted as counselor, somebody who offered an ear and listened to many, many problems.

"Many of these complaining witnesses that Mr. Tharp has indicated will testify are those who were most demanding upon Dr. Story in respect to utilizing his services that I consider extramedical. He was a friend to them. The evidence will show that many of them brought cookies to him and painted pictures of him, his family."

The lawyer closed with a palms-up gesture toward his client. "Dr. Story is going to testify. He *wants* to testify. This is his moment of truth. This is his ability finally to tell his side of the story." There was no mention of a conspiracy defense.

David Wilcock looked less rumpled than usual as he took the stand, followed by the strawberry blond Judi Cashel in her newest uniform and polished shoes. The two law officers outlined their qualifications, told how they'd located the victims and investigated the case, identified some of the state's exhibits, and laid the groundwork for the complainants' testimony. Aarestad's cross-examination was respectful and brief.

Rand Flory, a young obstetrician and gynecologist from the Yellowstone gateway town of Cody, took the stand and immediately brought Aarestad to his feet. At a bench conference, the blond defense lawyer renewed his motion to ban any testimony to the effect that Dr. Story's Ritter table "is one that is not found generally in a physician's office" and any testimony about Dr. Flory's personal preferences concerning nurses in the examining room. The judge denied the motion.

After Flory testified that he'd examined the medical records of the complainants, Tharp elicited a description of standard pelvic exam techniques. Metal speculums, the young gynecologist said, should be warmed because "women jump if they are not heated." The drape should be pushed down between the knees "so she can see me while I am working." The speculum portion of the exam should take two or three minutes. The bimanual exam, involving the use of the fingers, should be equally brief: "Find the cervix, find the uterus, go off to one side, go off to the other side and find both of the ovaries, and then it is over." The whole procedure, he said, should take about five minutes. The examiner's probing fingers, once inserted, should be left in place, not pushed in and out. There was no need to stand so close that trousers or coat brushed against the patient. And pelvic exams normally should not be given for ailments unrelated to the genital regions.

The county attorney pointed to the state's largest exhibit, sitting off to one side and topped by a mysteriously shrouded shape. "Have you ever seen a table like that before, Doctor?" he asked.

"Yes, sir," Dr. Flory answered. "We have one like this in our emergency room, or one very similar to it."

"Have you ever seen a table like that in a doctor's office?"

"I have not seen one in a doctor's office, but I haven't visited that many offices."

Tharp asked him to remove the sheet atop the table. The audience tittered as a skeleton came into view. "Now we didn't choose this to be funny," the prosecutor said brusquely. "There is a reason for it."

He asked Flory to place the skeleton in a "lithotomy position" and demonstrate some of the points he'd mentioned. The bones clicked in their wire armature as the young gynecologist moved the exhibit around.

Back on the witness stand, Flory testified that the only medical instrument that resembled a penis was a "vaginal dilater," for women who were too narrowly built for normal intercourse. The condition was called vaginismus, he said, and he'd noticed no references to it on the medical charts of the complaining witnesses.

He was asked if a woman could be sexually assaulted while lying on a Ritter table.

"Definitely," he answered.

In cross-examination, Wayne Aarestad underlined that the young doctor had graduated from medical school only eight years before, and asked, "Are you here today testifying that you have never conducted a pelvic exam without a third person in the examining room?"

"That's correct," Flory answered.

Q   Do you believe that whether or not a third person is in the examination room should be the option of the patient as well as the physician?

A   I personally do not believe that, no. The third person in there is there as much for my protection as they are for the patient's protection. . . .

69

Aletha Durtsche

AS SHE ENTERED the courtroom at 9:30 Thursday morning, the second day of testimony, the blond mail carrier felt an invisible barrier in place. The florist Beverly Moody and other Story supporters sat on the right side. On the left were a few friends and relatives of the victims.

Aletha was shaky but determined. Just a few days before, a girl friend had told her how Story had given her a pelvic and made her bleed when she was ten years old. My word, Aletha thought, he was deflowering little kids! She tried to keep that conversation in mind as she took the witness stand.

She recited her name and address in the same clear voice she used to direct the choir. Just when she was beginning to feel relaxed, she looked down at the table and saw Dr. Story taking notes on a long yellow pad. She thought, All those years I trusted you and we were friends, and now you won't even look at me.

The prosecutor said, "Calling your attention to the twelfth day of February, 1983, do you recall that day?"

She'd never been able to talk about her rape without crying. She still couldn't believe that it happened on her birthday. She opened her mouth to answer but couldn't talk. The courtroom swam out of focus through her designer glasses. She turned to the judge and saw a black blob. The next thing she knew, the lawyers were huddled around the judge, talking low. The one named Aarestad was saying something about prejudicing the jury. When they returned to their places, Tharp asked, "Are you able to go on, Mrs. Durtsche?"

She looked down at Judi Cashel, smiling from her seat directly in line with the witness stand. All the victims had been told to look to the red-headed cop for support. "Y-yes," Aletha said.

The judge leaned over and said, "Any time that you feel you would like a recess to regain your composure, just let me know." His voice was gentle, compassionate. She felt protected by his robes.

"Okay," she said.

A few questions later, she remembered something Dave Wilcock had told her a few days before. *They'll try to break you, Aletha. You'll be the first victim to testify, and they've got to make a quick impression. Don't let 'em use you that way. . . .* She thought. My lands, the bad guys haven't even started questioning me and I'm bawling. Well, it won't happen again.

She tried to tell her story calmly. Aarestad kept making objections, and she told herself to sit quietly until the judge ruled on each one. Tharp asked why she hadn't jumped up from the examining table after Story had abused her. "I didn't know what to do," she said, and the tears came again.

"Can you go on," the prosecutor asked, "or would you like a recess, Mrs. Durtsche?"

She sniffed and said, "I can go on."

She described what happened after she felt Story's hips shoving against her bare bottom. "I looked down at his face and he just stood there looking at me, and I knew he knew what I knew."

She felt herself slipping away again. Aarestad jumped up and said, "Your Honor, I am going to ask that we take a break at this point."

Tharp said, "Can you go on, Mrs. Durtsche?"

"Yes, I can."

The judge said, "Let's see if we can finish."

They were into the worst of it now. She testified in gasps and gulps as she stared at Judi Cashel through tears.

"Mrs. Durtsche," Tharp asked, "why, if you knew this was his penis being inserted in you, why didn't you kick him?"

Her answer was barely louder than a whisper. "I—I didn't know what to do. I was . . . afraid."

Aarestad jumped up again, his forehead pink under a wisp of blond hair. "Your Honor," he said, "I can't even understand the testimony of the witness. I object to continuing under these circumstances."

The judge declared a five-minute recess.

Judi held Aletha's hand in the hall and told her the worst was over. When court reconvened, the lawyers surrounded the judge again, and she heard both Aarestad and Tharp use the word "mistrial." She thought, Story will go free and it'll be my fault. . . .

Tharp resumed his questioning. She told about having to take her children back to Story because no other doctor was available, and telling Mike about the rape, and being interviewed by Chief Wilcock and Judi. Aarestad kept objecting and the judge kept overruling him.

There was another long conference at the bench as the defense lawyer accused Terry Tharp of trying to end her testimony "on a high emotional note." Once again Judge Hartman uttered the word "overruled."

Aletha said a silent prayer that she would hold up under cross-examination and not cause a mistrial. It was astonishing how quickly Story's lawyer came to the hardest question of all:

Q How old are you today, Mrs. Durtsche?
A Thirty-two.
Q So it would have been your thirtieth birthday February 12, 1983?
A Yes.

She thought, If I can get through that, I can get through the rest. But a few minutes later he began asking her about Mike's infidelity and the time she swallowed the aspirins. Tharp objected and there was another bench conference, with Aarestad doing most of the talking. She heard the judge say that he could ask about her relationship with Dr. Story, but not about any suicide attempts.

She kept her composure while she told about the incident in 1971 when she thought Story might have abused her and how she'd continued seeing him until her final visit on her birthday in 1983. She admitted that she'd baked him a loaf of bread and painted a picture for his office. Aarestad bore down:

Q Now has Dr. Story at any time ever restrained you in any fashion on an examination table?

A No.

Q Never tied your feet to the stirrups or anything?

A No.

Q . . . Did he have a weapon, a knife or any type of a device that caused you to be concerned about danger to your life?

A I don't know.

Q What did you think he was going to do to you? Kill you?

A I thought he might.

Q Did he say he was going to?

A No.

Q On what do you base your belief that he was going to kill you?

A If I came up off that table and asked him what he thought he was doing, I was afraid that if caught in a situation and knowing that he was caught, he might do that.

Q So you were just speculating at that time as to what might happen?

A Yes.

The lawyer ran her through minute details of the birthday assault. He showed her a diagram and asked her to point out where everything happened. The questions came like slaps and she didn't always think before she answered.

Q When did you hear this zipper?

A After he took his penis out.

Q You never saw his penis though, did you?

A No.

Q So did you ever hear the zipper prior to having this alleged penis inserted in you?

A No. He had the water running.

Heavy construction equipment banged and chugged outside the courtroom window, and the noise added to her distraction. No detail seemed to escape Aarestad's interest.

Q Now when Dr. Story comes back from the sink after leaving the speculum in it, what position between your legs is he in before he turns around?

A He is right—he is probably, oh, he is not real close when he turns around.

Q Would it be generally between the area of your knees and your ankles or in closer than between your knees and your thighs?

A More between my knees and my ankles.

Q So he would still be a foot or so away from your vagina?

A Yes.

Q   And now he is facing you?
A   Yes.
Q   As he stands there.
A   Yes. . . .
Q   Was your buttocks pretty close to the edge of the table?
A   When he set the table that day he had it—
Q   Yes or no?
A   Yes.
Q   Are your suspicions aroused yet that something improper is occurring?
A   Yes.
Q   Were you having any conversation with him?
A   No.
Q   Were you watching him over the top of the drape?
A   No.
Q   You were looking at the ceiling?
A   Yes.
Q   Do you remember what you were thinking about?
A   "I hope this is over quick."
Q   . . . Did you feel any poking sensation around your thighs?
A   No.
Q   Any type of hard object?
A   No.
Q   Was he looking down at you?
A   I didn't notice.
Q   Don't know what he was doing?
A   I didn't look at his face then.
Q   Okay. Then you feel something entering your vagina?
A   Yes.
Q   Describe that object to me.
A   It felt like a penis.
Q   And that conclusion is based upon your prior sexual experience, is it not?
A   Yes.
Q   Basically I assume that you are saying that it felt like your husband's
penis?
A   Yes.
Q   Was it a sudden entry, a slow entry?
A   Very slow.
Q   . . . You just remember it going in?
A   Yes.
Q   Slowly?
A   Yes.
Q   And coming out slowly?
A   Yes.
Q   You didn't ask him what he thought he was doing?
A   No.

Q   You just lay there?
A   Yes.
Q   Weren't you in a sense of outrage to think that someone would have the audacity to violate your person like that?
A   I was hurt.
Q   Offended?
A   Yes.
Q   Not angry?
A   Not at that moment. . . .

She thought, This is how they tear you down. Well, it won't happen to me. When he asked, "Do you want to take a break?" she proudly answered "No."

After lunch Tharp asked more questions, then passed her back to the defense. At last she heard the judge say, "You may step down, Mrs. Durtsche." She'd been on the stand for three hours.

70

Judi Cashel

ALETHA came reeling into the hall, and Judi steered her to a wooden bench for first aid. "Hey, it's over!" she said. "You did a good job. See, I told you we'd make it."

"I said some stupid things," Aletha said. She cried as she listed her mistakes.

"No, no!" Judi interrupted, wagging a finger. "You did fine, Aletha."

"I shouldn't have cried."

"You were believable. You sounded like what you are. We didn't want you to sound like a tape recording."

They walked downstairs and passed Aletha's husband Mike, on his way up to testify. He looked undaunted.

In the basement sequestering room, a deputy sheriff guarded the rest of the scheduled witnesses. "You're next, Emma Lu," Judi said.

"I'm ready," the wrinkled little woman said.

Judi thought, I hope so. Our side needs a boost. The truth was that Aarestad had beaten up on Aletha. She'd fallen into his rhythm, let him overpower her. Apparently his style was going to be to force the victims off balance, then highlight every contradiction and inconsistency. Aletha's emotional testimony had been honest, but some of the jurors looked unimpressed, especially when she admitted that she'd suspected Story of abusing her when she was a teenager and yet continued to see him. Fairly or unfairly, she'd come across as someone who'd worn a path to her doctor's office from the age of six. Jurors preferred strong, healthy types.

As Judi walked up the three flights with the seventy-six-year-old witness, she intoned her standard message of support: "Now remember, Emma Lu, give me a high sign if you need a Kleenex or water. If you think you're gonna pass out, wave your hand and we'll call for a break."

Emma Lu climbed the staircase like a young woman. "Remember," Judi went on, hustling to catch up, "you don't have to look at Dr. Story. Look at me and I'll smile. That's what I'm there for." *Yes,* she said to herself, *but I about wore out my smile on Aletha, and the trial just started.* "Remember, Emma Lu, there's plenty of folks on your side."

The cute old woman said, "The Lord will guide my words."

Judi took her own seat in the front row and smiled. When the witness was asked if she swore to tell the truth, she said "I do!" in a firm and fervent voice.

Her answers to Terry Tharp's questions were precise and direct. Did she go to Dr. Story very often? "Well, I have been very healthy so I haven't gone very many times." Was there a nurse in the room for her pelvic? "No, there was no nurse in the room." When she was asked for information that she no longer remembered, she simply said, "I don't remember," instead of fumbling for an answer.

Q What happened then from the point that he reentered the room?
A Well, he said, I am going to put a tube up you.
Q Up you? Where did he mean?
A Well, up my vagina, I suppose is what he meant. He says, I am going to use a tube.
Q Okay. What happened then?
A Well, then I began to hurt and I was looking at his face and I began to hurt. And then he got a real odd look on his face and in fact it looked like my husband did when he meant to enter me, and I looked down and there he was, and there was his penis.
Q You say you saw his penis?
A Yes, I did. . . .

Tharp held up State's Exhibit 20:

Q Is that a speculum?
A I guess it is.

Q Did that—I guess, this isn't what you saw on that day, is it?
A Heavens, no!

Judi looked at the jury. A few of the women were smiling. All seemed
attentive. Please, Lord, Judi said to herself, let her hold up on cross.

Tharp asked how she'd felt at the sight of Story's penis. "Like
kicking him!" Emma Lu said with a toss of her lank gray hair. It
seemed to Judi like a normal reaction for a pioneer woman who was as
tough and wiry as the greasewood roots she'd once torn out with her
father. The minor outburst only made her seem more believable.

Aarestad's first question was, "What is your date of birth?"

When Emma Lu said it was November 17, 1908, he asked, "So you
would have been approximately sixty-eight years of age then on October
3, 1977?" Behind the question, Judi realized, was another one: what
man would want to rape such an old woman? Few jurors understood
that a rape victim's age or appearance were meaningless to a typical
attacker. Judi had heard of women in their eighties who were raped
by teenagers. It was not a crime of love or lust. She'd watched defense
lawyers play on this ignorance before. It was a standard defense.

Aarestad returned the witness to the crucial scene and then
asked, "Did you observe him undo his trousers and remove this
tube?"

A I did not.
Q Did you hear a zipper come down?
A I didn't hear a zipper.
Q All right. Then you feel pain in vaginal area?
A Yes, I did.
Q And could you describe this pain to me, please?
A I don't believe I could. I think you have to be a woman. . . .
Q The next thing that you remember then is looking down and seeing
what?
A The next thing I remember was the look on his face . . . the look of my
husband when he penetrated me . . . a look of concentration. . . .
Q As I understand your testimony, you don't know whether or not he
entered you or not?
A It felt like it.
Q Okay. And then what did you do?
A I began to try to get out, get away from there.
Q How did you do that?
A I don't know. I'm quite agile. I'm in good physical shape. . . . I just got
out of the road as fast as I could.

Aarestad increased the pace, and Judi tried to project a message with her eyes: don't play his game, Emma Lu. Think carefully before you answer. Don't let him run you the way he ran Aletha.

Q   Would you describe this penis for me? How long was it?
A   I don't know how long. I only saw that much.
Q   About like that?
A   About like that, yes.
Q   A couple inches.
A   A little littler, less than that. Go littler. About like that. Up next to him, between him and me.
Q   So what you saw when you looked down was not the head of a penis?
A   No, it wasn't.
Q   What portion of the penis would it have been?
A   It would have been about two inches of him next, up next to—the root.
Q   I'm sorry?
A   The root up next to him.

Judi smiled. Emma Lu's bright green eyes were locked on the lawyer's. It was hard to believe that this was the same person who'd omitted information in her first two interviews because she couldn't say "penis."

Q   Did you see pubic hair?
A   How could you see—no.
Q   Was his zipper open?
A   Didn't see a zipper.
Q   Was his trousers pulled down?
A   I didn't see trousers pulled down.
Q   Was his lab coat unbuttoned?
A   Yes.
Q   So you could see through the opening of the lab coat?
A   Yes.
Q   Could you not then see whether his trousers were up or down or do you not recall?
A   I don't recall.
Q   What color was his penis?
A   Penis color.

The judge smiled as he called for order. Most of the jurors laughed.

Aarestad launched into a series of questions about Story's penis: its length, what portion she'd seen, how long she'd seen it. He asked her to use her hands to show its girth. Judi thought, *Don't let him embarrass you, Emma Lu. He's trying to upset you and make you look ignorant.*

She stole a glance at the jurors. They watched closely as Emma Lu refused to be bullied or led. Even when she misunderstood the questions, she seemed in control:

Q And I believe you indicated that [Diana Harrison] is your husband's aunt?
A No.
Q She would be your husband's nephew's wife?
A No.
Q She would be your nephew's wife?
A No. She is my nephew's wife.

Aarestad abruptly ended his questioning. Judi thought, score a round for us. The trial, she figured, was now about even.

A less emphatic Emma was next—Emma Briseno McNeil, a heavy, dark-skinned woman who'd moved to Maine two years earlier with her laborer husband Kenneth. She testified that Story had raped her while her two-year-old daughter Crystal played with the controls on his automatic table. ". . . He got mad and he said that I should have left her home. And then I guess he was mad, he backed up and then that's when I felt the penis come out. . . . He walked over to the washbasin and he started washing it off."

Despite the novelty of her story, the jury didn't seem attentive, maybe because her voice was too weak to carry over the construction din from outside, or maybe because she was less certain of her facts and nowhere near as angry as Emma Lu. To Judi, she seemed to lack the motivation of some of the other women. Maybe it was because she was isolated from the rest of them in her new home in Maine.

On cross-examination, Aarestad had no trouble mixing her up, and sometimes Tharp had to interrupt to keep the record straight:

Q (By MR. AARESTAD) In addition to the speculum portion of the exam—
MR. THARP Your Honor, I think that question—now she said, she never said anything about a speculum. . . . I object to that as misstating the testimony.
THE COURT Ask her, Counsel, if one was used that day.
Q (By MR. AARESTAD) For clarification, you do not recall a speculum being used by you on that particular day?
A No.

Once again, the tall defense lawyer dwelled on what seemed to be a favorite subject:

Q   Did you see his penis?
A   Yes.
Q   This is before he got to the sink?
A   Yes.
Q   Would you describe the penis to me that you saw?
A   Well, his pants were unzipped and it was hanging out and that's when he started to wash his hands and his penis.
Q   I take it his penis was hanging down?
A   Just a little bit.
Q   Okay. Was it erect and parallel with the floor? Was it drooping? Could you give me some indication with your hands?

While the embarrassed woman groped for an answer, Judi concluded that these repeated questions about the male organ could only be part of an overall defense plan to throw the women off and make them sound undignified and silly. Well, she said to herself, Story knows these women well. A month ago, before counseling, the technique might have worked. Now it just seems to be annoying the jury.

The last day of the first week of trial was Good Friday, and the only victim to testify was Julia Bradbury. She was now seventy-two, white-haired and neatly dressed in a black suit with red piping and a red blouse with a soft bow. She testified that she was a widow; her husband had run a store and she'd kept the books.

Tharp elicited her story in a straight line: a visit to Story for a flu shot, an unscheduled pelvic exam at the doctor's suggestion, a "tube," a rape. The jury perked up when she testified that semen ran down her legs after the exam, and "I was so stunned I didn't do anything."

When she inadvertently mentioned the Medical Board hearing, Aarestad objected and Tharp rephrased the question. When she mentioned it again, the annoyed lawyer threatened to move for a mistrial. Before he began his cross-examination, Aarestad arranged for the judge to remind the woman that the Medical Board proceeding "has no bearing in this criminal proceedings and we would ask that you not refer to it again." Judi thought that the elderly woman looked shaken and confused.

The cross-examination bore down on discrepancies between her testimony and her earlier statements, notably on whether she'd realized instantly that the fluid running down her leg was semen or only reached that conclusion later. Her anxiety showed in attempts to rush her answers, sometimes before the lawyer had finished his question. But Aarestad seemed gentler toward her than he'd been toward the others. From her front-row seat, Judi suspected that the North Dakota lawyer didn't want the jury to perceive him as a bully who browbeat old ladies. An image like that might rub off on his client.

Tharp took Mrs. Bradbury on redirect examination and wrapped up the questioning.

Q   I am going to hand you what is being marked State's Exhibit No. 15. Can you identify that?

A   Yes, I can.

Q   What is it?

A   It is my calendar for 1980.

Q   And calling your attention to the date September 23, is that the day you went to Dr. Story?

A   Yes. I had "Dr. Story, 3 o'clock" written on there.

Q   Is there anything else on that date?

A   I put a big red "R" . . .

Q   What does the red "R" on your calendar stand for?

A   Rape.

71

Terri Timmons

ALL THROUGH EASTER WEEKEND, she hadn't been able to get Julia Bradbury out of her mind. Terri had been waiting in the witness room with her husband Loyd when the elderly woman picked up her coat after testifying. Her face was as white as her hair. Terri had said to herself, What are they *doing* up in that courtroom?

Now it was 9:30 Monday morning and she was climbing the long staircase on her spindly legs. Judi Cashel clutched her thin arm and whispered that she was going to be fine, she was going to do just great, they were all so *proud* of her.

No sooner had she settled into the witness chair than her mind began to race. *Look at the jurors! They're so close I could almost touch them.* She wondered why two of the women wouldn't return her smile. *Are they against me already?*

While Terry Tharp shuffled some papers, she stole a glance at the audience. Every seat was taken and eight or ten people watched from the back wall. She thought, Why are all these people here? What business is this of theirs? *O Father in heaven, where's Loyd?*

She spotted his red hair in the middle of the standees. He'd given her a priesthood blessing the night before—such a comfort. She looked for more red hair and sighed when she found it. Judi was smiling.

"Would you please state your name and address?"

She opened her mouth to answer and barely made a sound. A clerk brought her a glass of water and she blurted out, "My name is Terri Lee Timmons I live at six fifty-eight North Bent Powell Wyoming."

Terry Tharp seemed unnecessarily grim as he guided her through a set of biographical questions while she gulped and tried to relax. She wished he would stop addressing her as "Mrs. Timmons." His tension was aggravating hers. She'd never felt as comfortable with Tharp as she had with Judi or the other women.

When he asked if she saw the defendant in the courtroom, she said, "Yes, I do," and pointed. Story looked antsy, as though he didn't know how to react. She had a momentary feeling of satisfaction. Let the little jerk squirm, she said to herself. She hoped that wasn't too awful of her.

As she was telling her story, the defense attorney kept jumping up to interrupt. He complained about her "narrative answers." She wondered how you could describe a specific happening without narrating. Then he griped that she wasn't being "responsive," or "he's assuming facts not in evidence," or "that's a leading question."

She thought, How am I supposed to concentrate? The other victims referred to Story's lawyer as "the devil's advocate." It sure seemed to fit. She wished he didn't have to be so rude.

After each objection, Tharp had to back up and start over. It seemed like boys playing word games. Her nervousness soon turned to pique. The judge gave her a good feeling, but both lawyers annoyed her. Tharp almost made her cry when he asked if she'd told her parents what Story had done.

"No," she answered. "I did not."

She hoped he had enough sense to drop *that* particular hot potato. The truth was that she hadn't told her parents about the rape because they'd been having awful fights and her father had been on the warpath and she didn't want to aggravate the situation. But the farm boy–prosecutor plowed ahead. "Why didn't you?" he asked.

"Because of how things were in our family," she said.

She blinked back tears as Tharp asked, "Were you concerned about what your father or mother's reaction might be?"

She gasped, "Yes," and started crying. He asked her if she would like a few minutes, and she said no. She thought, I'll have to go through this again when the defense lawyer questions me. He'll try to punish me with Mom and Dad's problems.

At last Tharp turned to Aarestad and said, "You may cross-examine."

Within a few minutes the two lawyers were toe to toe over another technicality. They gathered around the judge and argued back and forth and finally took a fifteen-minute break to cool their heads.

When they returned, Aarestad pumped her about Story's office layout, where the waiting room was, whether she had to pass the receptionist's desk, who ushered her in, a whole bunch of dumb questions that had nothing to do with whether she'd been raped. But his style gradually became more congenial, and she found herself relaxing. She thought, How strange. This blond guy's out to get me and yet he's being nice about it. But then he tried to trip her up and she disliked him more than ever:

Q Okay. The object that you describe now as very, very warm when it entered you—was it hotter or colder, if you recall, than when he had his finger inside of your vagina?
A Hotter.
Q Hotter?
A Hotter.
Q Much hotter?
A Much hotter.
Q Now perhaps I'm a bit confused. You have described this object as stiff and soft.
A Skin.
Q It felt like skin?
A It was skin. Bare skin.
Q You never saw that skin, though. Did you?
A No.

As the questioning intensified, she became aware of an occasional reaction from the audience. She thought, This is embarrassing enough without those folks acting ignorant. Some of the Story people seemed to think they were at a basketball game. She was relieved when the judge banged his gavel and said, "Ladies and gentlemen of the audience, I am going to have to admonish you. Please do not make any comments to each other during the course of the time the trial is in session. The remarks may be heard by the witnesses. They may be heard by members of the jury. . . . If this continues I may have to remove some of you from the courtroom and that I don't want to do."

The cross-examination passed the one-hour mark and Terri felt weak and tired. The LDS victims had been fasting together; she wondered now if that was such a good idea. She kept anticipating an avalanche of embarrassing personal questions about her mother and father and the trouble at home; she wasn't sure she could handle it. But she had no trouble describing the rape. She'd had eighteen years of the same horror film reeling through her mind.

When she told how Story had wadded up the bloody paper under her body and thrown it into a wastebasket that was "silver, with a pedal to lift the lid," the lawyer pounced:

Q   And from where you were lying on the table were you able to visualize that container?
A   No.
Q   This is a conclusion then?
A   Not that I remember.
Q   This is a conclusion then that you arrived at some time later than when he had allegedly ripped the paper off?
A   What are you asking? Where the wastebasket was?
Q   Yes.
A   I don't understand. I'm sorry.
Q   You just described a wastebasket that was silver in color, I believe?
A   It might have been white. I don't remember.
Q   Or it might have been black?
A   No. It was either white or silver.
Q   Did you—I guess what I am getting at, Mrs. Timmons, is at what point, before or after the paper was torn off the table, that you observed the color of that container?
A   I didn't see it. I couldn't see it when I was laying down. I mean my recollection would be from walking in the room.
Q   Okay. As you sit here today, you are not sure?
A   Not sure what? What color it was . . . ?

At last Terry Tharp came to her rescue. His high forehead looked boiled. "Your Honor," he said in a loud voice, "I am going to start objecting. We are plowing the same ground. He has already asked and that has been answered."

The judge said, "Sustained," and, a few minutes later, he added, "All right, Mrs. Timmons, you may step down." She was surprised. Aarestad hadn't tried to dredge out the details of her home life. She wondered if he'd forgotten, or if even defense lawyers had a little sensitivity. She cried with relief.

When she stood up, the courtroom went white. Someone grabbed her arm. "I'm gonna faint," she said. She was sobbing as Judi led her out the door.

72

Wanda Hammond

That little meatball Wanda, she looks like everybody's
grandmother, like a little old farm woman. And she cried
when she started her kinky little lie. . . . There was a gasp
in the audience.

—Cheryl Nebel

ALL WANDA WANTED TO DO was tell her story and get back to work.
A few days before, she'd told the owner of the Rose City Food Farm,
"If you want me to," she said, "I'll take a leave or quit." Poor Tom
Cornwall was losing customers in droves, and Wanda was afraid she
knew whose fault it was. Sometimes it seemed she'd been taking blame
all her life. That was one reason she cried so much.

Jan Hillman wasn't the only Story supporter who'd been avoiding
her checkout line, but she was certainly the loudest. For a while
Tom checked the large-bodied woman out while Wanda bagged,
but even that didn't satisfy Story's No. 1 backer. One day she
wrenched the bag from Wanda's hands and said, "Don't you touch my
groceries! I'll bag my own. I don't want you touching *anything* of
mine."

Jan's sweet mother LaVera had turned just as ornery. Whenever a
Story supporter entered the store, Wanda summoned Tom and busied
herself in the back, sweeping. But customers were still drifting away to
the Big Horn IGA.

Tom refused to let her quit. "It's my store," he said. "It's my
business who works for me." Wanda needed the $3.50 an hour. For
most of her life, she'd driven a school bus and grown beets, but at

fifty-five she was feeling her age. She'd already shrunk an inch from her four feet eleven.

She was surprised at the strength her Celestial Father gave her for the trial. She'd halfway expected to pass out and have to testify from a stretcher, but the prayers and fasting and counseling had helped. After she got over her opening jitters, she managed to answer Terry Tharp's questions with only an occasional sob or hesitation. But she was puzzled by the long talks between lawyers and judge. Right after she testified that she hadn't told anyone about the rape because "I didn't think anyone would believe me," the blond defense lawyer went up to the judge with Terry Tharp:

MR. AARESTAD   I would like to formally request that the Court remove from the courtroom one of the spectators who is sniffling and crying in response to the emotional statements or outbursts of the witness, simply because it is highly prejudicial, and the impact and detriment that it has towards the Defendant in this case has a potential of being considerable. And I might further state that when we have a courtroom that is apparently packed . . . that the Court is going to have to be extremely sensitive to comments coming from the spectators. And I would also note that there apparently is a young child in the courtroom . . . and I think that if this continues in any way that we are just going to have to simply ask that the courtroom be cleared. But I want the record to reflect what is occurring in the courtroom at this point.

MR. THARP   Your Honor, the woman in question doesn't look particularly discomposed. I see no reason to admonish anybody. I didn't see anything. I never heard any remarks. And the witness has been able to continue. I don't think it is so disruptive as to be prejudicial. And I see no sense in calling attention to it.

THE COURT   The Court has not seen or observed any women sniffling or crying or talking out loud after its first admonishment this morning. As Counsel well knows in this case, this case is a very highly publicized case. The Court also suggested to Counsel that since this was to be a very highly public interest case that perhaps this case should be moved out of Big Horn County. To date the Court has not received a Motion for Change of Venue. I think Counsel anticipated that this would be a large, packed courtroom if it was tried here. The Court sees no reason for admonishment of the people at this point.

The courtroom fell quiet as Wanda told how Dr. Story had dilated her, then lifted her hand "and placed it down around his thing." When she'd realized what she was feeling, she testified, she'd jerked her hand away and exclaimed, "Dr. Story!"

Someone in the audience laughed. Dr. Story looked up from his yellow pad with a faint smile. Aarestad brought the cross-examination to an end in a few minutes.

As Beverly Moody told her husband Larry, the stupid trial made her want to kick somebody where the sun don't shine. The judge was out for Doc's hide—you didn't need a law degree to see that. Every time one of the supporters made a sound, he banged his gavel. But over on the other side of the aisle, folks were oohing and aahing and faking tears, and not a word was said.

"That judge even climbed on me!" the florist told Larry that evening as he tended some tomato starts in their greenhouse. "I seen a conterdiction in one of the witnesses and I just went, 'Aaaahhhh,' and that dang judge said 'Order in the court!' three or four times. Seemed like he was picking on our side. And we weren't being ignorant ladies, ya know?"

Marilyn Story wrote in her journal: "John and Wayne and Scott [Kath] seem to be optimistic."

73

Hayla Fink Farwell

"I WAS all shook up when I got off the stand," Hayla told a friend later, "and Judi took me downstairs to the witness room." Hayla had testified that Story "dilated' her, then stepped back to reveal his erect penis, then went ahead and raped her.

"When I saw my husband Bill after I testified," the heavyset housewife went on, "I just came unglued. I kept telling myself, You can't cry like this in front of the other witnesses. You're gonna scare 'em.

"Bill said, 'I'm gonna go up to that courtroom and kill that little son of a bitch.'

"The deputy walked Bill to the window to calm him down. Somebody said, 'The Story people are looking for a mistrial. You go up there now and they're gonna have what they want.'

"A crew from Casper TV was out in front of the building, so Bill and I left by a side door. I was still shook. I heard somebody call my name, but I wasn't gonna turn around. A hand touched my shoulder and I jumped. It was Anna Parks, the columnist for the *Chronicle*. She said, 'Our prayers are with you and we believe you.' That made me feel better.

"My family always belonged to St. John's Lutheran Church in Lovell, and our pastor, Sam Christensen, showed up for my testimony. It felt good to see him there. At recess time, Dr. Story walked down the aisle and my pastor went up and hugged him."

74

Testimony

AFTER HAYLA FARWELL, the trial proceeded in spurts. Annella St. Thomas told about her rape thirteen years earlier and her futile attempts to get action. Her husband described his frustrating visit to LaMar Averett and how the old chief turned him away.

The sixty-eight-year-old Averett took the stand and rubbed gnarled knuckles across his eyes as he explained that he'd gone to Dr. Story for twenty-five years and refused to write up the St. Thomas complaint because "I didn't believe it."

Mae Fischer testified that she'd seen Story's erect penis after the rape and "I started backing up," whereupon he said, "You didn't know?" Her mother, Caroline Shotwell, no longer listed as a complainant, verified that Mae had come home and reported the rape. But Caroline made no mention of her own difficulties with the doctor a month earlier.

Diana Harrison drew whispers as she walked past the jurors. She was dressed in a gleaming white polyester dress-suit with off-white accessories. Her makeup was flawless, her hair coiffed. She didn't seem intimidated by the fact that most of the spectators considered her a turncoat. When the county attorney asked her to state her name, her voice carried to the back wall.

343

Her testimony went smoothly until Tharp asked if Story ever gave women pelvic exams for "nongynecological complaints."

Aarestad began a series of objections. "I am going to object to that on lack of foundation and incompetent on the part of this receptionist to testify as to what is or is not nongynecological examinations."

The judge had turned down most of Aarestad's earlier objections, but he sustained this one. A few seconds later, he sustained another, and then another. The questioning turned to the reluctance of Hayla Farwell and Julia Bradbury to pay their bills. Aarestad sat silently until Tharp slipped back to his original approach:

Q Did you ever notice any unusual behavior by the doctor during the course of any pelvic examinations?

MR. AARESTAD I am going to object again as to calling for a vague response and lack of foundation.

THE COURT Sustained unless foundation is waived.

Q (By MR. THARP) Would you observe the doctor during the course of your work as he was walking around the office?

A Yes.

Q And would you observe him as he might come out of an examination room?

A Yes.

Q Did you ever notice anything unusual in his demeanor when he came out of the examination room?

A Yes.

MR. AARESTAD I am going to object again on the grounds it lacks specifics and it is vague in respect to what day, what patient and time and place, et cetera.

THE COURT Overruled.

Q Go ahead and answer, Mrs. Harrison. What did you notice?

A Okay. On occasion we noticed he would come out of an examining room very fast, his hair would be ruffled, his ears were red, and he would go immediately to the bathroom.

Q Would this be from a room where a pelvic examination was scheduled?

A Yes.

After a few questions about Mrs. Bradbury's bill, Tharp asked, "Were you ever called upon to clean up an examination room?"

"Yes."

The defense lawyer stood up as Tharp asked, "Do you recall an incident—?"

"May counsel approach the Bench at this point, Your Honor?" Aarestad called out.

"Certainly," the judge said.

The agitated lawyer warned that Tharp was trying to elicit testimony about the finding of semen in Story's wastebasket, and called it "highly prejudicial . . . remote and irrelevant." His face showed disgust as he said, "That is so remote and so irrelevant and prejudicial that we can't even conceive of such testimony being allowed. . . . If Mr. Tharp were completely honest, what he would say is he is trying to use this witness to inject as much extraneous prejudicial information through this witness as he can to characterize the Defendant as some kind of a deviant."

The judge asked if there was any connection between the semen smelled by the witness and any of the complainants.

"No," Tharp answered.

"Highly irrelevant and prejudicial!" Aarestad interjected, and added several legal reasons why the testimony shouldn't be permitted.

The judge ran a hand through his white hair. "I am going to allow Mr. Tharp to make inquiry into this area," he said slowly, ". . . provided the proper foundation is laid in this matter. I believe that if the witness were to testify as to what Mr. Tharp has just revealed at the Bench conference that it does have probative value as to the Defendant's opportunity and, also, the Defendant's modus operandi."

Tharp resumed:

Q Mrs. Harrison, do you recall ever cleaning out an examination room in the Defendant's new office?

A Yes. . . .

Q Do you recall an occasion in 1983 when you cleaned out Room No. 2?

A Yes.

Q . . . Were you the first person to arrive at the office that morning?

A Yes.

Q . . . What did you do?

A I took off the lid of the garbage can. . . . I was going to take the plastic liner out of the garbage.

Q Did you notice anything about the garbage in that can?

A Yes.

Q What?

MR. AARESTAD I am going to object on the grounds that are set forth in our Bench conference.

THE COURT The Court will stand by its ruling.

Q (By MR. THARP) What did you see?

A A wad of tissue. . . . It was wet.

Q Well, did this arouse your suspicions in any way?

A   Yes.

Q   So what did you do?

A   I got a piece of plastic and I picked it up. . . . I smelled it.

Q   Do you associate the smell on that wad with anything?

A   Yes . . . semen.

Q   Did you shortly thereafter check the appointment book?

A   Yes. . . .

Q   Did you check for the previous day?

A   Yes.

Q   Was there any indication that a pelvic examination had been performed in that room?

A   Yes.

Q   Do you know what time?

A   Two o'clock.

Q   I believe it was your testimony that—well, you have testified that the Defendant—you made the remark to him about having a nurse in the room?

A   Yes.

Q   Now then, I take it from that there were occasions when the Defendant did not have a nurse in the room with him when doing a pelvic exam?

A   Yes.

Q   And did this practice continue throughout the time that you worked for him?

A   No.

Q   Did it ever change?

A   Yes.

MR. AARESTAD   I am going to object to this, Your Honor. Could we approach the Bench?

THE COURT   Okay.

MR. AARESTAD   I believe that we are getting awfully dangerous here. I believe that Mr. Tharp is attempting to elicit testimony from this witness as to the events of the Board hearing that stated that he was to have a nurse in the room. And if she even hints of that, I am going to move for a mistrial. I hate to do it on the last witness of the case.

MR. THARP   This witness will testify that in the spring of 1983 Dr. Story's practice changed and he began having a third person in the room because of the complaints they had received. That is as far as she has been instructed to go.

MR. AARESTAD   Those complaints stem from the hearing and all of that. And he wants his steak and eat it, too, that is he can bring it up to a certain point but prevents me obviously from cross-examination from determining the validity and the identity of the complaints. And I believe for the record at this point Mr. Tharp is trying to set up a scenario for a mistrial.

THE COURT   Well, the jury has already heard the testimony that Julia Bradbury had complained and, also, the fact that Mrs. Hayla Farwell had in fact complained to them as to the reasons for why the bill was not paid. I would, however, suggest, Mr. Tharp, you approach this very, very carefully and don't get into a situation that is going to cause a mistrial in this matter. We have gone a long way at this time and I'd hate to see anything approach that. Do you wish to take a recess to talk to this witness beforehand?

MR. THARP Maybe I can just phrase the questions so she can answer with a yes or no.

THE COURT All right.

Q (By MR. THARP) Now you stated, I believe your last answer was that at some point in your employment Dr. Story's practice changed. Is that correct?

A Yes.

Q When? Do you recall?

A Approximately a month before I quit.

Q This would have been in 1984?

A Yes. Maybe, sir, more than that.

MR. AARESTAD I'm going to object to the witness volunteering information.

THE COURT Sustained. Just answer the question.

THE WITNESS All right.

Q (By MR. THARP) At that point did he begin having a third person present in the room?

A Yes.

Q Was that because of some complaints that had been received?

A Yes.

After Diana Harrison testified that the examining rooms could be locked from the inside, Aarestad began his cross-examination with a series of questions about the layout of the clinic, her duties, her current employment, her relationship with the nine complaining witnesses, and Story's office procedures.

Q Isn't it true that Dr. Story had a standing order that any time the hospital called or another physician called that he was to be contacted immediately?

A Yes.

Q And who generally would go and inform him of that call?

A Usually whoever answered the telephone.

Q And did you ever go to an examination room in response to informing him of a telephone call and found the door locked?

A I cannot tell you I found the door locked because I never touched the door. . . .

Q You talked about [Dr. Story's] running to the bathroom. . . . Can you give us any type of estimate as to the number of times that you have observed this behavior?

A Twice.

Q Did that ever alert your suspicions as to any type of impropriety on his part?

A Not really. We just used to joke about it. Implying nothing.

Aarestad's nose crinkled as he returned to the subject of the tissue:

Q It is my understanding that you picked this wad up then and held it to
your nose?
A Yes, I did.
Q And can you describe the color of the tissue?
A No.
Q Can you describe the color of the substance that was on the tissue?
A The tissue had absorbed it.
Q So simply what we have is a moist tissue?
A Yes.
Q And it is that moist tissue then that you raised to your nose to smell it?
A Yes.
Q Why did you do that?
A Because I was suspicious.
Q Had you smelled semen before?
A Yes.
Q There was no doubt in your mind whatsoever that's what you smelled?
A None whatsoever. . . .
Q Do you know during this period of time whether Dr. Story ever did any
sperm counts in his office?
A No.

Tharp took the witness on redirect:

Q . . . When you were asked questions by Mr. Aarestad about the color of
the tissue, do you remember whether it was light or dark?
MR. AARESTAD Asked and answered.
THE COURT Sustained.
Q (By MR. THARP) Did it have any color at all?
A Yes.
MR. AARESTAD Same objection.
THE COURT Sustained.
Q (By MR. THARP) You said in response to Mr. Aarestad's question one
of the reasons you quit was because you started your business?
A Yes.
MR. AARESTAD May we approach the Bench, Your Honor?
THE COURT You may.
MR. THARP I am going to object to these Bench conferences.
THE COURT (AT THE BENCH) Counsel, confine your remarks to the Court,
not anything to the jury.
MR. AARESTAD Your Honor, the answer that in my opinion is being
elicited is a very dangerous one. It is because of the problems that she was
having with the Medical Board at that time, and again I have to state it for the

record that I believe that the Prosecution is attempting to set the stage for a mistrial through this examination. He knows that is the answer that is coming.

MR. THARP Well, Your Honor, I won't ask the question. I apologize to the Court for flying off the handle, but it seems that we have been having an inordinate number of Bench conferences. But—well, I'm not going to ask any more questions of her. . . . I will simply leave her alone.

Then the county attorney announced, "The State rests." It was 3:30 P.M. on Tuesday, April 9, 1985, the sixth day of trial. The defense estimated that its case would take two weeks.

75

Rex Nebel

Denial, O my Senators,
takes a random shape.
— Tess Gallagher,
*The Woman Who Raised
Goats*

HE WAS a complex man of thirty-seven—rebellious, compassionate, idealistic—but what was going on in the courtroom made him just plain angry. Friends said he looked like Grizzly Adams, with bronze and silver hair curling gently over his ears and a thicket of facial hair and a body as strong as a young bison's. For more years than he liked to remember, he'd clanked when he walked, as a Lovell cop, a Big Horn Country undersheriff, and a beer-swilling amphetamine-popping skull-cracking biker. Nowadays his major vice was chewing on Swisher Sweet cigars and smoking cigarillos.

Dr. Story and the Lovell Bible Church and Rex's own God-loving wife Cheryl had turned his life around. A year before the trial, he'd run a three-wheeler through a fence and Dr. Story had put him back together. Now they were like uncle and nephew, so close that the title "doctor" had begun to sound too formal for their relationship. At Marilyn's suggestion, Rex and Cheri started referring to him as "Doc," though never to his face. He was particular about his name and title. "It's my enemies who first-name me," he said. But Marilyn insisted that it was cumbersome to refer to him to their friends as "Dr. Story," and the compromise "Doc" had stuck.

From the beginning, both Nebels had felt that only a moron could believe the accusations against their beloved Doc. But as Rex liked to point out, the words "Mormon" and "moron" were only a letter apart. His LDS dad once told him, "Son, if you believe all the bullshit that you hear in the Mormon church, you're not as smart as I think you are. Stick with the Methodists like your mom. I'll go with you on Christmas."

Rex worked at a bentonite plant and helped Cheri raise their two boys in a small wooden house just off the highway at the east end of town. On the side, he sold Freedom Fireworks. It was a comedown. His pioneer ancestors had homesteaded a ranch at the confluence of the Shoshone and Big Horn rivers, but a half century later the government confiscated the spread for a park. "They lied to my father," Rex fumed. "From the handshake to the signatures, there were ten thousand lies."

Sometimes he soothed his unrest by hiking deep into the woods, not far from the old family farm, and just listening. "I go there at two in the morning, climb a tree, lay up and listen to the coyotes. It's something to be outside with everything around you alive—owls calling, foxes padding by. People think you're not supposed to be that free. It's my medicine."

Ever since the start of the trial, Rex had worked the midnight shift so he could watch over Doc in the daytime. He was assisted in his unofficial security job by a rangy old Big Horn deputy sheriff named Jack Doolan, "Deulin' Doolan" to his friends, who worked all night and protected Dr. Story all day without pay. As a deputy, Doolan could carry a gun into the courtroom. Since resigning as undersheriff, Rex had had to make do with a blackjack.

As Doc's courtroom ordeal went into its second week, Rex and some of the other Story supporters approached flash point. There'd been more slanted articles in the Casper *Star-Tribune* and the Billings *Gazette*. Diana Harrison's turncoat testimony outraged everyone on Doc's side. Rex had already been involved in one near-fight and several spitting matches. He'd spotted the claque of accusers chatting with Dave Wilcock in a basement room. "What the hell are you doing?" he yelled through the open door to his former law-enforcement colleague. "Discussing Dr. Story's case? You know you're not supposed to do that. You pigs make me sick. You call this a trial?"

When the police chief turned his broad back, Rex excoriated him till the door slammed. "Fat swine" was the nicest term he used.

Then he ran into an elderly relative who'd been sitting on the wrong side of the courtroom and cueing some of the witnesses. "What was all that headshaking about?" Rex asked.

"I was rooting," the woman said. "Yes, I'm for the victims, Rex. I've known Wanda all my life."

Rex said, "Does that justify you telling her how to answer, you stupid thing?"

At the end of the sixth day of trial, some of the Story people were picking their way down the steep steps when a flushed Bill Fischer made a subtle move toward Doc. Rex knew the guy. His wife Mae had testified earlier in the day—the usual bullshit about Doc abusing her but she hadn't mentioned it for ten or twenty years. Bill had been shooting off his mouth at the bentonite plant about punching Doc out, but no one took him seriously.

Rex made a head signal to Duelin' Doolan and the two guardians moved in. "It looked like Fischer was getting ready to throw Doc down the stairs," Rex told Cheri later. "I grabbed my Texas blackjack, and I'm thinking, I'm gonna brain this guy. If he touches Doc, I'm gonna choke him out, ya know? Doolan and I just kinda shoved Fischer out the back door. I said, 'Go ahead, make your move, sucker! Come on! I'll kill ya!' Fischer turned red, and he walked off like he didn't hear me."

Later Rex challenged Fischer to a fight at the plant. "I was just screaming at him," he told his approving wife. " 'Ooo-*oooh*! I want you out here!' I said, 'You lie, your mother's a liar, your wife's a liar! I want you outside with me in the gravel right now, 'cause you are a liar and your family's a liar and you're doing nothing but ruining this man!' "

In Rex's recounting of the incident, Fischer backed down again, and Rex finished him off by saying, "That little move you pulled over in the courthouse damn near got yourself killed. You're not messin' with kids on the block. You're messin' with a professional police officer and an ex-cop. I came *that* close to braining you. Stand clear of Dr. Story! *Stay off his back or I'll waste ya!*"

Rex figured that took care of one more wimp.

76

Marilyn Story

DRIVING toward the courthouse in their maroon air-conditioned '72 Chrysler, John nonchalantly mentioned that his accusers had told so many lies that he'd stopped passing notes to his lawyers. "Thousands of lies," he told her. "I can't keep up with them."

As a listed witness for the defense, Marilyn was excluded from the courtroom, and in his usual way, John hadn't been keeping her informed. But she'd heard enough to realize that there were problems. Terry Tharp had allowed John's lawyers to spend months preparing a conspiracy defense, then double-crossed the defense by dropping Minda and Meg and bringing in three non-LDS accusers. The only approach left was an all-out attack on the imperfections in the state's case, plus a parade of impressive character witnesses, of whom she would be first.

Her faith in the procedure was weakening. A few days earlier, she'd written in her journal: "I don't feel able to pray effectively any more, but we thought of the Lord Jesus as he stood before his accusers and false witnesses."

And still John acted unconcerned! From the beginning, he'd refused to believe that God would allow a good Christian to be punished unjustly.

His relatives had phoned to ask if they could attend the trial, and John had told them, "Stay home. It's a big nuisance—nothing." The Nebraska folks were still hurt about being kept in the dark at the twenty-fifth anniversary dinner, but John explained, "We didn't want to spoil the party for you. All doctors go through things like this."

His busy old bachelor uncle, still running the family store in Maxwell and playing an astute hand in the stock market, had told him, "Every cent I have is yours, John. From here on out I'll live on my social security." At the time, it had seemed like a symbolic gesture, but the total lawyers' fees had now passed the six-figure mark; if John was convicted and had to seek vindication in the higher courts, Uncle Howard's offer might have to be accepted.

Marilyn had spent so many days of deep anxiety that she was almost relieved to be sworn in. Wayne had stressed that her testimony could turn things around for the defense. Above all, she mustn't appear arrogant or vengeful. She was the dignified wife of a dignified physician, and she was there to draw admiration and respect, to convince the jurors of John's innocence, and to evoke their sympathy. It was no accident that one of his first questions was, "And I assume you have a deceased child?"

"Yes," she answered. She didn't have to fake a look of sadness. She'd mourned Annette for twenty years. She gulped and said, "We lost a little girl in an accident when she was two years old."

The lawyer asked a series of questions about the family, including what her children were doing now (Susan was a registered nurse in Fort Collins, Colorado, and Linda was taking her master's degree at the University of Maryland), where she was from, and what she did at the office. He spent ten minutes getting her to describe the exact layout of the office so that he could argue later that John would have been caught if he'd been abusing women in an examining room. Then:

Q   During the sixteen years that you worked full-time and the preceding years on which you worked a part-time basis, did you ever observe anything unusual about your husband's behavior that caused you any suspicions about improprieties with female patients?

A   Absolutely not.

Q   Did you ever observe your husband rushing from this room to either of these bathrooms with ruffled hair?

A No, I haven't.

Q Have you ever observed him rushing from this room to any of these bathrooms with red ears?

A No. . . .

She knew what was coming next and steeled herself. She'd heard how the Mormon women hated to discuss sex. Well, it wasn't one of her favorite subjects, either. She tried to smile pleasantly and act as though she were happy to chat about the most intimate parts of her life in front of a courtroom full of strangers.

Q What type of relationship have you had with your husband in respect to the thirty-two years that you have been married?

A We have had a very excellent marriage.

Q You have observed your husband in his relationship with women, have you not?

A Yes. . . . He is very—he is very much a gentleman. He respects women. He respects their privacy. He is kind and compassionate and sympathetic. . . . Our girls have a wonderful relationship with their father. They respect him and love him a great deal. They admire him. . . .

Q Now, referring your attention to a more specific part of your relationship with your husband and particularly the sexual relationship you have had over these years, can you describe to the jury what type of a relationship you have had in that area?

A We have had a very satisfying and normal, happy relationship.

Q Has your husband ever indicated a desire for what you would consider any unusual activities in that area?

A Never.

Q Have you ever observed him bringing home or even viewing or reading anything which you would consider of a pornographic nature?

A No. Just the opposite.

Q Has he ever asked you to attend any movies that you consider of a questionable nature?

A Absolutely not.

Q In your opinion . . . would you consider him abnormal in any respect concerning his sexual drive?

A No, I wouldn't.

Q How about off-color jokes or anything like that. Have you ever heard him tell them?

A No. He never speaks that way.

She was glad when the questioning turned to John's office practices. She testified that she'd interrupted him "many times" during examinations.

"I would go and knock on the door and wait for him to come to the door or say yes."

She would have liked to say that she often barged right in, but it wouldn't have been true. John had a strong belief in his patients' right of privacy. As she testified, "Whenever I was in any examination room in another doctor's office, I would not like to be in that position and have anyone stick their head in." She smiled, and several of the jurors smiled back.

They kept smiling as she described one of her husband's main problems. "He is the type of person that time doesn't mean too much to him. I think he kind of loses track of time. Patients would start talking to him about their troubles and it seems like a lot of times they would come in for supposedly one thing and they would end up asking him lots of other things and more or less counseling with him." She was thinking of Arden McArthur and Aletha Durtsche. "He spent a lot of time like that."

Wayne's direct examination ended on a key subject:

Q   . . . Were you ever privy to any discussions with him relative to having a third person in the examination room while pelvic examination was being performed?
A   No. We never talked about it.
Q   Was that ever a concern of yours?
A   No. Never entered my mind.
Q   Has any female patient ever complained to you during those twenty-six years concerning the fact that he did not have a nurse during the pelvic exam?
A   No.

She'd expected the skinny prosecutor to sound nasty or surly, or, at the least, to patronize her, but he seemed almost friendly. He was interested in the patriotic way she and John started the office day:

Q   You hang a flag up, you say?
A   Yes. Every day.

The rest of his questions were about procedures, her own duties, the daily schedule, and her husband's tendency to fall behind. She'd just begun to relax, happy to be of assistance, when the judge said, "All right, Mrs. Story, you may step down."

They drove back to Lovell together; John had a few patients to see. Before going to bed, she wrote in her journal, "My testimony was easy to give—it isn't difficult when you have nothing to hide."

77

The Defense

AFTER MARILYN STORY, Wayne Aarestad put on fourteen straight character witnesses, half of them nurses in starched white uniforms.

Hospital Manager Joe Brown testified that in "all my twenty years he has probably one of the finest behavioral records that I have seen in any physician." Brown denied that he'd taken an ad in the Lovell *Chronicle*—"To Doc and Marilyn, the angel of the Lord encampeth round about them that fear Him and delivereth them"—but admitted that his wife might have placed it.

Nurse Kathy Gifford observed that she'd worked for the doctor for seven years and never noticed him running toward the bathroom with red ears. She said he used Phisohex as a lubricant for pelvic examinations and that it could be mistaken for sperm. Did anyone leave his examining rooms "crying or tearful or in shock of any kind"?

"Maybe the babies," she answered.

Story's current nurse, Judy Gifford, the previous witness's sister-in-law, testified that he'd delivered her two daughters and had given her many pelvics and Pap smears. She'd frequently been in the examining room during other patients' pelvics and had noticed nothing unusual.

She described the typical examination in as much detail as the state's expert witness, the gynecologist Dr. Flory. She said the patient might be on the table for twenty to forty-five minutes, but the actual examination would take less than five.

Q . . . Has [Dr. Story] ever performed any pelvic examinations on patients who have come in complaining of headaches?

A Yes, that's quite common . . . because many times, in a menopause age type of lady, forty on up, headaches can be caused by their hormone levels, deficiencies in them . . . And by doing a pelvic exam he can note the amount of secretions and conditions that the vaginal wall is.

Q That doesn't strike you as unusual?

A No.

Q . . . During the course of these pelvic exams have you ever heard Dr. Story use the phrase "Can you take any more?"

A Yes. He is very conscious of the woman's pain . . . And if it is getting so painful that the lady can't tolerate it, he quits the exam. . . .

Q Have you ever heard him use the phrase "Can I go any deeper?"

A Yes. . . . Some uteruses are easy to palpate and some are very difficult.

On cross-examination, Terry Tharp asked if she'd discussed her testimony with anyone. "With Wayne," she answered. Then:

Q Are you familiar with or acquainted with the nine women who have testified here previously?

A I actually think that I really only know one of them.

Q You weren't in the room with any of them on the day they were assaulted, were you?

A Not that I am aware of.

Q So you don't know what happened or what didn't happen to them?

A Yes, I do. In my heart.

As she left the witness stand, Nurse Gifford seemed to be fighting back tears. She was known to be especially devoted to the Storys. Her daughter was a Down's syndrome victim and he'd always treated the child with extra care, including free drugs and medication.

When a hospital nurse, Jacqui Lynn Bischoff, testified that she'd noticed no difference between Story's pelvic exams and other doctors', Tharp stood up and objected that the defense testimony was becoming repetitious and irrelevant. At a bench conference, Aarestad's cocounsel, R. Scott Kath, explained, "The relevance is, Your Honor, to show that there is more than just one or two patients who have had a normal, uneventful pelvic, that there are numerous other patients out there who have no complaints. There is nothing else."

Judge Hartman said, "I hope you don't intend to draw every one of them into this courtroom."

MR. KATH No, we are not going to do that.

THE COURT Where are you going to draw the line on this?

MR. KATH . . . Possibly half a dozen.

THE COURT The jury and everybody else has heard the same thing.

MR. KATH We have heard from nine victims that there was something out of the ordinary going on. I think we have got to show that there is a number of people where this did not go on. That's the relevance. The State has paraded in front of this jury nine victims and I think it is very relevant to show that there is another story to this. . . .

MR. THARP . . . We are not contending he raped every woman in town. It is self-serving. It is like saying because there are more banks in town and he didn't rob all of them, he only robbed one, he is not guilty of robbing that one.

THE COURT I think we are getting into a cumulative situation. I will allow you to finish with this witness, but let's move on to something else.

Nurse Bischoff characterized Dr. Story as "very much a Christian." On cross-examination, she admitted that she'd talked to Story's lawyer about her testimony "last night and then two or three nights before that." She said her opinion of Dr. Story wouldn't change even if he were convicted. The judge ordered the remark stricken from the record.

Kaye Meeker, a family friend, testified that Dr. Story was "a very high principled, high moraled man," but she was silenced by more prosecution objections when she started to testify about her own experiences on the examining table.

The bearded Rex Nebel sketched in his police background and described the defendant as "the best."

Q Do you know what his reputation in the community of Lovell is concerning morality, integrity?

A Well, I believe that Dr. Story is one of the few people in Lovell that walks his beliefs and not just talks them. I believe he is of the utmost integrity.

Q During the period of years that you were in law enforcement, did you ever receive any complaints concerning any improprieties on his behalf?

A No, I did not.

Over renewed objections by Terry Tharp, substitute rural mail carrier Peggy Rasmussen described Story as "a very moral man who loves his family and always had good moral reputation."

Lynn Strom, a Lovell bank teller, said that she'd noticed nothing suspicious during her eight or nine months as Dr. Story's receptionist.

Wes Meeker, prominent Lovell realtor and Story neighbor, testified that there'd "just never been any doubt at all in Dr. Story's morality."

Barbara Shumway, another family friend and personnel director at the hospital, agreed.

Jane Keil, former Lovell hospital nurse, told the court that she'd never observed Dr. Story do anything improper. She denied writing a letter of support to the Lovell *Chronicle*. Shown the letter ("Dr. Story, we appreciate the many years of service and look forward to many more. Walt and Jane Keil"), she explained, "I think Walt wrote it."

Robyn Winland, a schoolteacher's wife, testified that Dr. Story had given her twenty pelvic exams in eighteen years, and that she'd sometimes felt him brush against her inner thighs but thought nothing of it.

Verda Croft, director of nursing services at the Lovell hospital, observed that Dr. Story had a communications problem—"He is a very intelligent man. But he tries to explain to the patient and he will talk a long time. And then when he is through he realizes and the patient realizes that a lot of times they don't know what he has said."

Another Lovell hospital R.N., Nina Elaine Strong, described Dr. Story as "much too trusting."

Story's onetime office nurse, Imogene Hansen, said that from 1965 to 1969 she'd never found his examination rooms locked or heard him tell off-color jokes.

78

John Story

Look at the way it thrashes around. The denial—so
stubborn.

—John Hersey, *Blues*

AT 10 A.M. on April 11, 1985, the eighth day of trial, the defendant
walked with slow dignity toward the witness stand. A low hum of
support rose from the right side of the courtroom but subsided at the
judge's frown. The defendant wore a conservatively cut gray suit, a
white shirt, a burnt orange tie and a light smile. As he was sworn in, his
voice was mild and respectful.

"State your name," Wayne Aarestad began.

"John H. Story."

Spectators in the back strained to listen as the doctor told how he'd
set up practice in Lovell because "they had a real need and I liked the
country. . . ."

Three minutes into the questioning, Aarestad sharply changed direction and asked if Story understood the charges against him. "Yes," he
said, "I understand them."

"In order to get them all out of the way once and for all, did you or
did you not commit any of those acts?"

"Those rapes? No. Totally not."

Q Do you recall your wife's testimony yesterday morning relative to the
quality of your marriage?

A Yes, I do.

Q Would you explain to the jury, please, your characterization of your marital relationship with your wife?

A Well, I think it is excellent. I am content to live with her my lifetime. She has satisfied me completely. . . .

Q Do you love her?

A Yes, I love my wife.

Q Very much?

A Ultimately. Extremely.

Still smiling pleasantly, he explained why he'd bought the Ritter table twenty-three years before. "I wanted an ear, nose and throat table, proctology table, and it is good for all those purposes."

Q . . . This table does not enhance your ability to perform a pelvic exam?

A No, it doesn't.

Q And can you approximate for the jury what percentage of your practice involves what would generally be considered obstetrics and gynecology work?

A In the past I would say maybe twenty-five, thirty percent. . . .

Q How many pelvic exams, Dr. Story, do you believe that you have performed over the years?

A I'd say thousands.

Q Do you have a normal routine procedure that you follow when you perform a pelvic exam?

A Yes.

For a half hour Story declaimed in medical terms—why pelvic examinations were needed, the positioning and draping of the patient, the use of the instruments, the two phases of the exam, the positioning of his own body and the movements of his hands and fingers. Aarestad asked how long a typical exam would take:

A Oh, five to ten minutes. Five to eight minutes.

Q Do you think you could do it in a total of one or two minutes?

A I could do a two-minute exam which would be different. It would be compromised.

Q It would not be a thorough exam?

A Right.

Story told about a survey that he'd conducted early in his career about the use of a third party in the examining room. "My first secretary asked the patients as they came in what they wanted . . . and it went on for a number of weeks. . . ."

Q And was it their collective opinion they did not want a third person in there?
A It was each individual. Every individual wanted to be alone.
Q Has anybody ever requested, over the years, to have a third person in there, as you recall?
A Not to me or my nurses that I know of.
Q . . . And isn't it true that you had some patients come to you specifically because you did not have a nurse in there?
A That was the word I received once in a while.

After the morning recess at ten thirty, Aarestad asked if there would be a reason for a patient to place her own hand in the genital area. Yes, Story said, to feel the string of an IUD or to point out a sore place.

Q And would it be possible for them to come in contact with your hand or feel your hand at that time?
A Yes, that happens.
Q . . . Would you have occasion to move around to either side of the patient with a glove still in your hand?
A I frequently want to feel something from the abdomen and I move around to the side to do that, rather than reach up between their legs. . . .

One by one Story refuted specific points in the complainants' testimony, using his memory and office records. He said he'd been wearing a lab coat, not a suit, on the date of Hayla Farwell's exam. He hadn't administered a pelvic to Terri Lee Timmons on the date in question but two years later, when she'd been approximately eighteen—"a virginal type vaginal-rectal exam."

Q . . . Could you explain that please?
A Index finger in the vagina and long finger in the rectum.
Q Why do you perform that type of a pelvic exam?
A Less pain. The other type exam might be impossible for somebody who needs a rectal-vaginal.
Q . . . And you are certain as you sit here today that you did not perform a pelvic exam on April 17, 1968?
A No, I did not.

Emma Briseno McNeil had been hospitalized three months before her pelvic exam on April 18, 1977, Story testified, for "acute abdominal pain, painful infection . . . venereal infection."

> Q   Now do you recall the testimony of Emma McNeil to the effect that you had paper towels in your room?
> A   Yes, I remember that.
> Q   And do you have or have you ever had paper towels in your examination room?
> A   No, I don't. I use cloth towels in there.

Story denied administering a pelvic to Emma Lu Meeks on Oct. 3, 1977, as she'd testified. He said she'd reported a mole on her left breast that day. No reference to a pelvic exam appeared on the yellowing chart.

Another chart showed that Aletha Durtsche had complained of pain in her head, ears, neck and back, a "minimal cough, sweat." No pelvic was shown on her birthday.

Wanda Hammond's records showed that she'd come in for insertion of an IUD, a sterile procedure which would have required the presence of a nurse.

Annella St. Thomas had testified that he'd performed only one pelvic exam on her, but office records showed that "over the three previous visits she had had a pelvic exam and they were over the course of several years."

The direct examination ended on the subject of mental health:

> Q   Dr. Story, have you ever been hospitalized for any mental or emotional problems?
> A   No, I have not.
> Q   Have you ever received any counseling of any kind for any mental or emotional problems?
> A   No, I have not.
> Q   In your opinion, do you have any?
> A   No, I don't believe so.

79

Terrill Tharp

As he assembled his notes for the cross-examination, the young prosecutor was worried that his case was slipping away. The jury seemed impressed by the slippery little doctor's command of medical jargon and technicalities. That was an advantage every physician had: instant respect, automatic believability. For himself, Tharp had regarded the performance as an attempt to obscure the issues. Story's testimony was like the first few snorts of a pumping jack when it went on-line in the oil fields: mostly noise.

He often found himself wishing that criminal trials could be scored like prizefights. At times he thought he was well ahead and at times he wished he'd never left the farm. Juries were so hard to read, especially this one. He'd wanted a jury of stable married men—they despised sex freaks and tended to be more protective of women than women were of themselves—but just about every husband in Big Horn County had been out calving or lambing or otherwise preoccupied.

So far, the only indication of this predominantly feminine jury's leanings had come when Story's faithful nurse Judy Gifford testified that in her heart she knew what went on in the examining room. The juror at the far end of the first row had shaped her lips into an exasperated "Oh, God damn!"

But what about the others?

Tharp still wondered if he'd weakened his witness list too much by dropping the McArthurs. Aletha Durtsche seemed strong till Aarestad tore into her on cross-examination. Dear old Emma Lu helped the state make a comeback, and so did Terri Timmons and Mae Fischer, but Emma McNeil's testimony proved weak. Several jurors had winced at Story's claim that she'd had a "venereal infection." Tharp was sure that the remark was hog-slop, as believable as earlier Story claims about "incest" in the Durtsche family. But did the jury know?

The doctor was a master slanderer—there was no doubt about that. With the aid of dubious medical records, he'd portrayed Wanda Hammond and Annella St. Thomas as liars. The Hammond chart showed insertion of an I.U.D., but Wanda swore up and down that she'd never even considered having one inserted. The St. Thomas chart showed post-rape visits on dates when Annella had been living in another state. Tharp wondered about the origins of the two charts; they hadn't shown up in the arrest-night sweep of Story's office. To the young prosecutor, the surprise exhibits seemed blatantly doctored. He thought he knew which doctor had done the job.

Tharp studied his notes till Story was sworn, then quickly forced him to admit that even by his own testimony he'd been alone with seven of the nine complainants and could have assaulted them "if you were so inclined." Then he turned to the subject of the bogus charts:

Q   Where were those charts the night your office was searched?
A   The safeguarding of the charts is not—that's delegated to other people. I have no idea.
Q   You have no idea where they were?
A   In the office. That's all I know. Someplace in the office.

Having sown some doubt, Tharp set about characterizing the "Lovell Medical Building" as a one-man pelvic mill:

Q   Will you find Hayla Farwell's chart there, please? . . . What is the first pelvic examination you ever gave her?
A   I believe it is June of 1967.
Q   The *first* pelvic examination, doctor?
A   Maybe I should take your chart apart.
Q   Take a look at December, 1962. . . . When is the first pelvic shown?
A   December 5, 1962.

Q . . . When is the next pelvic shown?

A Her next office visit. The seventeenth, I guess that is.

Q Then the next pelvic?

A Let's see. The next one is on February 20.

Q 1963?

A Yes.

Q Did you give her a pelvic on April 25, 1963?

A Yes. April 25.

Q Did you give her another pelvic May 4, 1963?

MR. AARESTAD I think I am going to object to this as irrelevant.

THE COURT What is the relevancy here, Counsel?

A Well, I want to ask him if he knows how many pelvics he gave her.

THE COURT All right. Overruled.

Q (By MR. THARP) Between 1962 and 1967, your last pelvic, how many pelvics did you give her? Any idea?

A I would have to count them up.

Q More than twenty-five be accurate? . . .

THE WITNESS I think twenty-nine is what I count, I believe.

The cross-examination slogged along as Story flipped slowly through his charts. He admitted that Julia Bradbury had had twelve or fifteen pelvic exams, Aletha Durtsche at least nineteen, Mae Fischer eleven. On the days specifically in question, the records showed that Aletha had complained of a cold, Emma Lu of a mole, others of various nongenital disorders. Tharp turned to the subject of Emma Briseno McNeil and her "venereal infection":

Q Now you stated that Mrs. McNeil had—what condition was it you described? . . . Pelvic inflammatory disease?

A . . . Yes, that's what I said.

Q Do the words "pelvic inflammatory disease" appear in the chart anywhere?

A No, they don't.

Q . . . There is no mention of pelvic inflammatory disease in these records, is there?

A Not—there is for me to see. I can see it, yes.

Q All right. Did you do any tests to determine that?

A Yes, I did.

Q Did she have some kind of a venereal disease?

A That was my diagnosis.

Q What kind?

A Do you want me to tell you what kind I diagnosed her as having?

Q Yes.

A I didn't put it on the chart. I protected her by not putting it on the chart.

Q Did you report this?

A If I can say one more—

Q No. Did you report this? Did you report the disease?

A No, I didn't.

Q Are you aware that you are supposed to report venereal diseases?

A Yes, I am aware of that.

Q You didn't report this, though?

A No, I didn't.

Q It does not appear on the chart, does it? Yes or no?

A To a doctor, yes. . . . A doctor who would read this would know what is going on.

As the cross-examination intensified, Story began drumming his fingernails lightly on the armrest of his chair. Tharp turned to another line of questioning, one which he'd prepared the night before with Dr. Rand Flory and two other local physicians:

Q . . . You did a pelvic on [Julia Bradbury] on that day?

A Yes, I did.

Q Did she ask you to do a pelvic?

A (looking at records) It doesn't really indicate. So often after—

Q Did she ask you? Do you recall her asking you to do a pelvic?

A I don't recall anything like that. That's been some time ago.

Q . . . What is a cystocele?

A It is a herniation of a bladder.

Q You are saying that was the reason for the so-called "stress incontinence" you talked about [in direct examination]?

A Yes.

Q Have you read any text on stress incontinence, Doctor?

A Have I read any text on it?

Q Lately.

A Oh, I'm not sure that I have recently.

Q Do you recognize any specific text as authoritative in gynecology?

A There are lots of texts. I have no specific one that I would name.

Q Would you consider a book called *Obstetrics and Gynecology* a clinical core of authority or at least reputable in the field? By Ralph M. Winn? He is a doctor.

A I have never read it. I don't know.

Q So you don't know?

A I have no idea.

Q Now you said she was having problems with stress incontinence?

A Yes.

Q   Would a cystocele cause that?

A   A cystourethalcele would, yes.

Q   We are talking about a cystocele here. That is what you have got in your records.

A   Yes. It is rather casually written.

Q   . . . Do you recognize that as authoritative, the text I just mentioned?

A   I am unfamiliar with that text.

Q   Are you familiar with any texts?

A   Well, I believe with some, yes.

Q   What?

A   Oh, Cecil and Conn.

Q   Would you recognize that as authoritative?

A   Oh, at least in some fields.

Q   What fields?

A   Oh, fields of medicine, internal medicine.

Q   What about gynecology? Do you recognize any text as authoritative in gynecology?

A   Well, I would—I'd have to use it and—

Q   You really don't know of any authority? That's what you are saying?

A   Oh, I have them in my library.

Story's voice remained calm, but his hands continued their little jerks and spasms as the prosecutor mentioned the times the doctor had ignored suggestions that he have a third party in the examining room. "How about Nelson St. Thomas?" Tharp said. "Are you aware of what he said in direct questioning?"

Story said, "Maybe you had better refresh my mind."

"Well, he said he turned you in to the Medical Board. Do you remember that?"

"Oh, yes, I do remember him saying that."

Medical Board proceedings were secret, and the St. Thomases had no proof that they'd written to the Board or received a reply. "Do you remember anything about that, the Medical Board?" Tharp asked offhandedly.

Story's fingernails clicked on the armrest as he said, "I have a letter, yes."

Tharp felt like grinning. Story had volunteered confidential information that couldn't have been elicited in any other way.

Q   And that was over a situation involving a pelvic exam, wasn't it?

A   Yes, it was.

Q   And you weren't concerned enough about that to get a third person in the room, were you?

A I think I understood the complaint.
Q But you didn't get a third person in the room thereafter, did you?
A I think I understood the complaint.

Tharp returned to the subject of Julia Bradbury, asking how long the elderly woman had been his patient before quitting him—"seventeen or eighteen years?"

"Maybe nearly that long," Story answered. "I can sure look it up and see for you."

"I don't want you to look it up, Doctor. Would you say seventeen or eighteen years?"

As Aarestad objected, the prosecutor became aware of muted catcalls from the Story side of the audience. They grew louder when he asked if Story had heard Mrs. Bradbury testify that she'd put a red "R" on her calendar.

"I was aware of that," Story said.

The judge slammed his gavel and said, "Ladies and gentlemen in the audience, I'm going to caution you against any outbursts or any snickering. If it continues I will have to clear the courtroom. I don't want to do that. But if it continues I *will* do that. Continue, Mr. Tharp."

Q Somebody might conclude that you did something improper in that examination, Doctor. Couldn't they?
MR. AARESTAD Objection! Argumentative and calls for speculation by this witness.
THE COURT Sustained.
Q . . . Did you ever single any of these women out?
A I beg your pardon?
Q Did you ever single any of these women out?
A I don't understand.
Q Well, because of a particular vulnerability, did you pay special attention to them?
MR. AARESTAD I am going to object. Counsel is trying to engage the witness in argument.
THE COURT Overruled.
THE WITNESS No.

Tharp expected a flat denial to his question about whether it was physically possible for a woman to be sexually assaulted during a pelvic exam. But Story surprised him again. "I would have to agree with

Dr. Flory," he answered, "that it would probably be possible." Tharp took the opportunity to underline the helplessness of the victims:

Q   It is a pretty vulnerable position up there, isn't it?
A   Vulnerable in several ways, yes.
Q   Hard to move. It wouldn't be easy to get down off that table, would it? If you needed to move suddenly?
A   I'm not sure.
Q   Have you ever been up there on that table?
A   No, I guess I haven't.
Q   What about the drape? These women have all testified that they couldn't see. There is a reason for that, isn't there?
A   They couldn't see, you mean?
Q   Yes.
A   You better—
Q   You don't know of any reason for that? Is that your testimony?
A   I don't understand your question.
Q   Is there a reason you draped the women in the way you did?
A   The way I do? Yes. I drape them for modesty and to cover them.
Q   How about so they can't see?
A   No. Untrue.

At three minutes to three, Tharp said he had no further questions and the judge declared a twenty-minute recess. On redirect examination, Aarestad set about repairing some of the damage:

Q   You indicated, Dr. Story, that you thought it was possible to have a sexual union on that table. Do you recall that testimony?
A   . . . Well, yes, words to that effect.
Q   Okay. Could you explain that, please?
A   Well, you would have to have, you know, a lot of cooperation to . . . We talked earlier about the vaginal inclination. It would take a lot of cooperation to have sex on the table.
Q   What is the vaginal inclination when a woman is on the pelvic or in the dorsal position?
A   If her knees are up, it is way up to thirty degrees or so. The higher the knees, the greater the angle.
Q   What if they are simply in the stirrups as in a normal pelvic exam?
A   Well, that increases the inclination up to closer to thirty degrees.
Q   And I assume you are familiar with the male anatomy?
A   Yes.
Q   Okay. Does the male anatomy point down at the direction of thirty degrees?
A   No.

On recross, Tharp asked, "You are not saying it is not impossible though, are you, Doctor?"

"To use the table for a place to have intercourse?"

"To insert a penis into a vagina with a woman lying on that table in the lithotomy position?"

"Without cooperation, yes—"

"How about by surprise?" Tharp interrupted.

"No, with cooperation."

Aarestad jumped up and said, "I would ask the witness be allowed to finish his answer before the next question is asked."

Story continued, "With an awful lot of cooperation it could be done."

Q (By Mr. Tharp) How about by surprise?
A That's not cooperation. I don't think so.
Q You are saying you could insert a speculum in there. Is that true?
A Yes.
Q You could insert fingers in there?
A Yes.
Q But you can't insert a penis?
A Not without cooperation. You couldn't insert a speculum without cooperation, I don't think.

Tharp pointed his tinted glasses at the witness box. "But the patient is draped as you have shown us?" he asked.

"Well," Story answered, "we are talking about with the knees up, aren't we?"

"Yes."

"That's difficult."

The prosecutor resisted the temptation to ask, How do you know it's difficult? *Have you tried?* But indirection was usually more effective. Juries liked to be treated as though they had reasoning powers of their own.

"All right," he said. "I have no further questions."

80

Experts

INSURANCEMAN CAL TAGGART, former Lovell mayor, flew up from his winter home in Sun City West, Arizona, to testify for his friend and personal physician. He called Dr. Story "honorable, honest, truthful" and said he'd never lied to him. "I have no qualms at all to stand up for Dr. Story."

Over objections from Aarestad, Tharp got the former state senator to admit that he'd interceded with the governor on Story's behalf.

Dr. Douglas Wrung, Story's friend and fellow churchman, sent embarrassed titters through the courtroom by testifying that a physician would have to have a twelve-inch penis to accomplish intercourse during a pelvic exam—"and I frankly don't know of any human being that has a penis that long."

On cross-examination, Tharp asked the physician to stand facing the head of the Ritter table. Over more defense objections, he instructed Wrung, "Could you touch the edge of the table with your clothes, please . . . ? Could you touch the foot pedal and raise that table to the level of your belt?"

Wrung complied.

"Thank you," the prosecutor said. "Now lower it to the level of your genitals, please. . . ." The table dropped into perfect alignment.

"And now could you stand there with your clothes touching the edge?" The jurors craned their necks to see. "Thank you. You can resume the witness stand."

Like several defense witnesses before him, Dr. Wrung denied writing a letter of support to the Lovell *Chronicle*. He explained that the letter had been written by his wife.

Just before 4 P.M., court was adjourned after the judge explained, "The Defense has indicated they have no more witnesses today. . . . There is a witness that will be flying in here and his arrival will be rather late, so we will start about ten."

That night, Marilyn Story attended a Bible Church prayer meeting for her husband and then wrote in her journal:

"Thursday, April 11, 1985: Today John is on the witness stand just about all day. Wayne said he did well. The prosecutor made him go through all the records and count the number of pelvics he gave. He took his time—Wayne liked that. He didn't get upset with Tharp even tho he had every reason to. Wayne had seriously warned him about that and prayed with him."

The delayed airborne witness turned out to be Dr. John E. Buster of Long Beach, California, a UCLA faculty member and board-certified obstetrician and gynecologist. Speaking slowly and distinctly, the expert witness gave a thirty-minute slide show describing the female organs and the proper technique of pelvic examinations.

Aarestad referred him to Story's medical records and asked if pelvics had appeared to be medically necessary on the days of the alleged assaults. Buster said yes. Speaking directly to the jury and sometimes smiling, he added that each of Hayla Farwell's twenty-nine examinations had been required by her condition, as had the many examinations of Wanda Hammond, Mae Fischer, Emma Lu Meeks and Emma McNeil.

On cross-examination, Tharp established that some of the records Dr. Buster had reviewed were incomplete and that he'd appeared as a defense witness in other criminal trials.

Q You are here as a consultant?
A Yes.
Q And I assume the defendant has paid your way?
A Of course.

Q   And he paid you a fee to be here today?

A   Of course he did. My time is valuable.

Q   But you are basing what you say today solely on your review of the records?

A   Yes.

Q   Okay. And you were not present at any time any of the complaints were alleged to have occurred?

A   No. I have never been here before.

On redirect, Aarestad countered, "Because you are being paid a consultant fee, Dr. Buster, would you come here and testify falsely?"

"No way."

"In respect to those specific dates and patients indicated by Counsel, does anything change your opinion that those examinations were justified?"

"No way."

The defense rested.

In the hall, Dr. Buster volunteered his opinion of the proceedings to reporter Catherine Warren of the Casper *Star-Tribune*. "Preposterous," he said. "A sham . . . obscenely stupid." The accusations, he said, were "patently stupid." He observed that "women are wonderful, but who in the world is going to do that in his office . . . where his activity is totally visible?" He said he'd agreed to testify only after Wayne Aarestad had verified that he sincerely believed Dr. Story was innocent.

Back in the courtroom, rebuttal witness Judi Cashel testified that a thorough search of the Lovell Medical Building on the night of Dr. Story's arrest had failed to produce the medical charts of Annella St. Thomas and Wanda Hammond.

Contractor Gerald Brinkeroff testified that he'd built the Story clinic and installed "privacy latches." He said that Dr. Story had wanted the doors rehung—for "more privacy, I suppose."

The judge recessed the day's proceedings at 11:30 A.M., and Wayne Aarestad confided to a reporter that "a conspiracy exists" to "drive Dr. Story out of town." He repeated that he was very happy with the jury.

On Monday, David Wilcock testified that Dr. Story had described his office procedures during interrogation and had denied that anyone ever suggested that he have a third person in the examining room.

Dr. Rand Flory, the young obstetrician and gynecologist from nearby Cody, repeated his contention that sexual intercourse was possible during a pelvic exam.

Q Why do you have that opinion, Doctor?

A Well, because when all this was going on, I had always assumed it would be possible, and so my wife and I went up to the office and tried it. It is rather, on my table—it is clumsy because I can't—I'm not the right height for my table, but it is a possible thing.

Q You don't have a table like this in your office?

A No, sir. I would assume it would be much easier on that because then I could adjust for the difference in height between me and my table.

Aarestad demanded that Flory's answer be stricken. "It is completely and totally unrelated to this case, and what the witness did with his wife has absolutely no bearing whatsoever on this particular table, these particular ladies and this particular circumstance."

"Overruled," Judge Hartman said. "His answer will stand." Aarestad declined to cross-examine.

Caroline Shotwell testified that Story's office procedures called for raising the lid on the garbage receptacle every night to "dry it out" and burning the contents in the incinerator in the morning. On cross-examination she admitted that she saw nothing unusual in the procedure.

After long wrangling, a Deaver woman was permitted to testify that Story had violated her. Then Wanda Hammond took the stand to deny the assertion that she'd had an I.U.D. installed. "I'm positive," she said.

Story was his own final witness on surrebuttal. Aarestad asked if there was any truth to the Deaver woman's story. "None whatsoever," he answered.

They were the last words of testimony. Just after 10:30 A.M. on Monday, April 15, two weeks after Judge Hartman had banged the case to life with his gavel, he gave the jurors the day off and suggested that they bring overnight bags the next day.

81

The Summing-Up

BY SUNRISE, a frieze of hopeful spectators waited under the pinkish tint of the county building's Grecian columns. Some blew on their hands or shuffled their feet. The temperature was expected to climb into the seventies later, but in the postdawn hours it was only a degree or two above freezing. A few of the curious carried Styrofoam cups from the restaurant down the block. There wasn't much talking. Feelings still ran high, and allegiances were better kept private. It would be time enough to take sides upstairs.

Everyone was seated, waiting for the judge and the lawyers to emerge from the back rooms, when Rex Nebel nudged his wife. Arden McArthur was about to make her first appearance of the trial. "She thinks she's a New York model," Cheri whispered.

The prominent Mormon woman wore a big hat and high boots. Before she found a seat in the left half of the spectator section, she whirled a cape over her shoulder and looked at the Story supporters. "Remember *101 Dalmatians*?" Rex said. "She thinks she's Cruella DeVille."

Dean McArthur had used every ounce of his authority as household leader to shelter her from the trial. "You don't want all the pointy fingers," he advised.

Of course Arden knew he was right. For months, the Story people had been tearing at her good name like woodpeckers. As fast as she tracked one rumor to its source and forced its originator to back down, another popped up. She realized that it would take a PR firm to put out the fire.

After the girls had brought their lawsuit and Story counterclaimed for $10 million, the harassment increased. A decent LDS woman couldn't repeat some of the words the callers used on the phone.

Now and then another victim had come forward to tell Arden her story, usually in strictest confidence. They thanked Arden for what she'd done but begged off active roles. Most were like the one who phoned and said that Story had abused her but "We don't want to take it any further. We can't afford to be sued."

"Land's sake," Arden had answered, "he can't sue you for something *he* did. It's just a tactic he's using." But the woman wouldn't give her name.

At the start of the trial, the ailing Dean had asked her to drive him to Kansas City to visit some favorite relatives. He'd been making trips like this lately—terminal trips, as though he knew his own timetable. Every night she called back home to Lovell for news of the trial. They returned the night before final arguments were scheduled, and she itched to go. She remembered the opposing lawyers in "Perry Mason," shaking their fingers at each other and hurling brilliant catchphrases as they argued on behalf of their clients.

"I'd rather you didn't go," Dean had said from the chair where he now spent hours every day, sucking in air a teaspoonful at a time.

"Dean," she'd said, "I've got to."

When Story turned from his seat to wave at his supporters, one of Arden's LDS seatmates remarked, "Well, he won't act like a tin god anymore."

Arden whispered, "He never did act like a tin one."

Another woman said she'd heard that Story's brother was drawing up charts to prove that the conspirators were related.

"If you go far enough back," Arden commented, "we probably are. Listen, let that guy alone and he'll do all your genealogies for you. I'm not very good at it myself."

Terry Tharp didn't believe in snake-oil oratory and doubted if he could bring it off if he tried. He was convinced that lawsuits were won by evidence, facts and trial prep—except, of course, on TV. A University of Wyoming law professor had said, "Keep it short. Then cut it in half." Tharp figured that any speech over thirty minutes wasn't worth the proverbial bucket of warm spit, at least to a Big Horn County jury. He knew these people; he'd grown up thirty miles south, raising sheep, alfalfa, beans, hay, and malt barley for Coors. He knew the locals. To some of them, "howdy" was a little long-winded.

There wasn't much left to say anyway. In two weeks of trial, every point had been made and remade ten times over. He'd seen jurors nodding off, and he'd had to fight sagging eyelids himself. He kidded his pretty wife that if he had to sit through one more lecture on female plumbing, he'd swear off sex forever.

The judge asked, "Mr. Tharp, are you ready for closing argument?"

"Yes, Your Honor. I am." He stepped to the front of the jury box and wondered why his bony knees weren't knocking. Some of Story's victims were in the audience, still pale and shaky. They would be marked for life. Sex criminals had that effect; they were the lowest order of life. He realized why he wasn't nervous. He had only so much space between his ears, and he couldn't be nervous and enraged at the same time.

"Ladies and gentlemen," he began, "since April third we have covered a lot of ground. . . . Lots of things have been tossed around and lots of things have been said. But I think this trial comes down to one basic question: who is telling the truth, these nine victims or the defendant? I think the reason for that is very simple. These are the only people in that exam room on the day these acts occurred. There was nobody else present."

He reminded the jurors that they weren't dealing with simple malpractice; "we are dealing with a crime: rape." He described these cases in short takes, a minute or so on each, emphasizing the common M.O. and circumstances, the women who'd gone in for colds and flu shots, their special vulnerabilities, the careful draping, the absence of a nurse, the odd remarks like "Didn't you know?" and "Can you take any more?"

He pointed to the exhibit table and picked his words carefully. "We have got the records. Now these records, as far as I'm concerned, are good for maybe a couple of things. They show the date of the visits. They show the last dates some of these women went to the defendant." He paused. "But I would ask you to scrutinize some of those records very carefully." The St. Thomas and Hammond charts hadn't appeared until the defense introduced them in court, he pointed out, nor had any defense witness explained where they'd been kept or why they hadn't been found earlier. "We never did hear a satisfactory answer to that question," he said.

He cautioned the jurors about pity. "[Story] presented his wife. Now she is not here because of what the victims did; she is here because of what the defendant did. You are not to feel sorry for him. What you owe him is fairness. You don't owe him pity.

"He presented two former nurses who actually worked in his office within the recent past. Examine their testimony carefully, because there was some difference between what one said were his office procedures and the other actually said. . . .

"What were the rest of the witnesses? They were character witnesses. Now these people saw the defendant in a setting, a certain setting—his public image. There wasn't one of them that was alone in the examining room with him when any of these assaults were committed. Not one!"

He turned to the medical experts. "Dr. Wrung has an obvious bias. He testified that it was physically impossible, but you saw him step to that table. You heard Dr. Flory's testimony. Dr. Buster had a lot of fine qualifications. He read the charts. But he never saw or talked with any of these victims. . . . He testified solely from paper. You can do anything you want with a pencil and a piece of paper. . . . With all due respect to his qualifications, he is a professional witness. He comes in, he testifies, he picks up his check and he leaves."

As for Story himself, "He skirted around the things that I, or I think anybody else, would reasonably want to hear. He was evasive on cross-examination. He could remember what he wanted to remember. The things that he didn't want to remember, he forgot. He tried to come across as a kind, caring physician, but yet he never cared enough to ask why Julia Bradbury, a patient for eighteen years, would quit him overnight. He never cared enough to ask—because he knew why."

He re-stated Story's three basic defenses: "He is a nice guy and he couldn't have done it. But if you don't believe that, it is physically impossible. And lastly, if you don't believe that, these women are all just mistaken. . . . I had a law school teacher who said in a criminal case if you have got more than two defenses, you don't really have any. And I think that's what we have got here. You have kind of got a grab bag, and that is what he is asking you to do—is grab."

He advised the jurors to take their common sense into the jury room. "You don't have to park it at the door. . . . There is only one verdict in light of the evidence and I think that is guilty. Thank you."

As he sat down, he looked at his watch. He'd spoken for twenty minutes. He wasn't worried about omissions. Since the burden of proof was on the state, courtroom rules permitted him to speak again at the end.

Wayne Aarestad stood up, smiled at the judge, and began with the gracious old legal formality, "May it please the Court and Counsel."

From his first words, the North Dakota lawyer seemed to be trying to take the jury into his confidence. "I believe that this case presents the starkest contrast between two sides . . . of any case that I have ever seen. Either Dr. Story is the most perverted sexual deviant physician probably to hit the face of the earth in years, if not for all times, or the State's case is completely and totally false and a fabrication."

In folksy tones, he agreed with Tharp; "you can't have it both ways. And I agree with him that either one side is telling the truth or the other side is."

He also agreed with the prosecutor about pity. "Mr. Tharp has asked that you not apply sympathy for Dr. Story into your consideration. We echo those sentiments. Dr. Story does not want your sympathy. He does not want your pity. He wants truth, because that is what is going to set him free."

The blond lawyer made a few eyes blink by admitting that his client was guilty—he paused for a few seconds—"guilty of practicing nineteenth-century medicine in the twentieth century. . . . His sin is failure to practice medicine with a law book in his pocket. He trusted his patients."

He called Story "patient-oriented to a fault." The women who'd had nine or ten pelvic exams, he said, had also had a total of anywhere from sixty to a hundred visits for "serious pelvic abdominal problems, longstanding." He warned against equating pelvic exams with guilt. "The only evidence that was presented in this stand was from Dr. Buster that testified that every single one of those pelvic examinations was justified."

He mentioned the "great disparity" in the complainants' descriptions of the exams. "In some cases . . . he, without advance warning and knowledge and while they were unsuspecting, inserted his penis in their vaginas. In other instances he seems not to care if they know or don't know. I mean he walks away and steps out alongside the examination table, pokes them in the breasts, allegedly—in one situation just standing for a minute or two—and exposes himself and then goes back in and incredibly enough reinserts his penis in a lady's vagina. Where is the consistency in that type of an M.O.?"

The jurors seemed to pay close attention as he alluded to a conspiracy defense. "Somebody either wants Dr. Story out of Lovell or wants him out of practice, but is out to get him. . . . Isn't Dr. Story, his family—aren't they victims if this whole thing is a hoax? Isn't he a victim? You can't just take and blindly accept and credit the testimony of those witnesses. . . . For a fleeting second, for a fleeting moment, they saw something that was flesh colored, this size, that size, whatever size. . . . That's what they saw. The rest, they offer up conclusions."

He took issue with Tharp's description of the three-pronged defense. "There are a lot of activities and actions and motions that are capable of being misconstrued in the course of pelvic exams, ins and outs and twists and arounds. We don't offer up a whole bunch of defenses to try to confuse anybody. Basically we only offer up one defense, and since I have been challenged to tell you what it is, I will. *He didn't do it!*"

A hum of agreement arose from the right side of the courtroom, and Aarestad waited for silence. Then he spoke of the jury's right to reject the total testimony of witnesses who lied on any point. He took issue with Terry Tharp's description of Story as evasive, but generously added, "Maybe he saw something I didn't see."

He reminded the jury that the state, in the county attorney's opening statement, had promised to call nurses, secretaries and receptionists who'd worked for Dr. Story, but instead "they offer you up Diana Harrison, a receptionist . . . and Caroline Shotwell, a non-medical-trained person who worked for him a couple of months more than a decade ago, whose daughter is one of the complainants. And they say these are our nurses, our secretaries and our receptionists. And I think you ought to hold them to that promise. *We* offered up the secretaries, receptionists and the nurses. And we didn't have to—the burden is not ours." He said the defense had presented "ten years of unbroken chain of testimony as to the consistency of his practice, his protocol, his procedures and everything."

Although he'd already talked five minutes longer than Tharp, Aarestad seemed to be holding the attention of the jury and the audience on both sides of the aisle. Reporters strained for usable quotes as he said, "What they would have you believe is that he walks into an examination room and sometime between when he hits that door and he hits between the legs, he has got this lust-obsessed act that he wants to perform on a patient. I don't think you can be that weird, that strange, and not have somebody notice it. Yet all the character evidence and testimony that came before this body was that he is a religious, devout, Christian believer. He has never had any problems in the past . . . none whatsoever."

He turned lightly sarcastic. "That's why I say he is an accomplished, successful deviate, because he fooled not only a wife of thirty-two years who works side by side with him in his office . . . but he also fooled his employees . . . the entire nursing staff at the North Big Horn County Hospital, director of personnel, hospital administrator, patients, and all the people that we put on that stand. And he fooled the public! I mean, this man is a genius if he can get by with that."

His deep voice became serious. "Every segment of society that he dealt with came in and delivered accolades of morality and truthfulness and the honorableness and the gentleness of this kind man. And offset with that, you have got these obscenities that the State offers up as to what went on in those examination rooms. That's why I say you can't have it both ways. You have got to find that this Dr. Story is demented in an unfathomable dimension in order to bring guilty verdicts through these bizarre allegations."

Tharp called out, "Your Honor, I am going to object to this line of argument. That's not part of the case."

"I believe that is correct, Counsel," the judge agreed.

Tharp said, "He is stating they have to find him demented."

Aarestad made a smooth retreat by reminding the jury that they could disregard his arguments if they were "inappropriate." Then he began his own victim-by-victim rundown, this time refuting each charge. He subtly discounted the state's expert witness. "Dr. Flory apparently had been in practice since he graduated in 1981. He apparently doesn't take very long on his pelvic exams. It doesn't seem to make much difference whether the women are subject to a particular physical problem or not, in respect to time. Weight doesn't seem to make any difference. Weigh that against the testimony of Dr. Buster, Dr. Wrung and Dr. Story. . . . Dr. Flory limits his practice to obstetrics and gynecology. He is not Board-certified but apparently it is an interest of his and he just limits his practice to it. . . . He tried it with his wife. I elected not to cross-examine him on that and I apologize for that, but I don't think that is terribly probative. At least he said it was difficult."

The defense lawyer walked over to a blackboard, smiled and said, "Now I'm gonna draw some pictures that if I caught my kids drawing, it would be a quick trip to the woodhouse." He sketched in an examination table and a patient in the lithotomy position, and pointed out that any sexual union would have to be "a long-range assault."

"The natural inclination of a woman's vaginal tract in this position is fifteen to thirty degrees in a downward area. . . . If you don't recall the testimony, at least rely then on some common sense and your own knowledge of the male anatomy that says that an erect penis points upwards, not down. Now when you weigh these two angles . . . what you will see is that they are ninety degrees off. So not only does this penis need to be rather lengthy . . . but it also has to have the capability of being converted from this angle to that angle. You would have to have some type of a U-joint or something like that in there to transfer that motion. *It is absurd.*"

And anyway, he said, sex isn't merely physical. "There is a mental component to an act of sexual intercourse, [but] where is the evidence of arousal? . . . Dr. Story is filling out the charts or doing some other medical procedure or working with the speculum, and almost coincidentally and at the same time with this act of lust-obsessed rape. How reasonable is that? . . . It is almost as if this male organ has a mind of its own. . . . It is as if it has the capability to almost strike at anytime, any place and anywhere, up here, down there, in the trousers here, out of the trousers here. . . ."

He brought Tharp to his feet again by saying, "Not one of these women caused him to fail in the sense of kicking him away or—"

"I object to that," the prosecutor called out. "That is a misstatement of the testimony."

"Well," Aarestad said, "I don't believe anybody did kick him away."

"Nobody kicked him away," Tharp said, "but there was testimony that they tried to get away from him."

Judge Hartman said, "I believe Mr. Tharp is correct, Mr. Aarestad."

This time, the defense attorney refused to back down, and the judge allowed him to continue along the same lines. "There is no testimony that any of them ran out into the hallway or anterooms. . . . Their reactions, as we have indicated, are remarkably similar—paralyzed with fear—went outside of the hallway. Several feet away are employees, perhaps a wife, patients. It isn't the situation where you are five miles out of town in a pickup or car, alone with an assailant with a weapon. . . . There wasn't even any threatening language."

The essence of rape, he noted, is "outrage," and yet one of the women "stops at the front desk and pays a bill. Some come back, continue to use him as their physician." At the time of the incidents, they didn't trust the legal environment "because who would believe them . . . [and yet] years later they all seem to not have that problem anymore, and now they trust the legal environment. It miraculously disappeared in each one of their cases. It will help explain why they are here. In that respect, their numbers defeat them."

He apologized for digressing and suggested that it might be time to break for lunch. It was five to twelve. The judge recessed the proceedings till one thirty.

The Nebels were exultant. "Did you see the jurors' faces?" Rex asked his wife during the break.

"It was like a great sermon," Cheri said. "Spellbinding." They agreed that Dr. Story had been wise to insist on a Christian lawyer.

"Wayne was so slow and deliberate," Rex said. "He came across as a nice guy trying to help out. It was a clinic on public speaking."

They agreed that Terry Tharp had been knocked from the box.

Meg McArthur Anderson still felt anxious after her sixteen-mile round trip to Greybull for lunch. The outside temperature was in the mid-seventies, and the courthouse air was warm and thick from body heat. Everything seemed so overpowering—the gloomy chamber in its dark wood tones, the judge in black, the defendant looking so eerie and detached, the blond lawyer smiling and trying to portray his client as another Jonas Salk.

All morning long, Meg had worried about the spectators on the right side of the aisle. The Story people stared, wisecracked, groaned when they heard testimony they didn't like. Several had giggled when the lawyer sarcastically referred to Story as "an accomplished, successful deviate." Meg didn't think it was funny. It was the tragic truth.

She walked into the courtroom after lunch and found that Molly Pratt and other Story supporters had deliberately moved into the left-side seats where she'd been sitting with her mother and Pat Wiseman, Dorothy Brinkerhoff and Terri Timmons. She didn't know how to react to the territorial intrusion. Was it a deliberate challenge or a mistake?

Molly was a lawman's wife, a former schoolmate, and once a good customer of the Kids Are Special shop. During a recess she'd been heard to joke about shoving Judi Cashel down the stairs.

My lands, Meg said to herself, these people scare me spitless.

As she took a seat next to Molly and the other supporters, she heard. "Oh, my Gawddddddd?" . . . "Lookee who's here!" . . . "Can you believe the *nerve*?" The voices were just audible.

She thought, I'm not gonna move. I have a little bit of pride.

Her mother and the others walked in a few minutes later and she joined them in the next row.

"For the record," the judge announced, "the Court notes the presence of the entire jury in the jury box. Mr. Aarestad, you may continue."

The lawyer returned to the witness-by-witness refutations that he'd interrupted before, but now his pace was markedly faster. ". . . And I would like to just quickly take you through that commencing with Terri Timmons who we have already briefly looked at. She claims that she was raped on April 17, 1968. Again, the chart shows no pelvic exam for that day. She said she had a pelvic exam for 1968. As a matter of fact, you will find one pelvic exam June 5, 1970. It says RV. It is a rectal-vaginal exam. . . ."

He quickly switched to Aletha Durtsche, then to Emma Lu Meeks. "She tells nobody, according to her testimony, until all of this comes out. Then she tells her good friend and neighbor, Julia Bradbury, who both of them state that they do everything together. And I think that when we take a look at both of them coming forward in this situation and testifying to the commonality of a sexual assault, they give new meaning to the word 'together' . . ."

He flicked a glance at his watch and turned to the subject of Hayla Farwell. Dr. Story looked bored. His supporters frowned and whispered. The judge studied the ceiling. The lawyer's words flew around the courtroom but seemed to land nowhere: ". . . She doesn't know if it is circumcised or uncircumcised, how long it is. She sees no pubic hairs. Doesn't recall seeing any underwear. . . ." After the ecclesiastical cadences of the morning, he'd seemingly turned to fragments. No one could understand.

He turned quickly to the desirability of the victims as sex partners. Emma McNeil, he insisted, had been hospitalized for VD. "You have to ask yourself how reasonable or likely it is that a rapist is going to pick as his target somebody with a communicable disease. . . . Again, she is a rather large lady. . . ."

When he claimed that Mae Fischer had a history of bladder problems, Tharp jumped up and said, "There is no evidence of bladder problems in the record."

The judge told the jurors that they could look at the medical records and make their own determination. He'd hardly completed his ruling before Aarestad hurried on. "She admits, and the charts indicate, that she is allergic to K-Y jelly as well as Phisohex. Again, how likely would a person like that be for a victim of a sexual assault since obviously you are going to have some problems with insertion? . . ."

He discussed Annella St. Thomas. "Again, she can't tell if he is circumcised or not circumcised. . . . No, she just passively lies there and waits for him to come back in. Again, she is Aletha Durtsche's cousin. And I suggest to you that you might consider the blood-is-thicker-than-water issue. . . ."

He had just started on Wanda Hammond when one of the jurors fell asleep. She blinked her eyes open during another objection from Tharp, then dropped off again.

Both sides seemed relieved when the defense lawyer said that Julia Bradbury was "the last one that I want to cover with you." He noted the elderly woman's long-standing bladder problems, the fact that she'd neither seen Story's penis nor complained to the nurse afterward. "Basically she has no concept or recollection of time. Never saw any instruments in the room. Confirms her relationship with Emma Meeks. Again, has some discussion with this same Diana Harrison. . . ."

Story rubbed his eyes and yawned. The judge covered his mouth and turned away. Then Aarestad regained everyone's attention. "Again," he said, still speaking of Julia Bradbury, "looking at her physical condition, we see that she has stress incontinence. . . . How reasonable is it that she would be a victim of a sexual assault? A lady who, to be quite frank with you, has a high chance of urinating on you and making a very messy situation out of you—you know, having to walk out, see other patients, be around."

Knuckles flew to mouths as he said, "It just becomes completely and totally absurd . . . bizarre."

Terry Tharp scribbled on his notepad.

Aarestad looked at his watch again and softened his tone to discuss Marilyn Story. "She is the wife and married for thirty-two years. And I think a wife gets to know her husband during that period of time. And I don't think she would be in this courtroom if he was the deviant that the State would have you believe. She was always there. He would have to have fooled her.

"I believe that women, especially wives, are given a God-given intuition really to know what their husbands are up to . . . She testified they had a good marriage, a good sexual relationship. He is anything but crude, off-colored. . . . She had constant access to his exam rooms. She was there full-time for sixteen years, never found a door locked. Kept an eye on him. . . ."

The lawyer discussed the other supportive witnesses—Joe Brown, the nursing Giffords and Verda Croft, Barbara Shumway—and as he spoke, his sentences became even choppier, telegraphic. "Imogene Hansen worked in his office. . . . Same story. No patient complaint. Uses him as her own physician. No jokes. All business. Totally professional. A completely total moral man. Nothing suspicious ever occurring. Known him for over twenty years."

He was still describing character witnesses in short bursts when Hartman interrupted, "Counsel, you have two minutes left."

Aarestad thanked the judge and rushed on. "Every indication is that he is a straight arrow, about as straight an arrow as you can find. Seems to have three interests in life: his family, his medical practice, and his relationship with God. He is a religious, devout individual. He answered a call to come to Lovell twenty-seven years ago. He raised his family; he has always been here."

He asked the jury not to buy "this obscene case that the State is putting on. Think it through. Weigh it. Come up with your own concept of truth. . . . I reiterate: he either did it or didn't do it. He either did all of them or he did none of them. And I ask that you bring in on his behalf a not guilty verdict as to each and every count. . . . And may God bless you, and may you have wisdom."

He had talked for 165 minutes in two completely opposite styles. The courtroom buzzed.

Terry Tharp's forehead was almost as red as his hair as he stood up for the last word. "Ladies and gentlemen," he said in a voice that snapped like a circus whip, "I won't keep you much longer. . . . First of all, I want to apologize for objecting during Mr. Aarestad's final argument. It's not often that I do that. I want to take this opportunity to counter a few things . . . the cheap shots, the insinuations, the distortions and misstatements made in that final argument.

"That drawing that you saw up there that he drew—that was distortion number one. That was Mr. Aarestad's concept of the pelvic examination. That wasn't a doctor's concept of the pelvic examination. You saw Dr. Flory position the skeleton. . . .

"The second thing he wants you to do, he wants you to nitpick your way to reasonable doubt. For example, if some dark night you see a cat cross the street ahead of you, you know it is a cat. You might not know what color it is, whether it is black, brown, gray, spotted, whatever. You might not know whether it is a tomcat or a she cat, a fat cat or a skinny cat, but you know it is a cat. Now Mr. Aarestad is going to say because we don't know whether it is a tomcat or she cat that there is reasonable doubt that it in fact was a cat. . . ."

The prosecutor noted that the defense had failed to address one subject: "Why would nine women come in here and accuse somebody of something like this when they stand to gain absolutely nothing? *Nothing.* On the other hand, what does the Defendant have to lose? *Everything!* Consider that when you consider the merits of the charges."

He said the victims had come forward when they'd realized that at last something was going to be done on their behalf. One had waited for eighteen years. "LaMar Averett didn't believe them. Joe Brown doesn't believe them. Cal Taggart doesn't believe them. The Wyoming State Medical Board didn't believe them in 1972. . . . It took a lot of courage for them to get up on that witness stand. Don't let anybody ever tell you that it didn't. It takes a lot of courage to make these kinds of accusations and get up on the witness stand and then go deliver mail to every house in town. . . . It takes courage because they have accused an important man. They have accused somebody with following."

His voice rose as he spoke in defense of his witnesses and their reputations. He noted that there was no indication in any of the medical records that Emma McNeil had had VD, nor had anyone other than Story ever made such a claim. Tharp called it "a cheap shot."

"I think it is also a cheap shot to make the reference to Julia

Bradbury that was made," he went on. "And then you wonder—then he gets up here and tries to tell you that these women are lying." He ran a hand through his thin hair and frowned in Story's direction.

"Just remember one thing as you go back in there," he said, turning back toward the jurors. "Be very careful, *very* careful, of the words of anybody who find themselves in a perilous position. Thank you."

The judge ordered the jurors to remain together and communicate only with the bailiffs. They were not to discuss the case with outsiders or accept "any other materials such as dictionaries, books or newspapers." He instructed the audience to stand while the jury was escorted out. It was 2:25 P.M.

When the last juror had filed out of sight, the florist Beverly Moody said in a loud voice, "What is the name for Terry Tharp? *Snake?*" The Nebels and other Story supporters rushed to the defense table.

Aarestad was talking to his client. ". . . So when I came back from lunch, the judge asked how much more time I needed. I said, 'An hour and a half or two hours.' He said, 'You got forty-five minutes.' It threw me out of my outline. I couldn't use my notes. I had to remember the salient points off the top of my head. Did I sound disjunctive?"

Rex Nebel was livid. "I watched the judge all day. He kept studying the jurors' faces. You were going too good, Wayne. That's why he shut you down."

The lawyer agreed. From the first witness to the last, the Story people had felt that the judge was proprosecution, that he'd treated the accusers like favorite daughters and vetoed defense objections willy-nilly. "Don't worry," the blond lawyer told the vocal group. "We're still on the right side. God won't let us lose this thing." Dr. Story wore the same small smile that he'd worn from the beginning.

The Reverend Ken Buttermore rallied two dozen of the faithful in the tree-shaded park next to the county building. "We'll pray here till the verdict comes in," he suggested. "Then we'll drive back to the church and offer thanks."

The anticipated acquittal hadn't come in by sundown, so the members drove north to the Lovell Bible Church to continue their prayers. At 10:40 P.M., word came by telephone that the jury had given up for the night and planned to return Wednesday morning. The prayers sailed upward till midnight.

Just before she turned in, Marilyn Story wrote in her journal, "It seems at every turn we get stopped." She was baffled by the way Judge Hartman had cut Wayne off. Wasn't it bad enough that John had to defend himself against satanic liars? The least an innocent man deserved was a fair trial.

82

Judgment

ON WEDNESDAY the jurors filed into the courtroom three times without a verdict. They kept wanting to look at the Ritter table, feel it, measure it, pull the stirrups up and down, even lie on it. The county building had turned from stuffy warm to hot; between morning and afternoon the outside temperature had climbed fifty degrees to an unseasonal 83. No one knew how to interpret the repeated inspections of the table.

Ken Buttermore sat on the hard wooden seat outside the courtroom, his large head bowed. He prayed that the jury lift the burden from Marilyn, her daughters Susan and Linda, and especially Elder Story. The pastor thanked God for giving him this opportunity to be of comfort to a suffering Christian family and for the honor of leading their church. There were bigger, tonier congregations and more prestigious pulpits, but none where the Lord's work was more appreciated or a preacher more rewarded with respect and love.

As he sat silently with his eyes half closed, reporters paced the hall and made strident phone calls from the clerk's office. "Naw, nothing yet," he heard them bark. The pastor had to draw on deep reserves of Christian charity to love these children of God. They'd written against Elder Story from the beginning. The busiest was Catherine Warren, a small-boned young woman who churned out daily articles for the Casper *Star-Tribune*. Just a few days before, she'd asked the Nebels to escort her to Bible Church services so she could write a feature article. Everyone knew what she was looking for: "smuts and gunk," as Buttermore expressed it. "She thought we were a bunch of freakos." He'd hammered the Book of Numbers at her and didn't utter a word about the case.

At 7 P.M. the jurors sent out a note that they intended to work late. Three hours later Big Horn deputies chauffeured them to a motel. Over two days they'd deliberated fifteen and a half hours. There were no hints that they were nearing agreement.

Before he went to bed, Terry Tharp drank some tea and tried to stay calm, but he kept remembering Henry Two Crows, a hulking Sioux who'd been charged with beating a hobo to death in Greybull. Tharp's fifth grade class had made a field trip to Basin to watch the trial, and he could still recall how impressed he'd been by the court-appointed defense attorney, Jim Sperry. But right now he wished he could get that old case out of his mind. Henry Two Crows had been acquitted.

On Thursday, the third day of deliberations, Rex and Cheri Nebel waited all day by the phone. At 6 P.M. it rang. "They've got a verdict," Marilyn told them in a quivering voice. She asked them to phone the others.

Soon a seventeen-car caravan was moving south toward Basin, with Doc in the lead in his old Chrysler sedan. Jan Hillman followed in her green two-door Thunderbird, with Rex sitting in front and his wife in back.

Cheri had forebodings. "It's no good, guys," she said as they drove past the entrance to the gypsum plant. "They're gonna find him guilty."

Rex told her to cool it. Jan said there wasn't a chance of conviction— the jury would have returned the acquittal three days ago but it wanted to look conscientious. At worst there would be a mistrial, in which case they would troop back to court and do it over again.

Doc drove at a funereal pace, even on the five-mile stretch of arrow-straight road across the desert floor. The orange ball of the sun touched the tips of the Rockies as they crossed the Greybull River and continued south toward Basin. "This isn't gonna be good," Cheri repeated. "I've got a feeling of impending doom."

Rex said, "The only problem we'll have is getting him home alive."
He'd stashed two loaded .44s in Jan's glove box but didn't intend to
take them inside the courtroom. He'd gone armed ever since a male
voice had threatened Cheri on the phone. Other callers had promised to
rape Dr. Wrung's daughter after he testified. The hotheads were
everywhere.

Deputy Sheriff Jack Doolan, armed and uniformed, met the caravan
in the parking lot and escorted Doc, Marilyn, their older daughter
Susan, and Wayne Aarestad through the side door. Rex had arranged
for Doc to be protected after the verdict was read. The Story people
planned to double back to the Lovell Bible Church for prayers and
exultation. A full house was expected.

When they entered the courtroom, they saw that the accusers' side
was almost vacant. "Those turkeys were tipped off to the verdict," Rex
whispered.

"Is that a good sign for us?" Cheri asked.

"Sure. Wouldn't they be here if they'd won?"

Cheri wasn't so sure. The light in the windows had changed to a
sickly yellow green. She wondered if it was the final rays of the afternoon sun sifting through the trees or a trick of her imagination. It
looked so . . . bilious. More supporters filed in, smiling and humming
hymns. She wished she didn't feel so bad.

"Okay," the judge said to the group in his chamber. "You're all armed,
right?"

Judi Cashel touched the small of her back, where her .380 five-shot
revolver pressed against her business-suit jacket. It was a popgun,
barely effective against ground squirrels, but she'd left her regular
weapon home in Casper.

Judge Hartman's chambers were crowded with lawmen, mostly Big
Horn County deputies, and the unrobed judge was telling them how to
deploy.

Judi had been down the street at the restaurant with Dave Wilcock
and Terry Tharp and a few others when the call had come in. Like most
of the others, she'd already concluded that the jury would hang and that
would be the end of it. Everyone was convinced that the victims would
refuse to testify at a second trial. Tonight most of them were attending
their regular support group meeting up in Lovell. Judi wondered if she
should alert them by phone when the verdict came in. If Story were

cleared, they'd be more upset than ever. But if he were found guilty—well, some of his supporters were dangerous, and it might be wise for the victims to drive straight home.

The shirt-sleeved judge was saying. "The jurors from the north end have requested armed escorts home." Judi's heart leaped. She thought, The jury's certainly not afraid of our side. We're not the ones who've been frothing at the mouth. Why are they asking for protection? She tried not to get her hopes up.

As she took her assigned position in the rear of the courtroom, she felt the hostile stares. Every seat on the right was taken, but the left was empty except for social workers and a few unknowns.

The jurors trooped into their box. Most of the ten women and two men looked haggard. Judi's ears picked up an undercurrent of sound from the right side of the aisle and realized that the Story people were humming a hymn.

"Good evening," Judge Hartman said calmly. "Please be seated." She wondered how he could sound so cool. In chambers, she'd watched him slip a pistol under his robes. "Ladies and gentlemen of the jury," he said, "have you elected a foreman or reached a verdict in this matter?"

The courtroom was silent as one of the women handed a slip of paper to clerk Bernice Argento. She passed it up to Judge Hartman, who perused it without changing expression, handed it back and said, "I would ask that the defendant please stand at this time while the clerk reads the verdict."

Judi watched as Story stood up. He looked so tiny. He claimed to be five-six, but when she'd stood next to him he hadn't looked much taller than her own five-two. She wondered if his runtiness had helped to fuel his anger and his crimes. Men had raped for stranger reasons.

The clerk's voice barely carried to the rear of the room. Judi caught the name "Durtsche" and then . . . "not guilty." She began to feel sick. Get it together, she told herself. No matter what happens, you're gonna walk out of here with your head held high.

Then one word soared above the others. There was no mistaking it. She heard it several more times before the wailing began.

At first, Rex Nebel wanted to fall to his knees in praise of God, but when the clerk came to the Emma Lu Meeks assault count and called out "guilty," he felt as if he'd been in another motorcycle crash. He heard Doc say a soft, "Oh, no," and watched as his small shoulders seemed to sag. Rex wanted to vault over the rail and drag him away. A few seats away, Marilyn and Susan embraced and cried.

He barely heard the remaining verdicts: guilty of first-degree rape against Mae Fischer and Terri Timmons, guilty of assault and battery with intent to commit rape against Wanda Hammond, Hayla Farwell and Annella St. Thomas, not guilty in the cases of Julia Bradbury and Emma McNeil.

The judge made Doc stand up again, and Wayne stood with him. "John Story," he said, "based on the verdict of guilty of these counts in this matter at this time, it is the order of this Court that you be taken to the Wyoming State Hospital in Evanston, Wyoming, and there be given a mental and physical examination by two disinterested and reputable and legally qualified physicians, one of whom shall be an expert in the field of psychology. . . ."

He ordered Doc jailed pending a presentencing investigation, and instructed the spectators to remain in place for five minutes "until Mr. Story has been removed from the courtroom."

Rex wished he could get his hands around the judge's neck. "*Mister* Story." What stupidity! All the kangaroo courts in the world couldn't change Doc into a mister.

Cheri Nebel shuffled toward the front of the courtroom like a sleepwalker. A red-faced Wayne Aarestad was leaning forward, his head down, his palms flat on the tabletop. He seemed compressed, squeezed, like a bull in a chute. His clear blue eyes looked flat and dazed. As far as Cheri could see, he wasn't even breathing.

Marilyn hugged Doc, then Cheri. "Justice?" Marilyn asked in a choking voice. "Where's justice?"

Doc managed a faint smile as one of his patients pinned a flower on his gray suit.

Rex held himself together till the last deputy had left the courtroom. The other spectators milled around, looking confused, forlorn. He opened the gate and marched up to the judge's bench. "The only rape that's happened in this county," he yelled, "is right here in this courtroom!" He spat a wad of Skol across the polished wood.

"Look at this!" he yelled, pointing to the left side of the courtroom. "Empty! Doesn't that tell you people anything?"

He stomped the floor and kicked the air. The judge was gone, but the clerk backed away and the court reporter grabbed for his machine. "This is a travesty of justice!" Rex called out.

He turned to the press row and said, "Can't you guys see what happened here?"

The journalists looked cowed. *"You!"* he snapped at a male reporter. "You had your nose in a slant from the first day! Wherever that Casper paper pointed, you stuck your nose in the same shit and went right with it."

Out of the corner of his eye he saw a TV reporter hugging the wall. The look in her eyes made him feel better.

Then he saw Jan Hillman holding her oversize glasses and rubbing her eyes. She'd been Doc's most effective defender. While others were wringing their hands, Jan and her mother had been risking their necks for Doc. Rex hated to watch this strong woman cry.

Someone took his arm and steered him into the hall. He felt as though he'd let down his church and his friends and his principles. He wished he could take Doc's place in the cell tonight. Behind him in the courtroom, a voice moaned in prayer.

Impromptu press conferences broke out. The Reverend Ken Buttermore said, "When all's said and done, God will get the glory, you watch. Lovell hasn't seen anything yet."

Wayne Aarestad told a reporter, "It was completely unexpected, and we will appeal." He said he doubted that his client would ever see the inside of a penitentiary.

Terry Tharp praised the jurors for having "a lot of guts."

Joe Brown asked someone a question and was referred to the prosecutor, standing nearby. "I won't talk to that man," the hospital manager said.

Cheri Nebel stumbled out on the front lawn to clear the stench of corruption from her nose. A cast-iron sky seemed to push down and flatten the unjust little town. Peaks and valleys had vanished for the night. Just as Marilyn walked through the side door, a meteor flashed across the Big Horns. For three or four seconds its phosphorescent tail lit up the ridge. To Cheri it had the same sinister quality as the bilious light in the courtroom.

"If Satan had fireworks," she said to her dear suffering friend, "they'd look like that."

"What a terrible blow!" Marilyn wrote in her journal. "We are all in total shock. None of the accusers were there which proves they knew what the verdict was before we did, AGAIN! Lord, what is your plan?"

83

Fallout

THE NEXT MORNING, Terri Timmons asked Loyd for the morning paper. The last word the previous night had been a brief call to the support group from the Lovell P.D., reporting that Story had been found guilty on some counts but not all. She'd gone to sleep convinced that her case was a loser.

Loyd perused the Friday paper and broke into a big smile. "There were only two guilties on forcible rape," he told her. "You and Mae. The rest were assault and stuff like that."

Terri started crying. "They believed me!" she said. "I can't believe it. *They believed me!*" It seemed the biggest miracle of all. She wasn't accustomed to being listened to, let alone believed. Loyd held her close and stroked her gypsy shag.

When she calmed down, they had a little talk and decided it might be wise to keep the kids home for a while.

Aletha Durtsche had mixed feelings about the not-guilty verdict on her count. She kept telling herself that she'd helped accomplish the important aim: an evil man was going to prison.

When her children's school called late in the morning, she had an idea what it was about. In the last few days, some of the Story people had turned vicious. Diana Harrison's daughter had gone home after one of her schoolmates said, "Your mother's a sperm-sniffer!" and others chanted the ugly word. There'd been a few fights, plus some pushing and shoving.

This morning the school reported that the Durtsche child wasn't seriously injured. She'd been hit over the head with a book, then flung down a staircase. Mike brought her home and they decided to keep her out for a few days.

One of Wanda Hammond's first checkout customers was the florist, Beverly Moody. The poor woman looked as though she'd cried all night. Wanda thought, Why can't she just accept the truth so we can be friends again?

"Wanda," the sturdily built woman muttered, "one of these days you're gonna pay for what you done. The Lord is gonna take care of Doc and you're gonna be reliable for the rest of your life."

Wanda swiped at the "total" key and missed. "Yes, I know," she said as she wiped her eyes with her sleeve. "The Lord'll take care of him."

When her shift ended, she rushed down Main Street to keep an appointment with Bishop Hawley in his office. She wanted someone in her church to confirm that she wasn't an evil person.

Bob Hawley was the swimming pool janitor at the school and popular with everyone. "Wanda," he said, "you did no wrong. Don't let those people bother you." The little round woman thought, Why, those are the only kind words I've heard!

Arden McArthur fed her two remaining schoolboys and told them to wait in front on their bikes. She'd already discussed the verdict with Meg and Minda. "He tightened the noose around his own neck," Arden told them. "Remember how we just wanted him helped? And he wouldn't admit he needed it?" The three McArthur women had agreed that true judgment would come later, not only for Story but for everyone.

When Mel and Marc were ready, Arden climbed on her bike and rode majestically ahead of them toward school. A driver swerved close and raised his finger. You just go right ahead, mister, she said under her breath. That's what I'm here for.

———

At noon, Rex Nebel still paced his yard. He'd been watching the highway, looking for the accusers or anyone else who'd spoken against Doc. Tears wet his beard. He and Cheri had cried all night, and he wasn't a man who cried.

When he recognized Gerald Brinkerhoff's truck, he ran out on the shoulder and shook his fist. "Pull over here!" he yelled. "I want to talk to you!"

The pickup sped past. "Hey, come back!" Rex yelled. *"Hey!"* He kicked a fence post. He wanted to beat somebody to death.

A few hours later, the phone rang in the pastor's study at the Lovell Bible Church. The caller was Deputy Sheriff Billy Joe Dobbs, and he needed to see Ken Buttermore right now.

At the sheriff's substation, Dobbs began, "I don't know quite how to tell you this."

"Let me have it," the preacher said. He was a former railroad worker, broad-shouldered and hard to intimidate.

"The sheriff says I'm to inform you and Rex Nebel and Joe Brown that you've been deemed potentially dangerous persons. He says if anything happens to any of these victims, you'll be in the same situation as Doc Story."

"Let me get this straight," the preacher said with less reticence than the lawman. "Are you telling me that without any witnesses, without any evidence, you'll throw me in jail?"

"I'm only telling you what I was told."

Buttermore left shaking his head. Later he learned that someone had called Mae Fischer at three in the morning and said, "This is Ken Buttermore. I'm gonna get you."

He didn't like this sort of nastiness one bit. He had a long talk with the editor of the *Chronicle* and was pleased to see some of his thoughts printed in the next edition. He was quoted as saying, "Don't get into hatred, backbiting, and all that stuff. It doesn't help." The article noted that he didn't condone threatening phone calls and certainly didn't make them. "If you talk to someone, be up front with them," he was quoted. "None of this behind the back stuff. That's not Christianity. I've been accused of doing it, and it's a blatant lie. . . . I want to work within the judicial system, not on the side. I respect the laws of the land. I don't want us to go to anarchy. Adults shouldn't revert to tantrums. . . . I'm not content with him being in jail, and I'll do everything in legal means to bring that right."

The young preacher disputed the easy claim that the Mormons were out to destroy the Lovell Bible Church, and he put in a word for his own parishioners. "We're not a bunch of idiots," he said.

The florist Beverly Moody swore to fight side by side with her pastor till Elder Story returned in glory. He'd been convicted only because he'd chosen to emulate Christ and follow the path of nonresistance. "Doc knows these women are sick," she explained. "That's why he didn't fight harder against 'em. He's been doctorin' 'em all their lives. Why would he want to hurt 'em?"

She admitted that there was no tangible evidence behind her belief. "*I just know.* You can't be around Doc and not know. If a man's gonna do some bizarre thing, you'd get a hint of it. You could look back and think of some strange incidents. But there was never! Doc is a rare breed of man that really cares about women's feelings."

When anti-Story people came into her shop, she unhesitatingly took them on. She landed on a Mormon customer who made the mistake of asking, "If he was so innocent, why wouldn't he let a nurse in the room?"

"Why should he?" Bev snapped back. "Because you stupid people told him to? Listen, I don't want a nurse in the room during a pelvic. Especially in a little town. I mean, you have that nurse in there and you're a little overweight like I am—I don't want some nurse looking me over and then going up and down the street and telling what I look like. Or have one standing there while I'm answering some of Doc's questions or discussing a personal matter with him."

The accusers and their backers, she decided, were just too danged ornery to understand a man like Doc and his ways.

84

Le Déluge

JAN HILLMAN was afraid she'd booked too small a meeting place. She and Story's neighbor, realtor Wes Meeker, had had only a few days to spread the word, and yet the Fire Hall was near bursting with Story supporters. She looked into the crowd and saw the Nebels, the Moodys, Tom and Kay Holm, city officials, bankers, nurses, businessmen, several doctors including Douglas Wrung, farmers, mineral workers, even relatives of the victims. Every religion in town was represented, every age from diapered babies to a man using a walker.

Jan usually felt faint at the sight of any audience too big for a row of bar stools, but she found herself calling the meeting to order with the élan of an auctioneer. When the last preliminary chatter died away, she cried out, "An innocent man has been put in prison!"

The audience yelled agreement. She reminded her friends that public pressure was important—"Doc could get bail or he could sit in jail. He could be sentenced to life in prison or walk out of court on probation. We can have an impact on that. Let Judge Hartman know that Doc Story doesn't stand alone." She closed her introductory remarks with one of her late father's favorite quotes: "All that is necessary for evil to prevail is for good people to do nothing."

The group was so unified that all business was concluded in less than an hour. Jan was elected chairman of the Dr. Story Defense Committee, which included among its charter members the Lovell city manager, Bob Richardson. Their only aim, Jan explained to a newspaper reporter, was "justice for Doc."

She went to work with the boundless energy she'd always reserved for the underdog. Within a few days, an ad appeared in the *Chronicle*.

> Contributions to the Dr. Story Defense Fund can be deposited in an account at Lovell National Bank or First National Bank of Lovell. Jan Hillman, chairman.

Two thousand dollars arrived almost overnight. Those short on cash pledged future payments. Farmers promised crop-shares and livestock, and townspeople offered to put up the deeds to their homes to get Doc out on bond.

Jan convinced Rex Nebel to channel his rage into a series of public pronouncements as incendiary as the M-80s he sold at his fireworks stand. More money flowed into the Defense Committee account as his polemics began appearing in Wyoming newspapers, sometimes in over-size type. He railed about "filthy gossip," "sleazy slandering," "a whispering campaign that grew to true conspiracy" and "a clear cut case of religious persecution." The trial, he wrote, had been "a parody." The prosecutor was a "rookie" who was "carried" through the trial by an "inexperienced" judge. As a former deputy and undersheriff, Rex explained that he knew rape, and "the only thing that was raped around here was justice."

One of his letters warned, "Right now a couple of women could file charges on a man in Big Horn County for the crime of rape and send him up with no physical evidence. You better fight this kind of ignorant garbage while there is still time! It is obvious no man is safe. The way it's going, it won't be long before they'll be coming for your guns or your family."

Through Marilyn Story, the Defense Committee contacted the doctor's relatives in Maxwell, and soon Judge Hartman's in-box overflowed with letters from Nebraska. Dr. Story's mother, Inez, wrote in the clear hand of someone who'd been educated in another era: "Dr. John H. Story is in jail for a crime he never committed. . . . A group of women have brought charges against the doctor. . . . They seem to want to destroy the doctor. . . . It seems they have formed a conspiracy against the good doctor."

A week later she added a businesslike character reference: "John is a man of impeccable character. . . . Search the world over, you will rarely if ever find a man of his equal in generosity and love for others and in their well-being. . . ." She requested leniency and asked the judge to "kindly do the right thing before God."

The next day, in a motherly letter neatly typed on parchment paper, she advised the judge that "you can ruin the life of an innocent man or return him to society to serve the people and care for their ailments." She suggested that Hartman "dismiss the trial and let Lovell start to heal its wounds. . . ." Below her neat signature she handwrote a plea: "I am Dr. Story's mother and 85 years old. Please let me see my son free from the awful charges which have been leveled against him."

A few of the Nebraska letters put the judge on notice that his soul was at risk ("At the judgment seat of Christ, all will be revealed, so give this serious thought that you will not pronounce him guilty and have that against your record in the Lamb's book of life"). Some listed Story's childhood accomplishments ("Star Boy Scout, never an off-color remark, respectful of women . . . an outstanding football player, undefeated his two years . . . always dependable"). Some were touching ("Sir I am 86 years old and am almost blind so please excuse mistakes") and some vituperative ("I can't imagine anyone stooping so low to get a person out of town").

Story's fifty-seven-year-old sister Gretchen, a teacher at Wheaton Christian Grammar School in Illinois, weighed in with praise of her brother and noted that their mother "has had two heart attacks during this stressful time."

A day or so later, the principal of her school followed up in a stern schoolmaster's tone, "I can assure you that there are a significant number of people in this western Chicago suburb that have an intense interest in seeing that Dr. Story is set free on bond in the near future. Please do what you can to expedite his matter."

Letters from Big Horn County tended to stress Story's skills as a doctor, his tolerance about delinquent accounts, his Christianity, his respect for women and children. A Powell woman's letter was typical: "When our son was born, when our daughter was thrown from her horse, when my husband broke his arm, when any of the boys we raised was hurt or ill, and during the loss of our baby this past January, Dr. Story was always there."

Marilyn Story wrote the judge, "I know beyond a shadow of a doubt that my husband is innocent." Daughter Susan added, "In my thirty years he has gained my ever increasing respect. Now I have been deeply hurt. . . ."

Other familiar names checked in with letters. Jan Hillman's mother LaVera told the judge, "I believe in his innocence. He has been my physician for 26 years."

Mrs. Douglas Wrung, "independent beauty consultant," wrote on pink Mary Kay Cosmetics stationery, "In the 2½ years that I have lived in Lovell, I have had nothing but pleasant and courteous experiences with Dr. John Story. He has always treated me in a very gentlemanly manner, even chivalrously."

Cheryl Nebel chastised the judge for "the rotten stench of corruption in your courtroom." Dr. Story, she wrote, "keeps himself pure in thought, word and deed by the power of the Lord Jesus Christ. . . . Dr. Story's innocence and deliverance will ring throughout this land. . . . Those who lied and dealt deceitfully will be revealed according to Matthew 10:26 and 27. . . . We that love this country are only in the embryonic stage of reconstruction but we will not be aborted."

North Big Horn Hospital manager Joe Brown quoted another biblical warning: "2 Chronicles 19:6 states, 'And (God) said to the judges, take heed what ye do: for ye judge not for man, but for the Lord, who is with you in the judgment period.' "

The Reverend Buttermore researched his own long letter for hours:

Your Honor, your position is very important to our great land for you represent God to all us by being elevated in the courtroom, wearing black showing complete acceptance of all light (truth, by your title of "Your Honor"), and by the fact that permission is needed to approach your bench. Because you represent God, I am reluctant to write this letter, but I do so only to assist you in your God-given trial position (Romans 13:1) . . .

Your Honor, the Bible says that to convict a man there must be two or three witnesses (Deuteronomy 17:6), but in Dr. Story's case there was only one for each alleged crime. Jesus himself would not condemn a woman on only one witness (himself John 8:11) and stated in John 5:31 that His testimony without witnesses was not valid. Based upon God's criteria for finding a man guilty, Dr. John Story is not guilty on any of the nine charges for there was no second witness nor actual proof presented. . . .

The pro-Story letters were augmented by petitions that had been left in public places by members of the Defense Committee. They began, "We the undersigned still believe in the professional and moral integrity of Dr. John H. Story." Hundreds signed.

Ironically, it was one of the most heartfelt communications that convinced the judge to deny Story's request for release on bail. After a defense attorney argued that the doctor had shown up at every court appearance and clearly represented no escape risk, Judge Hartman said, "The court . . . would like to read one letter which is from Linda Story. It states, 'As you can imagine, the outcome of the trial was quite unexpected and by the time I was able to come home two days later, my father had already been taken to Evanston' . . .

"What is significant to the court, however," the judge noted, "and I think it has been significant throughout the entire proceedings, is the fact that I do not believe that the Defendant nor his supporters ever thought that he would be convicted of any of the counts. I believe that had a great effect on the proposition that Dr. Story did in fact make all of his court appearances. I believe that when one is told by enough people as many times as he probably heard it that certainly he had to be innocent, that he could not be convicted, I suspect that he began to perhaps believe that in his own mind. . . .

"And I believe that the realization that a conviction was possible may have finally reached Dr. Story. I believe that in this particular case, if he were to be released on bond, that the risk of flight is very high. . . . Therefore, the Court believes that in this case that bail should be denied."

In the nine limbo weeks between verdict and sentencing, most of the complaining witnesses remained skittish and reclusive. Some refused to leave their homes, or spent most of their time and energy shepherding their children around.

The victims' feelings were expressed via the mails. Terri Timmons wrote the court that she'd "suffered through these 17 years of nightmare, anger, depression, humiliation and even now find it hard to trust others." She suggested that Story be made to suffer for the same length of time. Wanda Hammond informed the judge that she still felt "dirty and guilty." Annella St. Thomas said, "I have suffered for almost 13 years." Mae Fischer wrote that her husband's life had been threatened and she'd lived "in my own hell for eleven years." Emma Lu Meeks charged that Dr. Story "betrayed his manhood and the oath he should have taken as a doctor."

Hayla Farwell's oversized scrawl filled a page: "I would like to see John Story put away for life. I know that sounds terrible but I don't want him to be able to hurt anyone again. I feel if he gets out in a few years he would go right back to doing it again, even if he can't doctor anymore. . . . A few years doesn't change him. . . . The lives he has messed up, I feel he should have to account for that."

The National Organization for Women called for a grand jury investigation of public officials who'd refused to take action earlier. NOW asked, "Is it a crime to hinder, delay or otherwise prevent the discovery or prosecution of a crime . . . ?"

With weary detachment, Terry Tharp responded, "The man was tried, he was convicted. I'm not about to call a grand jury on the basis of what NOW is talking about."

Hardly anyone in Lovell was aware of an oddly related happening a thousand miles to the south. On the morning of May 30, six weeks after the trial and three weeks before John Story was scheduled to be sentenced, deputies cut a hanged man from a tree a few miles east of Mesa, Arizona. The body was swarthy, short, and slight. A single chain of footprints led to each of several trees, suggesting that the man had made a careful selection. A ring of rocks circled a dead fire, as though he might have performed some sort of ceremony. The soles of his boots lacked two and a half inches of touching the ground. A car was parked nearby.

It took several days to determine that the victim was Daniel Enoch Flores, the hard-drinking investigator who'd been hired to research the McArthur daughters' lawsuit. The last anyone in Lovell had heard, he'd gone to Arizona to interview a woman whose grown son was believed to be Story's. The young half-Indian had told a friend that the names of 121 victims were listed in files in the trunk of his car. But the trunk was empty, and no names were ever found.

85

Paul Sironen

Psychopathic personality: a disorder of behavior toward
other individuals or toward society in which reality is usually clearly perceived except for an individual's social and
moral obligations and which often seeks immediate personal gratification in criminal acts, drug addiction, or sexual perversion.

—*Webster's Seventh New*
Collegiate Dictionary

THE PRESENTENCE INVESTIGATOR was a calmly confident man
known for his exhaustive studies of criminals, but ever since the rape
doctor's conviction he'd felt uneasy. His report could be long or short,
but it had to explain John Story—his personality, his background, and
his motivations. The early word was that the task would be formidable;
Story was an expert at keeping himself private.

At thirty-eight, Paul Sironen had spent fourteen years learning that
no two Wyoming judges were alike. Some viewed the presentencing
reports as formalities, to be flicked through and ignored. Some slavishly
based their sentences on the PSI's findings. Two convicted felons had
been released on the spot as a result of Sironen's work, and dozens of
others put on probation.

The responsibility never weighed more than now. There were sub-
terranean forces at work to set Story free; only a fool could have missed
the signs. Sironen's bosses at the Wyoming Department of Probation
and Parole in Cheyenne had been as skittish as fresh foals ever since the
conviction. "Don't upset people about this case," one had lectured him.
"Take every precaution. Don't step on anybody's toes." Another executive admitted that he'd discussed the case with the judge and "others."
Sironen wondered what "others" meant. The governor? In the relaxed

Cowboy State, whose 97,000 square miles housed a population the size of Kansas City, Missouri, a telephone call to the right person could undo the work of a court or a legislature.

The presentence investigator always attacked his work in the same deliberate way. He was a burly brown-haired man, two inches taller than six feet, a Vietnam vet, a psychology graduate of the University of Wyoming, married, with one daughter. On both sides, he was descended from Finnish immigrants who'd worked the coal mines around Red Lodge, Montana. His own career followed the family continuum; he mined facts. The work was done in much the same way—digging hard, searching out rich veins, avoiding pitfalls.

In May, a month after the conviction, Sironen began the most important investigation of his career by scanning the psychiatrist's report prepared at the diagnostic center in Evanston. Breck Lebegue, M.D., had found John Story "alert, oriented and cooperative . . . shows a mild tendency for his thinking to jump from one subject to another, over-inclusiveness in an attempt to be accurate, and a great deal of projected blaming of others. . . ."

In a ninety-minute interview with Lebegue at the Wyoming State Hospital, the convicted man had insisted that he was the victim of "a vendetta against him by one woman whose request for a disability statement was denied."

As the PSI read, he thought, Here we go again. Certain offenders flatly refused to take responsibility for their actions, always had glib explanations, and, when one story didn't impress, blithely switched to another. Prisons and jails groaned with their weight. Once they'd been known as psychopaths, later as sociopaths, and now they were lumped under the category of "antisocial personalities." Whatever the term, Sironen knew them as conscienceless robots, incapable of feeling guilt or taking blame. Rape seemed to be one of their specialties.

Dr. Lebegue's report quoted Story as claiming that the complainants had falsely accused him after "a love/hate relationship that turned to hate." He charged that he'd been railroaded by a group of women, assisted by the state of Wyoming. His I.Q. was 135, there was no indication of major psychopathology or cerebral disfunction, he wasn't mentally ill, and he "wouldn't respond to treatment." Sironen had often read the same dreary conclusion in reports on antisocial personalities. Some neurotics could be helped; a small percentage of psychotics could be cured; but sociopaths stubbornly refused to admit they needed treatment and were impervious to it when it was forced on them. No therapist had ever learned how to create a conscience that had failed to form in earliest childhood, or to resocialize a person who hadn't been socialized at his parents' knees.

The PSI drove to Lovell from his home in Cody for a briefing by David Wilcock and Judi Cashel. Then he met for two hours with members of the Defense Committee at the Meeker Agency building on Nevada Avenue. It was a high-powered group. Wes Meeker had sold farm and ranch property for twenty years. Rex Nebel was a former undersheriff. Bob Richardson was Lovell city manager. A good-humored woman named Jan Hillman did most of the talking and came across as well educated and articulate. "We want Doc *out*," she stressed. "Here's a list of two hundred of his patients. We picked 'em at random from his ledgers. Maybe they'll give you a different slant."

"He doesn't belong in prison," the bearded Nebel spoke up. "It's a railroad job all the way."

Sironen thought how often he'd met good people like these. They were bright, dedicated and energetic, but for various reasons they suffered from tunnel vision. "Thanks," he said as he slipped the list into his briefcase, "but I think I should explain. My job is to provide background for the judge, to give him some alternatives. That's all. Unless you have new evidence, it doesn't do much good for people to tell me all the good things Dr. Story's done."

Jan Hillman said, "There's plenty of evidence, but the judge seems more interested in sending him away."

The PSI said, "Prison doesn't do anybody any good. That's my opinion. Let me see what I can turn up."

On May 21 he found himself interviewing Story in the Park County Jail in Cody, where he'd been transferred after the mental testing at Evanston. The 12- × 16-foot room was divided by a heavy steel mesh; Sironen's practice was to sit in the inmate's half of the cell so that he could read his face and body language. The only exit was a locked steel door that opened from the outside.

At first, he was annoyed at himself for being so ill at ease. Story sat in his royal-blue jail jumpsuit, blinking through his big dark-rimmed glasses, silently drumming the pads of his fingers on the side of the black chair cushion. He seemed to send out pressure waves of annoyed superiority. Sironen thought, He knows there's a lot of heat on me and he'll try to use it to his own advantage. This could be sticky.

For the first ten or fifteen minutes, the questioning was routine. There were vital-statistic blanks to be filled at the top of the Presentence Investigation form. The PSI switched on his Panasonic tape recorder and began asking questions. When he came to "height?" Story muttered, "Oh, about six-six."

The PSI held his pencil over the form until Story corrected himself: "I mean five-six."

Sironen thought, I'd have guessed five-four. "I'm not sure," Story added. "I haven't been measured lately. They might have measured me at the jail. I didn't pay any attention. My mind was on other things."

Sironen thought, Why so much chatter about height? It must be a real concern to him. He took note of the first break in the doctor's hauteur.

The next classification was "Family Background." Story acted offended that anyone would presume to pry into such a personal area, then sketched in an idyllic childhood: a loving mother who hadn't spanked him after age ten, a father whom he viewed with a combination of love, fear, respect, and awe, and never dreamed of defying; an older brother who had "gone his own way"; a younger sister with whom he'd had a "much closer" relationship.

Sironen noticed that the word "love" popped out several times, but with a curious lack of feeling. Story seemed to be saying one thing and showing another. Once he mumbled, "I should adjust my speech to what I think you are."

He all but refused to discuss his victims. His attitude was that he'd been oppressed by a pack of satanic Mormons. For a long time, he showed no animation except on the subject of getting out on bond. His theme word during most of the three-hour interview proved to be "normal." He spoke of his normal childhood with easygoing parents and siblings, his normal wartime service as a Navy Seabee, his normal friends and career, his normal marriage and normal outlook on life.

The PSI wondered, Is this for my benefit or his? The message was so obvious: *Everything about me is normal. How could I possibly be a criminal?* Sex offenders who were alienated from their feelings were a cliché, but this one also had a strong need to manipulate.

When Sironen admitted that he wasn't an active churchgoer, Story asked, "Then how do you expect to understand a Christian?" He suggested that the interviewer was also handicapped by his lack of medical training. "You can't possibly understand a physician unless you've studied medicine yourself." The PSI began to pick up on the doctor's subtext: *An ordinary guy like you couldn't possibly understand an accomplished person like me.*

As the interview continued, Story presented still other reasons why Sironen would have problems dealing with his case. The PSI noted later:

Mr. Story reported that he feels that he was unusually favored during his childhood. He went on to explain that by "unusually favored" he meant that he had a good family that he loved and who loved him and that he had a great number of positive influences in his life that allowed him to grow up in a good situation. He reported that he grew up in a time when, if you lived in your home town, you lived at home and you went home for meals every day. Mr. Story implied that since this writer was from a different generation and usually dealt with people with different backgrounds, I could probably not understand his family background. He went on to indicate that if the report indicated anything different about his background than he had reported to other people for many years, he would be offended.

Sironen switched off his Panasonic and called for the deputy to open the door. Sometimes it was wise to wait a few weeks and start all over again.

Back in his small office, the PSI did some research by phone. A policeman in Crawford, Nebraska, confirmed that a young doctor named John Story had once assisted Dr. Ben Bishop, now deceased. A few more calls produced the names of several Bishop patients and his veteran nurse, Rhea Jaffe. Sironen phoned and found the woman extremely close-mouthed. He was sure she was hiding something.

On a searing afternoon a week later, he cruised into Crawford after an all-day drive and began calling on the sources the local police had provided. One resident thought that Story had been in "some kind of trouble" as a young physician. Another said that a woman had made a complaint, but not with the police, and anyway she'd moved away years ago.

Sironen didn't bother to take notes on this secondhand hearsay. At the end of the day he drove to Nurse Jaffe's small frame house a few blocks from downtown. She was a gray-haired woman in her sixties, a heavy smoker, a firm believer in the ancient code of medical silence. It took her an hour to reveal that Dr. Bishop had died of diabetes, that she'd been his nurse till the end, and that Dr. Story, just out of med school, had indeed served as Dr. Bishop's assistant.

It took the PSI another hour to get up the nerve to ask if he could use his tape recorder. "Certainly not!" Nurse Jaffe snapped. "I don't want my name used and I won't testify. I will *never* testify. Do I have your word on that?"

On his solemn promise to shield her identity, she began to open up. Sironen reported later:

The information from Crawford indicates that in three or four instances, while examining teenage girls, Mr. Story's practices were questionable. It seems that his procedure was to require girls to disrobe completely, and lay on the examining table while draped with a sheet prior to an examination. Upon entering the examination room Story would yank off the sheet covering the individual, stating he could not do a proper examination if they were not totally nude.

Additional information suggests that he may have been involved in other questionable practices while administering pelvic examinations. The information suggests that he gave an unusually large number of pelvic examinations, the examinations lasted an inordinate amount of time and it appears that some patients were subjected to treatment that was not medically necessary. The observation was that during the long pelvic examinations, patients would be squirming on the table and forced to endure treatment that was not medically necessary.

Information from Crawford indicates that there was one instance in which a nurse's aide at the Crawford Hospital complained to nurses about Mr. Story's treatment of one elderly patient. The nurse's aide reported that during a supposedly routine examination, Story was "just playing with her."

The information from Crawford indicated that Dr. Bishop was advised of the alleged misbehavior by Mr. Story and Dr. Bishop confronted, or at least discussed the situation with him. Following the discussion with Dr. Bishop, Mr. Story's questionable practices ceased and only a short time later he left Crawford for Lovell, Wyoming.

Sironen now had the answer to a key question, one that was asked by every sentencing judge: Is there an established pattern, or is this an isolated case? It appeared that the formation of Story's M.O. went back almost twenty-eight years. Experience had shown that offenders who followed a pattern often returned to it on release, especially if they refused to admit their guilt or undertake a program of rehabilitation. Despite his medical degree and mild appearance, Dr. John Story was shaping up as a textbook example of the hardened criminal.

Three weeks after the first interview, the PSI found himself back in the Park County Jail. This time Story had several things on his mind. "You're not gonna talk to my brother Jerod, are you?" he asked.

Sironen said he hadn't decided.

"Well, he won't be any help. I'd rather you didn't talk to him." He paused. "Will you be seeing my mother?"

"I may," the PSI said.

Story looked ruffled. "When you talk to her, I think you should be sure to clearly explain what you're doing. Maybe somebody else should be there, because I don't know what you're gonna do to her."

Sironen thought, This man still thinks he can give orders. "I don't understand," the PSI said. "What do you think I would do to your mother?"

"I don't know, but she's eighty-five years old. Don't give her any false hopes."

They chatted for a while. Then the investigator said, "I haven't found anything to indicate that you're not guilty, or anything to suggest that you're interested in rehabilitation. If you keep on denying everything, you'll give the judge no choice. You're not crazy—that's been established at the state hospital—so he can't send you down there. He can't put you on probation, because you're not treatable. How can you be treated when you won't admit you have a problem? Now let's talk about this and see if we can come up with alternatives. If we can't give the judge some options"—he paused for emphasis—"you're going to the pen."

Story began a lengthy peroration. The PSI described it in his final report:

Mr. Story reported that he believes the present offense resulted from a conspiracy involving one Arden McArthur and the Mormon Church. Mr. Story reported that he believes that because he refused to join the Mormon Church at the repeated urgings of Mrs. McArthur, she has gone on a personal campaign against him. He reported that Mrs. McArthur alleged that her two daughters had been assaulted by him in the past and she is the one that stirred up all of the other individuals in the community to come forward and falsely accuse him.

When asked repeatedly and directly for any information substantiating his beliefs about Mrs. McArthur and her church connection, Mr. Story was only able to give vague descriptions of how Mrs. McArthur had a great deal of power and influence over a majority of the women in the community.

Mr. Story further reported that he believed the conspiracy against him was more widespread than just within the community of Lovell. He reported that due to his lack of cooperation with the State Medical Board over the years, particularly concerning welfare patients, people at the state level were also in a conspiracy against him.

When asked to provide specific information, Mr. Story again was unable to provide details of any type of conspiracy. When questioned specifically about how one woman in a small community such as Lovell could somehow influence a statewide conspiracy against him, Dr. Story was unable to provide any explanation.

The two men discussed the "conspiracy" for another hour. Story asked, "Do you know the connections on the Lovell police department, how many are related to my accusers, how many are Mormons?"

Sironen replied, "In any group in Lovell, you're gonna find relationships like that."

He tried to get Story to discuss the cases on their merits, one by one, and this time elicited a few comments. Story said he felt sorry for Hayla Farwell; "she had marital problems and medical problems." Both Farwell and Mae Fischer, he said, were "easily led." He made vague charges about Terri Timmons' reputation, called Wanda Hammond "unattractive," claimed that Annella St. Thomas had made her accusation as a result of "family problems" and that Emma Lu Meeks's late husband had had "quite a reputation." It was the same sort of character assassination he'd attempted on the witness stand. He seemed jittery as he ran down the list, repeatedly clearing his throat and shifting in his chair.

After two hours, the PSI asked, "What about your strange examining room practices in Crawford?"

Story turned pale. Several times he started to talk, then finally said in a voice just above a whisper, "You went to . . . Crawford?"

"Yeah."

"Who'd you talk to?"

"I don't think that's important. What's important is the indication that you were doing the same kind of thing."

"I never raped anybody in Crawford!" Story said, raising his voice for the first time. His color went from gray to pink, and his brown eyes flashed. "Who said that?"

"I didn't say you raped anybody. I just said you were doing strange things in the examining room."

The conversation deteriorated. Finally Sironen said, "Look, I'll sit here for three more hours if you want me to, but we're not getting anywhere. Unless you've got something else to tell me, I'm done."

Story glared. The PSI flipped off his tape recorder and called for the guard to open the door. Back at his office, he dictated his conclusions:

Mr. John Story appears to have established a very definite pattern of criminal behavior which includes humiliation, victimization and sexual assaults on select female patients. It appears that this behavior has progressed from its initial stages of simply humiliating women in the examining room as early as 1958 in Crawford, Nebraska, to actual sexual assaults on female patients in Lovell as recently as 1983. He appears to have been quite selective concerning his victims in that, for the most part, he selected only those women who were particularly vulnerable at the time. It appears that Mr. Story used a wide variety of methods to select his victims and to increase their vulnerability.

First, it appears that he used his position of authority as a doctor to intimidate patients. It appears that he then based further actions on individuals' responses to his position of authority as a doctor and if they seemed particularly easily led or influenced, he continued with his victimization. Throughout the police department investigation and this investigation are references to Mr. Story's view of himself as a doctor. He did not like to be questioned about his medical decisions or, for that matter, any decisions, and he made that quite clear with people he worked with. Additionally, he did not volunteer information to his patients or other individuals concerning medical decisions.

Second, Mr. Story has a good command of the English language. He has a substantial vocabulary and a good understanding of semantics. It appears that he has developed a pattern of using the language to help intimidate, confuse and humiliate other people. Again, during the investigation it was learned that it was widely known that Mr. Story could talk all around a subject or talk over people's heads and did so regularly. It appears that when he combined his command of the language with his knowledge of medicine and medical terminology, he easily confused and intimidated a good number of people.

Finally, it appears that Mr. Story believes that he is superior to most other individuals in society. This seems evidenced first by his criminal behavior in the present offense and additionally by his attitude toward various social programs, rules and controls suggested by the state of Wyoming. It appears that he has the attitude that the laws and rules apply to all other individuals, but not to himself.

With such an attitude, it seems quite understandable how he could continue to humiliate, intimidate and victimize his patients with probably a relatively clear conscience. Throughout the trial on the present offense and his incarceration pending sentencing, he has steadfastly maintained his innocence and proclaimed he was convicted as the result of some grand conspiracy against him. It would appear to this Writer that the idea of a conspiracy would be the only way he could allow himself to view his situation, as he is far superior to other individuals and only a conspiracy could have resulted in his conviction.

In this writer's opinion, Dr. John Story does not appear greatly different from other rapists this writer has dealt with, except that he has a better education and has committed a larger number of offenses. His attitude toward the present offenses appears to be that he is above the law, the laws are for other people and that his only mistake was in getting caught. He appears to have somehow made the determination that it is okay to sexually assault his patients in the examining room, but it is probably not okay to have an affair with his neighbor's wife or to murder someone. It is not clear, however, how he has made that distinction and what would stop him from going even further in his victimization of people.

In his report, Sironen noted that there were twenty-two confirmed victims, seventy-five unconfirmed, "and perhaps more."

Shortly before the sentencing hearing, a copy of the PSI's observations was turned over to Story and the defense lawyers. Next to the information from Crawford, the doctor scribbled, "Lie . . . lie." He sprinkled question marks throughout the document and underlined numerous passages. In the repeated references to "Mr. Story," he overwrote each M into a D.

86

Sentencing

MARILYN wrote in her journal: "John has now been in prison 55 days. The sentencing will be June 18th. John is so strong. Lord, protect his mind, his body, his spirit. . . ."

The Defense Committee spent weeks preparing for the sentencing hearing. Jan Hillman and her mother stitched up boxfuls of white armbands and painted big banners:

FREE DR. STORY

SET MY DR. FREE

WE BELIEVE IN DR. STORY

WHO'S NEXT, ARDEN?

A week before the hearing, Committee members began a telephone campaign, urging Story supporters to attend and bring as many others as they could round up. The plan was to fill the small courtroom, shut out the prosecution groupies and the whiny victims, and make an impression on the judge.

At daily prayers in the Bible Church, Reverend Ken Buttermore continued his message of nonviolence: "Don't get angry. Moses got angry and failed to believe. The people angered and provoked him and he struck the rock twice. We cannot let people provoke us to anger. We must keep our eyes fixed on Christ in praise, and thank *Him*, despite what Dr. Story's accusers are doing."

Parishioner Rex Nebel recruited two of his biker friends from Billings. "Hey, one of these guys looks like Bluto in the cartoons," he told a friend. The other muscleman wore a T-shirt with a black widow spider across the front. Both were veterans of Vietnam and the North California marijuana wars. Rex outfitted them in black baseball caps with "WAR" inscribed on the peaks. The letters stood for "Won't Accept the Rapes."

"In case things get out of hand," he told his imported centurions, "we'll just kick ass. We'll tear that place apart. We'll stomp those little husbands through the walls."

On sentencing day, the sun came up in a cloudless June sky. Picketers arrived hours early. They wore white armbands and flowers to symbolize Dr. Story's purity and innocence. Jan Hillman handed out her placards and was pleased to see some new ones appear:

ASK GARY DOTSON—WOMEN *DO* LIE

WYOMING LAW—EVIDENCE APPRECIATED, BUT NOT REQUIRED

The conservative Wes Meeker marched under the weeping birch in front, his grandchildren following him with placards. "If anybody had ever told me I'd be carrying a sign," he called across the lawn to Hillman, "I'd've had their brains examined!"

"Hey, Wes," Jan bantered back, "I've done it before. It's no problem. You'll feel right at home!"

The Defense Committee's new watchword was passed from mouth to mouth: "Don't Let the Flowers Wilt." No one knew exactly what it signified, but it had a nice ring.

As cars drove up and parked, Defense Committee members photographed the license plates and occupants for future reference. Cordons of placard-waving supporters formed along the walkways to the front and side doors. The judge walked past Nebel's security force and said, "Good morning, gentlemen." The big men stared through mirrored shades.

By eight thirty the county building was jammed. Two deputies with metal detectors flanked the entrance to the second-floor courtroom.

When Judi Cashel walked down the hall toward a side office, a woman put out a foot to trip her. The petite policewoman sidestepped and continued as though she hadn't noticed.

Just before 9 A.M., a titter went through the crowd. Staffers from the Lovell Behavorial clinic had arrived, and the crowd wouldn't let them through.

Waiting in Judge Hartman's chambers with Wayne Aarestad and other officers of the court, Terry Tharp was feeling nervous. He didn't like mobs and he dreaded turning his back to some of these characters in court. He cringed as they chanted, "We want Doc. *We want Doc . . . !*" He wondered how much more of this holy-roller display the judge would tolerate.

Two deputies escorted the convicted man into the courtroom. Story was wearing his gray polyester suit, accented by a white armband. He smiled and gave a two-fisted wave like a boxer, and his backers responded with cheers. As he took his seat, a new chant began: "We love Doc!" There were whistles, cheers, war-whoops, high-pitched screams of adulation. Raised fists pumped the air. The grinning Story faced the bench and wigwagged behind his back for silence, but his fans refused to obey.

After four minutes of the din, Judge Hartman told Story's attorneys, "Go out and get those people calmed down. If there's one more outburst, I'll clear that courtroom."

On the drive down from Lovell in Chief Wilcock's car, Terri Lee Timmons had felt her anxiety growing. "Quit worrying," her husband Loyd had told her. "The county building's right next to the sheriff's office."

She'd just been appointed Culture Refinement teacher in her ward's Relief Society, assigned to tutor other women on forgiveness, courage and love. It was an honor, but she didn't think she would last. She still seethed with resentment of males—her ex-fiancé, her father, the punk who'd raped someone close to her, any male who'd ever done her an injustice, sometimes even including her beloved Loyd. She'd written in her journal: "I feel so much anger inside of me so much of the time that there isn't much room for love. My heart is full of pain. At this point I am a selfish, ugly person. I need to forgive and repent." Her bitterness was polluting her marriage. The counselor at the Behavioral Clinic had advised her to attend the sentencing as therapy. At least she would see one male get what was coming to him.

The Timmonses arrived a few minutes late and picked their way across a lawn littered with placards. Terri read: SALEM MASS. 1692—BIG HORN COUNTY 1984.

Inside, they were blocked by the crowd at the foot of the staircase. "Excuse us," Loyd said. "We're supposed to be upstairs in court."

"So are we!" someone called out.

Terri saw a face from years back, when she'd washed dishes at the hospital. It was her old boss, Margaret Anselm, a white band on her arm. Terri smiled; she dearly loved the woman. She didn't understand why Margaret turned away.

All around her were Saints she'd known from childhood. She thought about the angel Moroni and his message that God's truth would be manifested through the Holy Ghost; that's what was meant by "a burning in the bosom." Had all these brothers and sisters felt a burning that Story was *not* a rapist? Was that their idea of revealed truth? She'd never felt so confused.

Judi Cashel offered to escort her and Loyd up the stairs to the courtroom. At first the crowd wouldn't part. "Please!" Judi called out.

Someone shouted, "They're no better'n us!"

A woman who resembled Grace Kelly stuck out her elbows and growled, "Hey, we're in line!"

"Please," Judi repeated. "We have to get to the courtroom."

"No!"

Terri and Loyd followed the persistent policewoman inch by inch to the court entrance. Standees were four deep. Furious faces turned to stare. Inside, a female voice said, "You're not sitting by *me*!"

They managed to squeeze into standing room space just behind the Nebels. Terri had read some of Rex's letters in the newspapers. She said to herself, He looks just as mean as he sounds.

She heard Mrs. Nebel say, "I brought my sword with me!" Terri clutched her throat, then sighed with relief as the heavyset woman waved a Bible.

A big man in mirrored sunglasses stepped next to Loyd and stared down at his red hair. Terri grabbed Loyd's arm and turned to leave, but the exit was sealed off by folks in armbands. Now she knew why the other victims had stayed home.

She craned her skinny neck to see. Seated close to Story were LaMar

Averett and some of his relatives, all wearing armbands. A few seats away sat a bishop who'd written the *Chronicle* that the charges were "filthy lies." Next to him was a pregnant LDS woman who'd asked permission to enter the jail so Dr. Story could deliver her baby. Terri thought, O Lord, what am I doing with these people? *Where are the other victims?*

She didn't know what she and Loyd would do if Story were freed on probation. She thought, His people will go wild. They'll carry him off like a football star. It'll be my worst nightmare come true. As she stood in the back of the courtroom, she kept trying not to scream.

In all his years as a presentence investigator, Paul Sironen had never known a defendant with backing on so many levels, from laborers coughing up bentonite phlegm to fellow physicians in pin-striped suits.

A friend came out of the judge's chambers with disquieting news. "Somebody from Cheyenne just called the judge to apologize," the friend said.

"For what?" Sironen asked.

"Your report."

The PSI was annoyed but not surprised. There was plenty of support for Story in Cheyenne. The higher-ups had probably been pressured by some heavyweight politico—maybe Cal Taggart, or maybe even Taggart's friend, the governor. Or maybe a Story supporter had threatened a lawsuit. The Wyoming Department of Probation and Parole lived in fear of litigation.

Waiting to testify, Sironen sat on the wooden bench outside the courtroom and wished he were safely home in Cody. He wondered whom the protesters would attack first. Placards, chants, hymns, white armbands, flowers—he was surrounded by the totems and talismens of the basic lynch mob. He wondered who'd orchestrated the performance.

The PSI was relieved when a deputy stuck his head out of the courtroom and said, "Mr. Sironen?"

He squeezed through the massed bodies, held up his hand and swore to tell the truth, then gazed into the somber face of Wayne Aarestad. The tall blond defense lawyer went through a few preliminary questions, then asked with exaggerated courtesy, "Could you tell me whether or not you interviewed any of those alleged girls or ladies who you claim were mistreated sexually in Crawford?"

"No," Sironen said. "I did not."

The audience gasped.

Aarestad went on. "And then let me ask you what the source of your information is then that enabled you to make these statements?"

"An individual in Crawford who wished not to be identified."

"Hoo-boy!" someone stage-whispered. Groans went up, soft whoops of derision, outright laughter.

The judge slammed his gavel. "Ladies and gentlemen," he said, "let me tell you, we will not tolerate any type of outburst in the courtroom. If we have any additional outbursts, we will clear the courtroom. I don't want to do that. You are entitled to stay. We want you to be here. But we can't tolerate this."

He stared hard from one face to another, then said softly, "Proceed, Mr. Aarestad."

"Thank you, Your Honor."

Q I assume that as you sit here today you are going to continue to honor that request for anonymity on the part of this individual?
A Yes, sir.
Q At this particular time, Dr. Bishop is deceased, is he not?
A As I understand it, yes.
Q In the course of your investigation, did you ever learn that this Dr. Bishop, after Dr. Story had left Crawford and came back to Lovell where he set up his practice, asked Dr. Story to return in the practice with him in Crawford?
A I was not advised of that, no.
Q Okay. If you had that knowledge at that time, would that, in your opinion, have influenced some of the comments you made under "Prior Offenses" relative to Crawford?
A No, sir.

Aarestad asked how many of the twenty-two confirmed victims and seventy-five unconfirmed victims had been interviewed. Sironen acknowledged that he'd talked to none. His sources had been police records.

The lawyer asked, "For my own edification, why did you not obtain any other statements from either Dr. Story's family or anybody else relative to their attitudes towards sentencing? In other words, why did you just concentrate on them?"

"On the victims?" Sironen asked.

"Yes."

"Because they are victims."

Aarestad turned to the judge and asked if he'd read the PSI's report. The gray-haired jurist said slowly, "The Court has."

The lawyer moved that Hartman disqualify himself from the sentencing, since major portions of the presentencing report were "*totally* hearsay," their prejudicial effect was "obvious," and now that His Honor had read them, he could no longer be fair or impartial.

The county attorney took issue. "This Court sat through the trial," Terrill Tharp argued. "This Court is in as good a position or better position than any other court or judge to decide what happens to this defendant. And I think that the court can take cognizance of the things that went on at trial, and I think if there is any hearsay or anything in that that Mr. Aarestad complains about, I think the Court is perfectly capable of separating that from what went on at trial, and sentence accordingly."

The judge declined to remove himself but promised to ignore the hearsay portions in determining the sentence. Sironen was free to return to Cody.

There was a stirring in the courtroom as the young prosecutor called for sentences of six to ten years each on the three counts of assault and battery with intent to commit rape, and fifteen to twenty-five years each on the single count of second-degree sexual assault and the two counts of forcible rape, all to run concurrently. "I think this is just," he said. "I think it is fair. Twelve people convicted him. That is as close as we can come in this society to the truth."

The judge asked for Aarestad's recommendations. "We would reserve our judgment," the big lawyer said, "until we have had an opportunity to put on a few witnesses." He called the defendant's mother.

The tiny woman walked to the witness box with steady steps. At eighty-five, she looked like a healthy woman of sixty. She had lively brown eyes like her son's, and her gray hair was arranged in neat waves and intertwined with dark strands. Her voice was strong as she stated her name, "Inez Story," with the accent on the first syllable: EYE-nez.

Aarestad asked if she knew the defendant, and she said briskly, "That's my son. I know him very well." The spectators smiled as she added. "He is very mild and kind and good and never an evil thought about anyone. Always bent on doing the best he could for his companions, his fellow man."

The lawyer asked if she'd seen him display violent tendencies. "None whatever," she said.

"Do you believe even today that in any shape or form he poses a safety hazard to society?"

"Of course not!"

When Aarestad turned to the happenings in Crawford, the testimony took a less predictable turn:

Q Do you have any knowledge that you would like to share with this court relative to what Dr. Bishop's attitude towards your son was?

A It was very good. And he—may I speak more?

Q Yes.

A After John had left there several years to come to Lovell, Dr. Bishop called in my home by telephone to ask where John was—Dr. Story. And I told him that he was right there in my home on vacation. And he asked to talk to him and he wanted him to return to Crawford to practice there. As he said, they needed another good doctor. . . .

Q The information that you have just relayed—is that a result of what? Your conversations with your son?

A Partly. And partly with Dr. Bishop.

The old woman's testimony finished with a ringing rebuke: "I think men so interested in the welfare of others, that has given the best of his life to the people up here, to the good of the community, that it would seem almost impossible that they would want to destroy his life. But they *have* ruined it and that of his family, and ruined him financially and his medical practice and disrupted his home. It is time for justice in this community! I believe many lies have been told here that would destroy him. Full of lies." She asked that the court suspend her son's sentence "by all means, in justice."

Another small woman identified herself as Gretchen Story Stevens of Wheaton, Illinois, a fourth-grade teacher at Wheaton Christian Grammar School. Her brother, she testified, "has always been very self-disciplined. He has high moral standards. He has never had the outward display that some adolescents have had. And he has always been courteous, kind. . . . He is a well-balanced person. He played football, went out for track." She said he'd been the role model for her family, and "Society is the loser if he is not present."

Linda Story told of her father's "love and concern" and the quality time he spent with his family. "I have never even heard him raise his voice to any of us," the younger daughter said. She was certain of his innocence "because I know his character, his stability, his dedication to

God, and his principle. And I would think that placing him among murderers and thieves just makes no sense at all."

The University of Maryland graduate student suggested that the Court sentence her father to Ethiopia, "where he might take care of the people that are suffering and dying." Like her grandmother, she showed no false humility and no deference to the judge's robes. She looked straight at Hartman and said, "To deny him his quality of life and to deny he and my mother their later years together greatly compounds the injustice that has been done to him by this court."

Susan Story, a registered nurse from Fort Collins, Colorado, defended her father in a torrent of words: "I just can't stand the thought of him being treated like a criminal when he is the most wonderful man. . . . A wonderful doctor. . . . A rare doctor. . . . Not many doctors showed respect for individual persons the way he does. So medicine is very important to him, but it is not his whole life. . . ."

Aarestad asked, "Do you feel that he poses in any way, shape, or form any type of a safety risk to society?"

"Are you kidding?" the older daughter said. The answer brought a laugh from the spectators.

Marilyn Story testified that women had always been envious of her because her husband was "the most gentlemanly, courteous, considerate man that I have ever known, and many other wives have even made that comment that they wish that their husbands would be so kind to women." She swallowed hard as she spoke of "those false accusations [that] have totally ruined our lives."

Her husband would never hurt anyone, she testified. "He never has. He deserves to be out with us. He has already—he is the victim. . . . He is our counselor and our guide for us, for me and my daughters." She dabbed at a tear as she concluded, "I just can't bear the thought of him being away from us any longer."

In a final plea for leniency, Aarestad stressed that he was personally convinced of his client's innocence. Like the others, he didn't hesitate to attack the court and the judicial process. "We believe that the injustices that have been perpetrated to date are great enough without compounding them at this point. We believe this case cries out for justice, and we believe the case is far from over, and we believe that a day of vindication will come."

He brought dismayed groans when he informed the judge that Dr. Story had voluntarily turned in his medical license "in order to prevent any concern that he would return to an environment under which these allegations occurred." Without the license, the lawyer argued, there was no evidence that his client posed a threat to society. "And he has removed himself from that environment just to eliminate any confusion whatsoever on that issue."

He asked for a suspended sentence or release on bail.

Judge Hartman thanked the North Dakota lawyer and turned toward the defendant. "John Story," he said as a hush fell over the courtroom, "do you have anything that you would like to say to the Court prior to passing sentence in this case?"

Clothes rustled as the spectators leaned forward. Story made no effort to stand. He said, "I think not."

The judge said, "Is there any reason why sentence should not be pronounced at this time?"

"I am aware of none," Story said.

"John Story, would you stand, please?"

The judge acknowledged that he'd read over a hundred letters and petitions, "and I must say that the overwhelming number of letters that I did receive, of course, were in your favor." He confirmed that he'd looked into the possibility of probation. At the mention of the magic word, hopeful sighs arose from the crowd like vapor.

The judge went on. "I also considered, among other things, your age, your intelligence, your training, your background, your lack of criminal record, your present attitude. I have also considered the number of lives that you must have saved in Lovell, the many calls that a physician is called upon to make at all hours of the day, the number of persons that you have healed and those that you have treated, and for those persons that you have been both a counselor and a confidant for. I have also considered the tremendous amount of training that you have received and your God-gifted talent for being able to heal the sick and care for those who are in need of your services."

As he spoke, the courtroom mood seemed to lighten. The Story family, seated side by side in a single row, stared intently at the judge, but their truculent air had changed to mild expressions of hope. Why would the judge spend so much time in praise of the man he was about to sentence? Did it mean . . . could it possibly mean . . . *probation?*

The judge's tone darkened. He spoke of "the seriousness of these crimes" and noted that the possible penalty on two of the counts was life imprisonment. He mentioned the "vulnerability of the victims . . . the psychological and emotional havoc that you have visited." He said he was certain that "the scars that you so inflicted cannot measure, by any stretch of the imagination, any type of sentence that I could impose." He admitted that he was distressed to have to impose a sentence "on a man of your abilities and with your training. It is a waste."

He paused for a sip. It was ten o'clock. For the first time all morning, not a cough or a whispered aside was heard from the spectators. They seemed cut in stone, faces tilted upward, brows furrowed, eyes narrowed to slits as though it would help them to hear.

The judge continued. "The Court notes that there has been no admission by you that any of those crimes have occurred. Also, the Court has taken into consideration the question of whether or not any incarceration would deter the general public from committing these types of crimes, or specific persons from committing these crimes.

"The Court has also considered the factor of incapacitation, whether you need to be separated from society. And finally, the Court has considered the question of retribution, that one who breaks the law must pay the penalty or receive his just deserves."

He picked up a sheaf of papers, then sentenced Story to six terms ranging from ten to fifteen years on the lesser charges and fifteen to twenty years on the rapes, all to run concurrently.

Story didn't react. A moan came from the front row as the judge intoned, "I will remand John Story to the sheriff of Big Horn County for transportation to the Wyoming State Penitentiary located in Rawlins, Wyoming."

This time there were no good-byes or hugs, no spitting on the bench, no imprecations. Marilyn Story glared at Terry Tharp and ground a fist into her palm. The other spectators milled about like survivors of a train wreck.

Deputies steered the prisoner toward the back door. Someone called out, "It's not over, Doc," and another said, "It's just the beginning." The steadiest sound was the crying.

Sergeant Judi Cashel decided she'd been putting too much stock in omens lately. On her way up from Casper, she'd flogged her new Fierro, a black one this time, to 70 mph, and been awarded a speeding ticket, an embarrassing blemish in the personnel jacket of a supervisor who often wrote tickets herself.

After that, she'd expected the worst. She was afraid that the judge would be snowed by Story's clean record and his prominence in the community and his Mr. Peepers persona, and let him walk. Which would be too bad, she'd said to herself, because it would mean more rapes. She knew enough about antisocial personalities to know that they didn't change.

She was happy with the verdict, but not happy enough to smile or laugh or otherwise exult in front of the upset audience. She felt strong compassion for the relatives and friends and supporters. At heart, she considered them decent people, no better or worse than the victims.

Standing in the well of the court, she saw two women sidling toward her. She recognized Janet Buttermore, the pastor's wife, and Rex Nebel's wife Cheryl. They stood just behind the rail and muttered, "Are you satisfied?" "You've ruined this wonderful man." "What an un-Christian person you are!"

Judi had no taste for a fight. Story was a manipulator, and he'd manipulated these good women just as he'd manipulated the others. "Look," she said softly, "the way you're acting now isn't very Christian, either. Why don't you just go home and sleep on it?"

They were still fussing at her as she picked up her purse and walked through the door to the back.

Even after the main players had left the stage, Terri Timmons couldn't stop shaking. The crowd's grip had loosened, but she still attracted stares and whispers. Nila Meeker, Wes Meeker's daughter, stared at her. In the far corner of the courtroom, three women held hands and looked sideways at her, then started praying aloud, as though her soul required immediate intervention.

As she teetered down the stairs with Loyd, Terri tried to collect her thoughts. Well, she thought, the sentence was fair. He deserves it. He put me through all those bad years; let him serve fifteen of his own. She wondered if the judge had read her letter. It made her feel good that his sentence had approximated her own formula.

In the lobby, the Reverend Buttermore approached. She disagreed with him about Story, but she'd been grateful for his public stand against violence. He spoke past her to Loyd: "It's not over yet. We've just begun to fight."

"Fight?" Loyd snapped. "The next time you see him, he'll probably be dead."

Buttermore turned away, and Terri heard him tell a newspaper reporter, "We're picking up more and more out-of-state support. I think this thing will get very big by the time it's all said and done."

Terri asked her husband, "What made you say he'd be dead?"

"I just blurted it out," Loyd said. "I was thinking that convicts don't like child molesters."

Child molesters. Yes, she thought, that's exactly what he is. In spite of all the phony words of praise by his family, he's a plain ordinary sicko creepo child molester. O Lord, she said to herself, why has that always been Lovell's special problem?

When they went outside, she saw the supporters marching around on the grass, still clutching their placards. They seemed to have recovered their spirits. Apparently they were waiting for a final glimpse of their hero as he was walked to the jail next door. There were a few fierce looks.

Dave Wilcock came out to drive them home. As they headed for the parking area, Bev Moody called out, "Are you happy now?"

Wilcock whispered, "Ignore it!"

In the parking lot they passed an official Wyoming vehicle with an "S" license plate. Someone had run a nail along its side. They guessed it was Sironen's.

Terrill Tharp decided to wait in his office till the last of the supporters were gone. Passing the time, he opened a letter from a woman in Colorado. It said that she'd read about Dr. Story and wanted the authorities to know that her daughter had gone to him for a Girl Scout medical exam and been given a pelvic.

Tharp shook his head. Ever since the arrest of Halloween night, he'd been receiving phone calls and letters like this. He said to himself, Some conspiracy!

He leaned back in his polished wooden chair and thought how seldom it was that criminals paid their accounts in full. Crime was one of the last great bargains. Burglars committed fifty or sixty break-ins and went to jail for the one time they were caught. Arsonists, larcenists, child abusers, car prowlers, cattle thieves, bunco artists—hardly any of them got as much as they gave. Story was only the latest example.

He wondered how many victims were still keeping quiet, how many children Story had fathered, how many teenagers he'd deflowered, how many girls had been too embarrassed to go home and tell their parents that he'd complimented them on their "buds" and fondled them, how many skittish old ladies like Emma Lou Meeks and Julia Bradbury had fled his clinic and been ashamed to tell what he'd done to them till events had left them no choice.

It was a numbers puzzle, a game of educated guesses. Dave Wilcock guessed there were at least 150 victims. Judi Cashel estimated 200. Tharp remembered his first interview with Caroline Shotwell. He'd thought at the time that she was a prime candidate for the Burlington Liars Club. She'd said that she firmly believed that the rape doctor used his penis every day during his one thirty appointment, sometimes during his final appointment of the day around five or five thirty, and occasionally in evenings and off-hours. Mrs. Shotwell had estimated his victims at over a thousand, and told Tharp, "You can just stand outside our church on Sunday and you'll see very few LDS women who weren't victims."

Whatever the truth of the numbers game, the young prosecutor was convinced he'd put a fiend away. Now, he said to himself, if only we can keep him there.

87

Pressure

REX NEBEL relayed the first word from the imprisoned doctor. In a note published in the *Chronicle*, Nebel wrote, "Doc recently stated in a letter from 'the joint' as he calls it that it would be better to leave Lovell than stay here and hate these people. Doc stated that it is our job to love these even though we don't understand the reason why. . . . Doc continues in his love and concern as always; as our example, as the Holy Bible instructs!"

Nebel added, "There are some of you who hold back information that is vital to Doc's freedom. I know who several of you are."

The newly formed Dr. Story Defense Committee moved to the attack. Fruit sales were held, bake sales, auctions; doorbells were rung, arms twisted, old debts called in. Jan Hillman, master telephonist and committee chairman, worked the phones. Assisted by her mother and Bev Moody, the robust bar owner soon had $20,000 in the coffers. LaVera Hillman also helped the cause by auctioning off her late husband's gun collection and other personal possessions.

Defense Committee sleuths hounded the jurors for an explanation of their verdict; most refused to talk. Pressure was applied to state witnesses in the hope that one would admit that there'd been a conspiracy and provide details. Just when they needed bucking up, the Story forces were strengthened by Ed Herschler's statement that the victims' testimony had been "hogwash." If the governor was on Doc's side, could justice be far behind?

Wanda Hammond, never far from tears, was publicly labeled "a fat whore" by a Committee member. The roundish little woman took so many abusive calls that she was afraid to answer her phone. Lifelong friends cut her dead. High priests turned away when she came through their handshake line at church. Customers pulled up to the Rose City Food Farm, looked through the window to see if she was checking, and squealed their tires to get away. Wanda was a wreck.

Over at the IGA Thriftway, the Bob Negro family remained staunchly pro-Story. Mae Fischer waited for ten minutes before she realized that the manager's wife didn't intend to check her out. Diana Harrison called "Hi, Mitch!" to the owner's young son and was ignored. The former receptionist was already hurt by the whispering campaign against her. Schoolchildren spread word that she was "the best come-sniffer in Big Horn County."

"We're catchin' hell," Nelson St. Thomas complained in his Montana cowpoke accent. "The hardest part is going down to the IGA. They turn us away like we had leprosy. I'm working in the oil fields, and some of those damn fools out there spend half their time complaining about Story. He's in jail and they still don't believe he did it! Meantime, 'Nella's back at our house, where anybody could walk right in. All day long I worry about her. She's been through enough."

A few friends and relatives of the victims finally reached the end of their tether. A Story supporter taunted Gerald Brinkerhoff on the street. "Who're you Mormons gonna go after next?" he asked.

"You, you dumb son of a bitch!" the feisty carpenter exploded.

Brinkerhoff was the husband of one victim and the father-in-law of another, and he was rubbed raw on the subject of Dr. Story's innocence. He'd heard that the second ward bishop had publicly asked the brethren to play down the case, and that the third ward bishop, Larry Sessions, had called for a more tolerant attitude toward Story and his backers. "You're hurting our missionary effort," Sessions was quoted as telling some of his people. "They're getting too many doors slammed in their faces."

The morning after Sessions made his plea, Brinkerhoff asked him, "Are you trying to tell us that it's okay to let this man have his way with our women? It's okay for our wives to be raped? You tellin' us *that*?"

"You weren't there, Gerald," the bishop said. "You don't know what happened."

"I wasn't there," the carpenter agreed, "but my wife Dorothy has never lied to me. If she says that he bothered her, I believe it. There's a hundred women sayin' so. Why can't you people see the truth?"

The Story forces stepped up their campaign to bring him home. Week after week, paid ads appeared in the *Chronicle*:

IT'S NOT OVER until it's over.

WE KNOW THE REAL DOC!

Official-looking information packets were bound in clear blue plastic and sent out with an appeal: "Make checks payable to 'The Doctor Story Defense Fund' and mail to First National Bank, Lovell WY 82431." Jan Hillman added her money pitch to a newsletter, *The Real Story*. The first edition contained a folksy message from the prisoner himself:

> I wish I had scales. I think I'm in a battle with my stomach. I'm outdoors quite a bit more here. Pretty good sun tan. Working on weights a little bit. Everyone here seems to have a Bible or something religious. . . . I saw 5 antelope out in the sagebrush meadow. They ran a little then grazed back into view.

In a letter to the Lovell *Chronicle*, daughter Linda called for her father's vindication. "We should take a lesson from history," she wrote. "In 1939, the Western nations, desiring peace more than justice, sat idly by as Nazi Germany crushed Poland in less than a month and the Holocaust began. How many lives (6 million, at least) would have been saved if 'moral' nations had acted immediately on their principles of right over might—and numbers?"

Linda complained to the prison warden when her mother was chastised for using the wrong telephone during a visit. After the offending lieutenant was peremptorily transferred, word passed among the guards that the runty doctor in medium security wasn't to be taken lightly.

Letters to the judge gradually turned from wheedling to stern. Defense Committee charter member Kay Holm, identifying herself as a University of Minnesota alumna and daughter of a Lutheran pastor who'd counseled rape victims, wrote the judge that Dr. Story "is hated in a very deep and dark way because of his stand (boldly) for Christianity in a very non-Christian area. . . . I'm sure you wish with all your heart Dr. Story would admit to something, anything. Unfortunately, you picked the wrong man. Dr. Story will never admit to anything nor can he show any remorse for something he hasn't done. . . . Mr. Hartman, the disgust in my town is the very strongest for you than anyone. It was obvious from the beginning that Terry Tharp didn't have much between the ears, but there was hope for you. . . . You are a coward among cowards. . . . I cannot in good conscience refer to you as an honorable judge. You are not."

The day after the Holm letter arrived, former Lovell physician Henry R. Eskens was deposed under oath in an unrelated case in Casper. He testified that he'd practiced in Lovell for seventeen years.

Q And why did you leave there?
A The number one reason was John Story.
Q Why was that?
A . . . When I have patients coming into my office and into my living room seven days a week, crying and complaining . . . "Dr. Eskens, I felt some spurt in my vagina, and when I looked up, I saw him zip up his pants." And when I found out he examined twelve-year-old girls' tonsils with his penis, but nothing was done about it all these years. Year after year after year. I wrote to the Board of Medical Examiners. Nobody answered. "Henry, how do you dare to talk that way about your colleagues," etcetera, etcetera. This went on and on, and that was the number one reason we left Lovell, Wyoming. I just couldn't stomach that filth.

The Medical Board repeated its denial that any such charges had been recorded. "We don't lose those types of things," the executive secretary said angrily. He announced that the Board was considering libel or perjury charges against Dr. Eskens.

The Casper *Star-Tribune* took note of the squabble in an editorial cartoon suggesting a new motto for state medical officials: "Curamus Nostrum. We take care of our own."

88

Yellow Ribbons

I thought we were rid of him when he lost his license. I
thought we were rid of him when he was convicted. I
thought we were rid of him when he was sent to Rawlins.
Gol, am I stupid or what?

— Minda Brinkerhoff

THE APPEAL PROCESS promised to be expensive, and the Defense
Committee paid a $19,000 retainer to the newest addition to Story's legal
staff, Gerald Mason of Pinedale, Wyoming. In his first public statement, Mason said he'd conferred with Wayne Aarestad and assumed the
convictions would be reversed by the Wyoming Supreme Court. He
promised new evidence "of a signficant nature."

When Judge Hartman refused to release Story on bail pending appeal,
his lawyers turned to a friendlier jurist in the penitentiary town of
Rawlins. Judge Robert A. Hill admitted that he knew "very little" about
Story's background but authorized his release on $50,000 surety bond.

Within twenty minutes, the Defense Committee collected the money
from Wes Meeker's well-to-do brother Earl. Jan Hillman began cutting
up spools of yellow plastic. An ad was phoned to the Lovell *Chronicle*:
"WELCOME HOME Doc! We've missed you!" Everyone was invited
to the homecoming.

Terri Timmons read the ad and thought about buying a gun. "Story's
people'll act more ignorant than ever," she told her husband Loyd. She
ordered her children indoors. Her lymph glands swelled and a pinching
pain in her stomach signaled the start of an ulcer.

On her thirty-fourth birthday, she looked in the mirror and saw her first gray hair. Loyd perked her up with a big bouquet. She wrote in her journal, "The flowers made me feel that maybe I am of some worth to Loyd and the children. It helped so that my heart didn't hurt so bad. The flowers were daisies, two white, yellow and purple ones with an orange carnation and greens. It helped bring some peace. . . ."

On Sunday night, August 18, ten weeks after her husband had been sentenced, Marilyn Story wrote in her journal, "Arrived in Lovell late last night to a beautiful sight! Yellow ribbons—all over the yard, plus posters saying Welcome Home Doc, signed by the children—his little patients.

". . . People started arriving for an open house in the backyard which was planned and served by the Defense Committee. What a wonderful, happy, heartwarming day! Probably 200 people there. . . . O Lord God! Behold, Thou hast made the heavens and the earth by Thy great power and by Thine outstretched arms. Nothing is too difficult for Thee! Jer. 32:17 Look up!"

Two months later, she wrote, "Beautiful fall days with my beloved. Hours out in the hills and up on the mountain cutting firewood—precious times here at home, cherishing each day and hour together, knowing that one sad day it will likely come to an end."

Occasionally the idyll was interrupted by the phone. "Why don't you and your husband get out of town?" a woman's voice challenged. "Your husband has raped people behind his coat."

Callers hung up when she answered, or let the recording machine's tape run out. She was horrified by a call from two sweet-voiced little girls, one talking, one prompting in the background:

> "*Suck my come.*"
> "Suck my come."
> "*Suck my penis.*"
> "Suck my penis."
> "*And your vagina.*"
> "And your vagina. G'bye."

She and John talked more than they ever had, but seldom about the case. He explained the origin of some of the earliest rumors about him, and she repeated his explanation to a friend: "When Doc was getting started, there was a school of medicine that held that when a sick child came in, no matter what was wrong, you got 'em used to the tongue blade, the auroscope in the ear, things like that. And you gave young girls one-finger pelvic exams to get 'em used to it."

For herself, Marilyn never asked or required explanations. She knew John's problem: he was too straight, too good, too naive. He'd trusted his patients, thought more of them than he did of himself and his family. "You know, Doc's always the same man," she told Cheri Nebel on the phone. "Gentle and concerned. That's why so many of these women have crushes on him. He never flirts, but he's interested in women in a happy, teasing manner. He tells 'em they look nice, etcetera. I like that in him."

She explained to other friends that he'd set himself up for persecution by helping to found the Bible Church and being too critical of the Mormons. "He couldn't stomach that business, 'As man is, God once was. As God is, man may become.' Whenever he talked to a Mormon, he'd bring that up. He'd say, 'Hey, do you really believe that?'

"And they'd say, 'Yes.'

"And he'd ask 'em, 'Well, who do you think Jesus was?'

"They'd say, 'Jesus was just a man, like we are.' That rankled Doc. He'd ask 'em where the Book of Mormon came from, and they'd tell him how Joseph Smith sat behind a blanket up in his room and looked through his magic spectacles, etcetera, and all about the Urim and the Thummim, and how he translated the buried plates from Palmyra, reading through a blanket to three men who wrote it all down. Doc just bristled at that kind of stuff. The Mormons saw him as a threat. It took twenty-six years, but they finally got him."

Pastor Ken Buttermore saw the same evil scenario. "The Mormons were tremendously jealous of Doc as a successful businessman, parent, and husband," he explained with his robust eloquence. "There's a quote in 'Mormonism's Temple of Doom' that women are like butterflies in a jar—and men control the lid. That's why you find so many Mormon women with mental problems. They want a meaningful, rich marriage, and instead they're slaves, total bonded servants, trampled on. So they look at this doctor who treats 'em very graciously, opens car doors for his wife, a gracious, kind man, and something develops."

Buttermore felt bad that he and the Bible Church had helped to worsen things for Elder Story. "We made waves, we bucked the system. I'd co-officiate at big funerals at the LDS Church, and I'd speak right out for biblical Christianity. It didn't set well with the Mormons. They had to lash out at somebody. Doc consistently refused to convert. He was a perfect target."

The pastor also had it in for the women's movement. "Look at the women at the thrust: Kathy Karpan and Judi Cashel. Karpan wants to dominate. Cashel's overly sensual. They both show anger toward men. Doc can't fight back. He's a 1950s doctor. He doesn't understand that in the 1970s, people began to use the law to their own benefit. He didn't change with the times, and it caught up with him."

Arden McArthur had her own theories about Story's problems, but she was much too busy to join in the lengthy exegeses. She had a pair of failing businesses on her hands and a husband too weak to help.

Late on the morning of October 14, 1986, she was working on cap transfers at the dry cleaners when fifteen-year-old Marc phoned from home. "Mom," he said, "you better come! Dad's laying here in the chair and I can't tell if he's breathing or not."

Arden raced out the door. Dean had spent most of the summer in a Billings hospital. When they'd sent him home with a portable oxygen pack, he'd insisted on another long driving trip, this time to see their children in Wyoming and Utah. Arden had had a good idea what that meant.

She ran inside her house. Meg's husband, Lovell Patrolman Dan Anderson, was administering mouth-to-mouth on the floor. Arden picked up Dean's cold hand. "Danny," she said, "he's gone."

"No he's not!"

It took the ambulance thirty minutes to make the run from the hospital, and five minutes for the return. Arden and Dan followed in the police car.

When Dr. Welch came out of the operating room, his lab coat was covered with blood. He said Dean's heart had burst.

89

Appeal

WITH STORY'S APPEAL pending, the Defense Committee scrambled for exculpatory evidence. Volunteers pored over the 1,600-page trial transcript and analyzed thousands of pages of police reports and other documentation, looking for leads and contradictions. Private detectives stepped up their surveillances.

In a typical move, Lovell's Avon Lady was prevailed upon to sign an affidavit saying that on one of her sales visits, Arden McArthur had "expressed anger and frustration" about Dr. Story.

Back in Maxwell, Nebraska, the scholarly William Jerod Story began massive genealogical research on his brother's behalf. First he used the voluminous Mormon files in Salt Lake City to trace the Story family lineage to Pepin the Short, Eleanor of Aquitaine, the Viscomte d'Avranches, and an unnamed Irish king of 340 A.D. Then he searched out ancestral connections on the prosecution side. "Everyone's related to someone," he explained. "That helps us to understand why these people behaved the way they did toward my brother." He had no trouble showing interlocking family trees, but made no progress on his highest priority: "to show that the judge is related to the accusers."

Jerod soon amassed boxes full of "family group sheets" and other data. "Look here," he showed a visitor. "Five generations back, Richard

Harrison was one of fifty-two Mormon assassins who committed the Mountain Meadows massacre. They killed a column of Arkansans on orders of Brigham Young. And he's in a direct line with Emma Lu Meeks!"

His file card on Judi Cashel began, "Judith Ann Cashel, 1141 Freden Blvd., Mills, Wyo. With Casper Police 7½ years, came to Lovell 27 Sept. 84, set up office in Town Hall Building on Nevada. Used search warrants. Didn't know the word 'surreptitious.' Specialist in sexual cases. Penchant for wearing Dolly Parton wigs. Gave a lot of lectures— 'I am woman, hear me roar' . . ."

His complete file on the Casper policewoman included her marital history, the churches she'd attended, her "hangouts," closest friends, personal habits, and ancestry for six generations.

Jerod also drew up an enemies list of corporations and businesses which he believed to be antagonistic to his brother. The list included Osco Drugstores, General Mills, General Foods, Beneficial Life, and the Pizza Hut in North Platte, Nebraska.

The sheer bulk of his research material began to tax the hand-hewn cedar walls of the old family store in Maxwell, where he'd lived since 1974 after retiring as a college language instructor. His trove included every edition of the Lovell *Chronicle* back to 1940, listings of prominent Lovellites and businessmen by religion (and Mormons ward by ward), and deep biographical and genealogical studies of every personage in the case.

Searching for legal references, he accumulated thirty lawbooks to go with his 800 works in German, his 300 volumes in French, his seven volumes on the Basques, his Bibles in English, German, Hebrew, Greek and Latin, and his works in Middle High German, Old High German, Frisian, Old Frisian, Old Saxon, Gothic, Chinese, Russian, Greek and Hebrew—10,000 volumes in all, just inside the old grocery's door bearing the faded Rainbow Bread logo.

In the course of the research, Jerod dredged up unexpected nuggets. "Meg and Minda are both liars," he informed the Defense Committee after reading a paper on psychology. "They look down and to the left. Psychologists claim that is a sign of lying."

When he wasn't flexing his scholarship, Jerod worked late into the night with his eighty-six-year-old mother, getting out the latest edition of *The Real Story*. Inez functioned as label paster and folder and some-time proofreader, often working for six and eight hours at a stretch.

"Look at this!" the meticulous matriarch complained late one night. " 'Ridiculous' is misspelled three times."

The former undersheriff Rex Nebel nosed around the country on Dr. Story's behalf, but came up short on his most ambitious caper. He flew to Michigan to interview Terri Timmons' ex-fiancé and try to settle the delicate question of who dismantled Terri Timmons' virginity. But the man wouldn't budge from his claim that in three years of dating, they'd never touched below the belt.

After a few such setbacks, Rex felt waves of helplessness and frustration. "It doesn't do much for your peace of mind to know that a great and innocent man is in the penitentiary and you can't lift a finger to get him out," he explained. "It's like one of those bad dreams where you're running from something and you can't move.

"I try to forgive the accusers," he went on. "I asked the Lord on my knees, 'Lord, show me how to love 'em.' I don't want this hate inside me 'cause it keeps me awake nights. I got so mad I broke our cordless telephone, just winged it outside. I've been taking baking soda and eating Rolaids, but I still got bad guts. I never had anything affect me like this."

His wife Cheri added, "Rex feels deeply. He hates hypocrisy. I do, too. I believe there's a constant battle for the souls of men. I believe there's a realm of evil with principalities and powers and rulers of darkness that battle against true men of God, men that refuse to be involved in sexual sins, refuse to be dishonest. Doc was one of those men."

Financial contributions picked up as Defense Committee members began appearing on talk shows to recount the railroading of an innocent man of God. Soon *The Real Story* was able to inform its thousand or so readers that "Wheaton, Illinois; White Bear Lake, Minnesota; Deaver, Wyoming; Kremmling, Colorado; Rockford, Minnesota; Worland, Wyoming; North Platte, Nebraska; are just some of the places that contributions keep arriving from."

The Committee responded to every slur on Story's name. The merest mention brought a flurry of corrections, counterclaims, and threats of legal action, usually by Jan Hillman herself. Phone calls and letters went to Judge Hartman, Terrill Tharp and Paul Sironen. The *Ladies' Home Journal* drew an attack after it referred to the case in an article on doctor-rape. Patricia Wiseman of the Big Horn County Behavioral Clinic was threatened with a libel suit. Wyoming State Penitentiary officials walked on eggs.

Traps were set for the unwary. When Diana Harrison asked to meet old friend Marilyn at the Story clinic, Rex Nebel hastily installed a tape recorder in a heating vent. Marilyn's assignment was to put on a friendly face and pry out the inside story of the Mormon conspiracy.

But Marilyn proved to be a poor manipulator. "You're saying he's guilty," she said angrily, "and he isn't! And you *know* he isn't, Diana. . . . You have put an innocent man in prison."

"No, I haven't," Diana said meekly.

"Yes, you have! I'm sorry, but you have! You've hurt us more than anyone possibly could. . . . I am amazed that you are the kind of a person who knows us as well as you know us and would believe Julia Bradbury, Emma Meeks, Wanda Hammond, Arden McArthur—the whole mess of people. I can't believe that you would take a side against us."

As Diana sighed, Marilyn remembered that the tape was running and sweetened her voice. "There's something more to it, don't you think?" she said. ". . . Did someone ask you to come here today?"

"Absolutely not. You know me better than that."

"No, I don't!" Marilyn snapped. "I don't know you at all."

As though to stress John's guilt, Diana asked, "Why did they take his license?"

"I'd like to know," Marilyn answered. "There is something more to this than meets the eye."

"What?"

"I'd like to know from you . . . and I'm not the only one to think that."

Diana turned the conversation to "things that you confided in me, that I have never told anyone."

"I don't know that I confided in you," Marilyn said.

"Well, listen—things that, you know—your depression. That has to mean something—"

"Oh, no."

"—with the way he treated you."

"Oh, no! He was never more than a perfect, beautiful, wonderful husband to me. . . . Depression comes with middle age. . . . If you're trying to get something out of me about my marriage, you'll never, because it was a perfect marriage. *A perfect marriage!*"

"Okay."

"I never once suspected him. I never will in all of my life. . . . No, absolutely no! You'll never convince me. . . ."

Marilyn took a final stab at finding the smoking gun. "Does it have to do with family ties? . . . Has Arden got to you? The whole bunch?"

"No."

The meeting of the two old friends broke up after Diana asked sarcastically, "Marilyn, where did your prayers go? What happened to your prayers?"

"You don't have any idea what God has in mind for us," Marilyn snapped back. "Christians have gone through persecution and suffering for many, many years. And your fasting and prayers and your burning in the bosom and all that—I would be very careful about that. . . ."

Diana mumbled, "There's no hope. . . ."

"Did you come to twist the knife? Is that what you're doing? Well, you did, when you said there's no hope."

On the way to the door, Marilyn stressed that she felt no hate toward anyone.

Argument on the appeal was scheduled for a week before Christmas. Early that morning, two dozen demonstrators sheltered against the knifing winds in front of the State Capitol in Cheyenne. One carried a cardboard effigy of Story locked in stocks under black letters: "RAPIST JOHN STORY, convicted by a jury of his peers." Some wore buttons: "Trust Me, I'm a Doctor." A few circulated NOW petitions demanding a grand jury investigation.

Minda McArthur Brinkerhoff couldn't stop crying. "It's taken a long time," she told a reporter. Her youngest child, Shanardean, rode her shoulders in a snowsuit.

The biggest crowd in twenty-five years crowded into the Wyoming Supreme Court to hear Story's new lawyer, Gerald Mason, stress judicial errors, the "overzealous" prosecutor's "239 leading questions," Diana Harrison's claims about the sperm-stained tissue, Dr. Flory's inflammatory testimony, and the impossibility of having to defend against charges that went back seventeen years.

An assistant attorney general argued that the defense was asking the Supreme Court to retry the facts of the case. He also reminded the justices that Wyoming was one of two states without a statue of limitation. The court took the appeal under advisement.

Six months passed without a ruling. Then the court reversed Hayla Farwell's count on technical grounds. The other five were affirmed. Later the United States Supreme Court declined to review.

Arden McArthur heard the news by long-distance telephone. Her husband's death had sent her on a frantic odyssey, visiting with old friends in Texas and Utah, moving in with one or another of her children, then running off again. "I'm afraid of what I'll find if my feet touch the ground," she explained to one of her daughters.

She'd been trustful all her life, but no longer. She regretted the hardening in her outlook and fought against it. Sometimes she was able to summon up a twinge of pity for her old friend Dr. Story. Three years back, she'd come to the reluctant conclusion that he was sick, like Bob Asay, like the Rose Doctor, like so many other sad and dangerous men. She thought, This could have worked out better, but Story wouldn't let it. All we wanted was a nurse in his examining room, but he always said no. *I'm the doctor here. . . .*

She'd read somewhere that sociopaths or antisocial personalities or whatever they were called never admitted guilt and enjoyed taking risks. She'd also read that they adapted well to prison life. For her old friend's sake, she hoped it was true.

On August 4, 1986, seven weeks after the Wyoming Supreme Court ruling, Marilyn turned sadly to her journal. "Today John entered the Wyoming State Prison for the second time," she wrote. "This time he drove himself up to the gate and reported in 'returning from bail.' Susan and I said good-bye to him while a guard quietly stood by. He picked up his few personal items, slung his 'prison' boots over his shoulder and walked alongside the guard across the compound and through the doors without looking back (our last view of him). His last words to us— 'Head for [Susan's home in] Colorado and don't stop until you get there.' We obeyed."

90

Prison

PENITENTIARY OFFICIALS were quickly reminded that the new man was important. His first visitors were former Senator and Mrs. Cal Taggart. The three old friends chatted for several hours.

Taggart returned to Lovell with a confidential message for his friends on the Defense Committee: "I don't think Doc wants to get out of the pen. He's always been very naïve about the whole situation. He asks for advice and doesn't take it. He only wants you to agree with him. I feel sorry for Marilyn."

Soon Taggart received a letter from Story asking for an affidavit affirming that he'd been victimized by an unfair judge. Taggart replied that he hadn't attended the trial, "but I still think you're innocent." Privately he took the position that he'd done enough.

Inside the walls, the first blowup came after prison officials took letters addressed to "Dr. John Story," stamped them "no such person," and returned them to Lovell. A small package was sent back to Jan Hillman in damaged condition that suggested tampering. Before the long-distance phone calls and incendiary letters stopped flying back and forth, Story and Hillman had involved the warden, the Lovell postmaster and a team of U.S. postal inspectors. The prisoner put out word that he wouldn't accept mail that lacked his title. After that, all mail addressed to "Dr. John Story" or "John Story, M.D." went through untouched.

There was more friction when a prisoner staffer mentioned "Dr. Story" and was told by an annoyed guard, "There's no Dr. Story here."

"There sure is," Story piped up. "I'm him."

When another guard addressed him as "John," Story instructed him, "You call me anything you want here, but save my first name for my wife and my mother."

He took a fellow prisoner aside and said, "Pass the word to the others. You're no friend of mine unless you call me doctor, especially if there's a guard around. They think they can erase my degree. They don't understand. Nobody in the world can take it away except the University of Nebraska."

He refused to respond to a guard lieutenant who called him "John." The officer repeated his first name, and Story walked away. For weeks afterward, prison personnel went out of their way to use his first name. At night, guards would peek in on him and say, "How ya doing, *John?*"

The psychological warfare raged. Story told Marilyn, "A counselor warned me, 'You better not let anybody call you doctor or you'll end up in the hole.' I just smiled and said, 'Well, I've never been to the hole.' I kind of challenged him to put me there. I'm one of Solzhenitsyn's prisoners that don't change. In here, they know the guys that are tough enough to go to the hole and live there for months. I'm one."

He confided that prison officials were "Kennedy-type people. They would first-name the Queen of England." He insisted that there was an important issue involved. "In prison, all you need to do is say you're guilty and they'll smile at you and treat you fine. The worst thing you can do is be innocent and say so. You're a dirty dog then. Everybody frowns, the counselors are down on you. They'll never destroy me. I won't change."

He admitted that prison was an incongruous place for an innocent man, but G. Gordon Liddy had toughed it out and so could he.

Marilyn went home and wrote in her journal: "Separation—something so rare for us—so foreign and distasteful. But 'I will lie down in peace and sleep, for tho I am alone, O Lord, You will keep me safe.' "

Dutifully she added the scriptural reference, "Ps. 4:8," as she'd always been taught as a child.

Epilogue

1

The Supporters

By the blessing of the upright the city is exalted: but it is
overthrown by the mouth of the wicked.
                              —Proverbs 11:11, quoted by
                              Cheryl Nebel

FOR A LONG TIME after her hero went off to prison, florist Beverly
Moody tried to reconcile her anger with her need to earn a living. "In
my business I can't be ignorant to people," she explained. "But I'm not
gonna put my arm around Aletha Durtsche and Arden McArthur and
say, 'Hi, how are ya?' There's no 'Hi, how are ya' when an innocent
man's in prison."

She maintained that Lovell was dying because too few of its citizens
lived their beliefs. "That's why I admire Doc so much. I've told my
husband Larry over and over: there's not enough men in this world
that'll stand up for what they think is right. You could never say that
about Doc."

Shunned and boycotted by the accusers and their sympathizers, the
Moodys talked about starting over in Worland.

Pastor Kenneth Buttermore looked out on his thinning flock and announced, "Volunteers will now collect the offering." He was at a loss to
explain where the Bible Church's regular ushers were on this beautiful
Sunday morning when the air flowed down the mountain slopes like
melting ice. "Are those guys on strike today?" he asked with a mischievous
smile. "Are they striking for more money? For better sleeping conditions?"

The congregation had to laugh. Someone called out, "They're working at the sugar factory."

"Oh, yes," Buttermore replied. The sugar tramps were working around the clock these days. A white cumulus cloud hovered over the refinery at all hours, and the hum of the centrifugal separators hit the ear like the lowest note on an organ. The pastor said he would expect to see his missing ushers as soon as the campaign ended.

He led the group in song, his own jubilant voice soaring above the others. He'd always tried to maintain a joyous church, even in these difficult days when its most prestigious charter member was serving time for unspeakable crimes.

In the second year of Elder Story's incarceration, Pastor Buttermore reduced the schedule of special prayer sessions and finally halted them entirely, but his personal fidelity remained as solid as his belief in God. Had he ever wavered about Dr. Story's innocence?

"*Never*. In my wildest dreams I couldn't imagine him guilty." Nor had he given up hope that yellow ribbons would fly again in the Story front yard.

"Doc might die in the pen," he said in a moment of frankness, "but the case is not closed, because God is gonna do some marvelous things." He said he just hoped the accusers would "accept the Lord and become part of the family. Then I could hug 'em and love 'em."

Lovell's senior pastor had greater expectations for Elder Story than for his failing community. Church attendance was down all over town. "The sexual abuse and sexual sin here is staggering," Buttermore said with a glum shake of his head. "It will always be that way, till folks return to God."

Rex and Cheryl Nebel went through changes of their own, but their belief in Doc's innocence remained as constant as their pastor's.

"My letters to the editor were the only thing that saved my butt," Rex mused. His philippics also revealed a hitherto undeveloped talent for writing. He enrolled in the community college in Powell and began pulling straight A's. Some day he hoped to be able to write for a living.

He told friends that he doubted he would return to law enforcement. "I lost every cop friend I had. Good riddance! I don't want these Lovell pigs around here." He spat the word again: "*Pigs!*" "One of 'em stole the nameplate off Doc's office. One of 'em's a window peeker and a weirdo. Another's into porn. This case was right up his alley; he got to talk dirty to women."

Like the Reverend Buttermore, Rex and Cheri saw a doomsday scenario for their hometown. "These fools never learn, never change," he said. "Things just get worse. Crack cocaine is the big deal in Lovell now. I see dopers that are skin and bones. Sex and dope—that's their life. The other day a guy beat up his wife 'cause she left a party before he did. When he woke up the next morning, his right hand was Superglued around his penis and they had to take him to the hospital. I saw him the next day with his hand in a bandage. That's Lovell for ya."

Rex, Cheri and a few of Doc's other supporters liked to sit up late in the warm Nebel living room and share gleanings from the case. "She started when she was sixteen, and I can prove it" . . . "She wore a filmy nightgown in the hospital and just threw herself at Doc" . . . "What can you expect of pea-brains like Hartman and Tharp?" . . . "That guy calls himself a Christian attorney. Isn't that a contradiction in terms?"

The Mormons were highest on their verbal hit list. "There's ten church high councils scheduled in Lovell right now for polygamy," Rex confided. "What does that say about those Latter-day quote unquote Saints?"

But the former biker also found an unexpected mellowness within himself. One might he was sitting in a saloon when someone accused the Mormons of ruining Lovell's only good doctor. Another customer responded, "I'm sick and tired of the LDS being blamed for everything!"

Rex clenched his fists, then walked out. "I would have said too much," he explained to Cheryl.

He still considered himself Doc's strong right arm, but he was no longer disposed to throw folks through walls or sit up till six in the morning writing invective. Doc put him to the test by trying to involve him in a half-baked jailhouse scheme to pry a partial refund from Wayne Aarestad. Doc wanted Rex to sign an affidavit that Rex and the lawyer had been out partying on nights when Aarestad should have been preparing for trial. Doc wrote from his cell, "It could mean 32 to 42M in dollars for Marilyn instead of living off borrowed money. Do you know the extent of Aarestad's deceit? Now—the time is now or not later. *We're all accustomed to my years in the penitentiary by now.*"

"See?" Rex said when he read the letter aloud. "He's so damn sarcastic, trying to jab me."

Rex wrote that the plan was too dangerous. Doc replied, "It's come to a point where you're just gonna have to feed everything to me and let me be the judge."

Rex complained to Cheri, "See? Doc's judgment has got him into some pretty deep water. I'm not letting his judgment rule our future."

Doc pressed on. He gave Marilyn a note to be hand-delivered to Rex: "Would you please quite soon write to me a description of all things that you know as soon as possible. Could refer for security to him [Aarestad] as Alice. . . . This would be critically valuable unless I am reading you completely wrong. . . ."

Rex refused. "I've got three kids and an old lady and a future in this state," he explained. "I've got to think about that, too." He hoped his old friend and mentor wasn't trying to use him. That certainly wouldn't be like the Doc he'd known before.

Jan Hillman was the only member of the Defense Committee willing to admit that she'd ever questioned Doc's innocence. Fortunately for her peace of mind, she'd been able to resolve her doubts and continue her buzz-saw campaign to win his freedom.

"When I take a stand I'm not about to back down," she explained in her pleasant voice, "but I do try to be intelligent about it. When I first read the trial transcripts and the Medical Board hearings, I thought, Can I be that dumb? Am I being blind? But no, I'm not. I'm still convinced. Do you know what Aletha Durtsche wrote the Medical Board? 'I dearly love Dr. Story. I don't want to hurt him.' Now that woman has *not* been raped!"

Two years after the conviction, Jan was still sending out press packets, attacking the accusers, pruning and correcting the record, threatening lawsuits. She instigated a portrayal of the case on TV's "60 Minutes." After the CBS airing on March 1, 1987, letters and checks poured in. A woman in Massachusetts wrote, "I have never been so ashamed of our judicial system." A letter from Montana said, "What kind of monster is your county attorney?" A New Jersey nurse asked, "How can I help?" A Seattle man said, "Everyone at Boeing Aircraft was talking about '60 Minutes.' Almost unanimously they agreed that Dr. Story was railroaded."

Jan found herself in demand on the broadcast circuit. She swore she wouldn't rest till Doc was freed. But she refused to let the case squelch her natural sense of humor. "In the Lovell area," she quipped, "sexual harassment will not be reported. But it will be graded."

2

The Storys

Death—I used to sit here and she used to sit over there and death was as close as you are. . . . The opposite is desire.

—Tennessee Williams,
A Streetcar Named Desire

MARILYN'S CRUSHED SPIRITS were revived by "60 Minutes." In her regular Saturday phone conversation with John, he told her that he was receiving better treatment from guards who'd seen the show.

"An excellent job!" she wrote in her journal. "So many saw the truth—know John is innocent! Sue and I feel it is a miracle! . . . Many who thought Doc was guilty have changed their minds after watching those women and their lies."

She began to join Jan on radio and TV interviews, defending her husband's honor and reputation. Every morning she drove the two blocks to the clinic, hoisted the flag, then rattled around the halls keeping busy. She studied the file on the case and pointed out flaws and inconsistencies. "Meg Anderson was a schoolteacher," she commented, "and yet in her letter to the Medical Board 'penis' is spelled 'p-e-n-u-s'! Jan and I laughed so hard when we read that. It's unreal!"

Once every month Marilyn made the six-hour drive south through the Wind River Canyon and across the mountains and gulches and sagelands to the sunny town of Rawlins. There she checked into a motel and tried to get a good night's sleep so she would look fresh and rested for John in the morning. Visiting hours began at 8 A.M., and she always pulled up at the blocky guard tower on time.

The low-slung penitentiary was surrounded by sere hills, spotty clumps of sage, bare brown rocks and a few misshapen trees in a scrub-desert basin just south of Rip Griffin's Truck Stop off Interstate 95. Rabbits and ground squirrels nibbled on cheatgrass by the side of the road. The two-lane blacktop served only the prison, and a half mile from the gate a solitary sign warned:

PROPERTY OF WYOMING STATE PENITENTIARY.
YOU MUST HAVE OFFICIAL BUSINESS BEFORE ENTERING.
NO TRESPASSING.

At each sight of the chain-link fences and glittering coils of razor wire, Marilyn felt nauseated. The prison seemed like a continuing test by the Lord. It was simply unimaginable that her gentle husband was living without her in the bowels of this awful place.

Inside, John's smile would show up in a window adjacent to the visiting room as a guard patted him down. He was allowed to carry a Bible and a pen, and sometimes his hymnal. After one trip, Marilyn wearily described the scene to Cheryl Nebel: "It's such a tiring place. And so noisy—*bang! crash!*—all the clanks and screeches, kids crying and running around, people going in and out to smoke, crashing the electric doors. Sometimes it's bitter cold. We sit on plastic chairs and shiver. All around us men and women try to see how far they can go, grunting, making animal sounds. John and I sing to shut them out."

Early in 1988, the warden ordered a crackdown on overaffectionate displays, and John and Marilyn were admonished for a simple hug. "You don't shake your head at *my* wife!" John told the guard through gritted teeth. He'd always been so overprotective. He threatened to make a personal complaint to the warden.

Marilyn was surprised at the ease of his adjustment and recalled Cal Taggart's strange remark that he didn't think John really wanted his freedom. He'd enjoyed his World War II service in the Navy Seabees and claimed that prison life wasn't much different.

"It's good for me," he told her and a tearful Susan at the end of a visit. "This is the place I've got to be, the best place for me to be right now." Of course he didn't cry. No one had ever seen him cry, even as a child. He admired stoic heroism, read books about prisoners of war, and considered himself one of their number. His anger was directed at the bureaucratic apparatus that had landed him here—the lawyers, the

Medical Board, the Mormon hierarchy, all of them as united as a twisting of rattlesnakes. "Don't be too hard on the accusers," he advised Marilyn. "They're just pawns."

Except for the lunch hour, the Storys huddled together from 8 A.M. till 5 P.M. on four days of every month. As always, he was full of well-intended advice. "When you go downtown to shop," he instructed his wife, "dress up. Look your best. We're not criminals and we shouldn't carry ourselves like criminals."

Sometimes, after a visit, Marilyn drove on to Maxwell to see his mother, and John always reminded her to stop by Annette's grave in the family plot in Plainview Cemetery. Left to her own instincts, Marilyn would have avoided such painful side trips, but she obeyed her husband as always. John also urged her to visit the Fort McPherson Cemetery, scene of so many of his childhood joys and ceremonies. He was pleased when she brought back rubbings from the graves of Spotted Horse and another chief.

Visiting Maxwell, she still found herself uneasy about the Story family's attitude about death. They grieved, but in their own way. They talked animatedly about Annette and other lost children. At fourteen, John's youngest brother Tom had been killed by a swerving truck while hitchhiking to North Platte, and when the family discussed him, it was always in vivid, cheery tones—what a neat boy he'd been, his sense of humor, his imitations and jokes that had made the family laugh. You'd have thought old Tom was coming for dinner with the wife and kids.

Marilyn returned from one Nebraska trip and told a friend, "Inez's sister Lola died, and they talked and talked and *talked* about it. The day I got there, John's mom says, 'We're gonna eat, then we're gonna go up to the mortuary.' So we all pile into our cars and follow little banty hen Inez into this cold room. She says, 'Oh, doesn't Lola look *so* nice! She looks better than she did when she was teaching Latin!' And she pats Lola's hand and stands there looking at her and talking about her hair and her glasses. John's sister Gretchen and his brother Jerod came, too, and *nobody* cried. I'm standing back and kinda gulping and I just— *oooooh*, I thought I was gonna faint. It was about the only dead body I'd ever seen."

Every four months the penitentiary permitted a conjugal visit in one of the three mobile homes parked just inside the razor-wired perimeter. Marilyn's first visit was on Christmas Eve 1986, and she cried all the way down and back. Old friend Wes Meeker had loaded her car with a tree and gifts, but the guards wouldn't let them in. The parting was on Christmas morning. John tried to comfort her, but she was so upset she could hardly say good-bye.

She didn't fare much better on later overnight visits. The red tape drove her to tears. A guard would call out her personal possessions—"one nightgown, one underpants . . ."—while another checked them against a list of acceptables. She always brought John's favorite meal—meat loaf, baked potatoes and salad—and the guards removed each piece, unwrapping, sniffing, handling her creations. By the time they were finished, she wanted to dump the food in the dirt.

There was friction with the woman who presided over the conjugal area. Checking in, Marilyn insisted on writing "Dr. John Story" on the line marked "inmate's name," which invariably precipitated a brisk order: "Number and last name only!" At John's stern insistence, Marilyn refused to yield. After a few visits, the clerk began obliterating the word "Dr." with Liquid Paper.

Marilyn was happy to do her small part for her husband's dignity. But the partings never became any easier. She wrote in *The Real Story*:

> It seems like a bad dream as I walk away from there. It is especially hard to bear when they lead him away in handcuffs. . . . Our sustaining hope is that this "lifestyle" of ours will not go on much longer.

With each trip, the hope dimmed. She was living off borrowed money and handouts. The legal billings reached $200,000, wiping out their life savings after twenty-six years in medicine. The Defense Fund helped with legal fees, but the flow of contributions was down to a trickle.

After John's second full year of confinement, Marilyn still went to the clinic daily, but no longer raised the flag. "I won't fly it till he's home," she said. Nor did she put up Christmas trees or other ornaments.

One by one, friends accepted the status quo and lost a measure of their solicitude. She didn't expect them to grieve as she did. Ignoramuses gawked when she went downtown. She spent most of her time alone.

Sometimes the former cowgirl wondered what it would be like to move back to her home state of Colorado, but John kept insisting that he was going to resume his old practice. She couldn't bear to spoil his dream, even as it became less and less realistic. They'd married "till death do us part."

She still saw a heavenly hand in everything. She'd always known that God had taken Annette for some reason or other, and now the reason came clear. "Annette would have been a high school student when all this came down on us," she explained patiently. "It would have been *so* hard on her. It was hard enough for Linda and Susan, and they weren't living here anymore. I don't think Annette could have taken it. God spared her. God's in control of everything."

With her husband in his third year at Rawlins, uncharacteristic hard touches crept into Marilyn's voice and manner. When a friend mentioned that some of the accusers had switched to a doctor in Powell, she snapped, "I hope they get raped up there."

Her friends knew it was the pain talking.

One cold winter night Inez Story told her daughter-in-law, "People ask me how we're getting along, what with John in prison. I say, 'I'm a-hangin' in. We're tough, our family.' I always tell 'em, 'We're gonna win. It may take time, but we're gonna win.' Maybe the Lord'll come before then and take us Christians. It could be anytime. I'm gonna be ready. The Scriptures tell us it'll happen in the twinkling of an eye."

The spry old woman still exchanged Bible verses with her son. To her, John was the victim of a Mormon plot. "They were afraid he was some kind of guru," she explained. "They thought, If we can convert a deacon in the Bible Church, that'll give us good points in Salt Lake City. But John stood as a Christian. So they had to put him away."

William Jerod Story, retired instructor in Germanic languages, considered himself the main defender of his younger brother and every other Story through the ages—their names, honor and reputations. He batted down any hints of a bad seed and bristled at suggestions that his father's cool detachment might have had a detrimental effect on John's personality.

"Dad was preoccupied with business, not mollycoddling me or John," the oldest brother recalled sixteen years after his father's 1971 death. "He got up early, made his own breakfast, and we wouldn't see him again except for lunch and dinner. Then he'd go back and work on the books till we were all asleep. He was always in a hurry to get to the next customer. One day I heard a farmer say, 'Look at that young feller go up them stairs!' Dad was forty then.

"Of all the generations that ran our store, Dad was the most professional. It was like Thomas Mann's story of the Buddenbrooks: the third generation is best. Of course, our business is down to a few customers a day now, folks that drive miles to get something like an old-fashioned castellated screw, but that's because Maxwell is on its last legs and everybody around here shops in North Platte.

"Whatever Dad did, he studied up on it. It wasn't enough for him to sell poultry medicines; he practically had to become a veterinarian so he could advise the farmers on the right medicines. He wouldn't stock a new brand of peas till he'd made a study of it. He was the most thorough man I ever knew. You might say John got that from him, but not much else. Dad was neat and John's sloppy. In most ways, John's like our mother. They're still so close they finish each other's sentences." He paused and smiled. "But then she does that with nearly everybody."

One day the diminutive Jerod was photocopying a newspaper story about his brother's case in the University of Wyoming library when a retired state supreme court justice looked over his shoulder and said, "They should be a lot harder on those fellas."

"Some of them are unjustly accused," Jerod snapped back. "Dr. Story's not guilty of any crime."

The old judge looked surprised as Jerod continued, "Those wicked Mormon women told lies. They're guilty of slander."

Relating the story later, Jerod said, "I kinda felt as though we were about to get into a bout of fisticuffs, you know? I was pretty close to him, looking at his ugly nose. He says, 'Oh, well, that's a different point of view.'

"I said, 'That's a *true* point of view.' "

3

The Prisoner

It is also characteristic for the real psychopath to resent punishment and protest indignantly against all efforts to curtail his activities. . . . He is much less willing than the ordinary person to accept such penalties.
—Hervey Cleckley, M.D.,
The Mask of Sanity

AT FIRST John Story rebelled at a counselor's advice to "get off your ass and make something of yourself in here," but later he became law librarian in the penitentiary's medium-security unit so he could research his way to freedom. Once in a while he pecked out a contribution to *The Real Story* (e.g., "We have the power and capacity to correct this terrible injustice") on a Smith-Corona memory typewriter donated by his backers. He made a few jailhouse friends, gave advice, even counseled some of his fellows as he'd counseled his patients back in Lovell. He carried himself more like a guest than a prisoner. Unlike the others, he wore no number on the shirt that stretched tightly across his expanding physique. His weight climbed to 146.

He seemed put out that prison officials didn't utilize his medical abilities. "It's an old tradition in American prisons," he observed. "Dr. Mudd practiced. There's a lot to be done." But he had no intention of volunteering. "I wouldn't work without pay. Not after what the state's done to me."

He talked softly except on the subject of pet hates like the Mormon church or "liberals," a word he used as a pejorative long before the Bush Republicans. As he spoke, he rubbed his neck, fiddled with his collar or his hair, tapped a pen or rolled it in his fingers, shifted positions and tugged his trousers over his knees. His voice was flat, unstressed, his delivery devoid of spark or metaphor. He dropped his terminal g's and chirped dry little laughs at the absurdity of the charges against him.

"As a child I loved the outdoors and people," he told an inquiring visitor, dismissing his childhood with a wave of his small hand. He confirmed that he'd been the first "Christian" in his family and that his mother, brother and sister had followed his example. "My dad didn't go to church," he added.

Did he recall tagging behind Jerod when they were boys? "No," he said, adjusting silver-rimmed trifocals. "I don't remember things like that." In the same breath, he added, "Basically I'm the most private person anybody's ever known. I don't even want my name in the paper for good things. Once I was quoted as saying that prison life reminded me of the army. But I was actually in the Navy. I said 'Army' instead of 'Navy' to throw people away from the truth about me. It depersonalizes me. I do that a lot."

He said he saw no point in discussing the influences that steered him toward medicine. "That's more of that man-worship," he said disdainfully. His mother had named him after a physician and he'd admired his namesake, but "I don't have anyone to thank for becoming a doctor except myself and God." He made it clear that humanism was the greatest vice and love of God the greatest virtue. In that context, he noted, there could be only one true hero.

After a silence, he offered a seeming non sequitur: "Do you have any idea what causes sexual perversion?" He shifted position on the straightbacked wooden chair. "Refusal to believe in God. It's in Romans, first chapter. People who refuse God and deny Him are at risk of becoming perverted. It's epidemic now."

He rattled off a bill of particulars against his accusers. One had been "a slut all her life." Another had sneaked off to Billings with a journalist during the trial. One attended orgies. One was a pornographer. One smoked weed. One had been seen in Rock Springs with a woman. One of the husbands had been involved in bestiality. One of the older accusers had fornicated with her male classmates in high school. Hardly anyone on the other side was spared his soft invective.

When Story was told that Rex Nebel had spat on the bench after the verdict came in, he produced a rare grin and said, "Good for him. Good for him!"

His enemies list seemed to include half the citizens of Lovell, but he insisted that those evildoers paled into insignificance next to the most satanic force of all. "The state certifies that Doc Story is a liar and a rapist," he said as he drummed on his notebook. "And people believe the state. But there's nothing believable or trustworthy about it. If this experience has given me a mission, it's to pull the plug on the state."

His first parole hearing was scheduled for 1991, "but the state gets $17,000 per year per inmate from the federal government, so I'm not expecting to get out on my first attempt. Maybe the second, or more likely the third. If they make me do my bottom number of fifteen years, I'll have no life left. I'll get out just in time for the nursing home."

He was firm about resuming his practice in Lovell. "Where is there to go but a place where people know me and I have good friends and where Marilyn and I have love?" he asked as he stretched his pant legs over his kneecaps. "I figure I have maybe four hundred enemies in Lovell, but at least that many friends. No, I wouldn't allow any of my family to be buried there. Eventually we'll all go home to Maxwell.

"I'd like to be around my mother for a year or two before she dies. And I'd like to be with Marilyn for the rest of her life. She's the only hold the prison has on me—the way they treat her."

He beckoned toward the warden's office. "If she should suddenly die, these state and prison people couldn't do a thing to me. I wouldn't give in on *any*thing." His brown eyes narrowed and his pen drummed faster. "I could live in the hole forever."

4

The Accusers

ALONE of the women involved in the case, Aletha Durtsche felt improved by her ordeal. "Somebody said, 'I bet you just hate Story so badly.' I said, 'I don't have any feelings about him. The way he is—that's his problem. I'm too busy with my own life. And it's better than ever.' "

She mourned her Uncle LaMar Averett. The old farmer-chief had said that if Story were convicted he'd be the first to apologize to her, but they never spoke again. After he died, one of his relatives claimed that Dr. Story could have kept him alive and therefore the accusers were all murderers. Aletha found such thinking too convoluted to be taken seriously.

Most of the time she concentrated on better memories. "My LDS visiting teacher was in her eighties, a strong Story supporter, and after the trial she didn't want to come into my house," the letter carrier recalled. "She'd hand me a little card and say, 'I know you're busy, so I won't give you the lesson today. Have you read it?'

"I'd say, 'I'm *not* busy. I'm off work, ya know? Come on in!'

"She'd say, 'No, no, you're busy.' Then she'd run out to her husband's car.

"A year or so after Story was put away, she came to me and said she'd talked to Dr. Croft in Utah. He was old and nearly blind, but he told her, 'I knew years ago what Story was up to. He's right where he belongs.'

"She knew that Dr. Tom wouldn't lie. She said she was ashamed of the way she'd treated me. A few things like that have helped make me feel better about Uncle LaMar."

Emma Lu Meeks was shunned and insulted on the street, but she just grinned and called out "Hi!" as she'd done for years. She was proud that she hadn't shed a tear over that man—not when he'd abused her and certainly not later—but she did wish the nightmares would stop. She kept seeing him behind the drape, moving in and out of her body, smiling his dirty little smile. The dream made her feel ashamed all over again.

At eighty, she was glad she would never have to explain or apologize to her husband. Ted was waiting in the Celestial Kingdom, where all things were known. She said she doubted that the subject would come up.

Her friend and fellow victim, the widow Julia Bradbury, never discussed the case, and Emma Lu didn't press her. There wasn't much to be said, anyway. The two old friends knew the truth and the whole truth.

Whenever Annella St. Thomas mentioned Story, her small voice took on a halting stammer, as though she were short of breath. Fifteen tainted years had passed since she and her husband had made their first official complaints to Police Chief Averett and then to the Medical Board.

"I just feel lucky that Nelson stuck with me," she said. "Other husbands have disbelieved their wives. Some got divorced. Nelson, he's my strength. I'm sure glad he didn't use his double-barrel that night."

Hayla Fink Farwell hired on as a baker at the Big Horn Restaurant, grew a few petunias and roses at her old farmhouse out on the Emblem road, and tried not to feel too lonely when the coyotes howled or the diesel horns blared up from the tracks running south to Casper.

She didn't return to the Lutheran church for a long time and neither did fifteen or twenty other members of the big Fink clan. "I missed church real bad," she recalled. "I went into town for counseling one night and when I got home my husband had left me for another woman.

I needed the Lord more than ever. I have such peace in church. It was awful hard, not going."

After the departure of Story's backer, the Reverend Sam Christensen, Hayla slipped into a rear pew and was so overcome with emotion that she barely heard the new preacher's sermon. The first time she took Communion, "I kneeled up there and bawled." A few of her fellow worshipers slid away, and no one apologized for backing her rapist, but she drew her comfort from the cross.

Emma Briseno McNeil, the only Roman Catholic complainant, returned to Maine and wasn't heard from in Lovell again.

Terri Timmons couldn't seem to shake her powerful anger at males. Soon after Story was handcuffed and taken to Rawlins, she told her husband Loyd, "If they would leave it up to me, sex crimes wouldn't be a problem. They'd just take a gun and go up and down the line shooting those guys. That's how a lot of Indian tribes and Orientals rid themselves of diseases. Why was somebody like Ted Bundy on Death Row for ten years? *Why?*"

She was proud that she'd stopped being a doormat, and she even talked back to her father and Loyd. One night her father said that he didn't want to hear another word about Story, and Terri put her hands on her hips and said, "Well, Dad, that's just too dang bad about you! I've lived with this for seventeen years, and I'll talk about it whenever I please."

She didn't understand the process, but somehow a therapeutic dream seemed to guide her back to the path of forgiveness and love, even toward the opposite sex. It opened as a nightmare. "Story was shopping at the fabric store in Powell and I was in the back where he couldn't see me. I shook and started to faint, but then I found a gun in my hand and I walked out and said, 'Okay, you little son of a bitch, strip!' I made him walk down Main Street naked. I yelled, 'Now everybody's gonna see what they think they've been missing!' A cop took me away, and I laughed and said, 'This has been worth it!'

"That dream helped. I needed to have that power over him, to control and humiliate. I began to feel better. My lymph gland stopped swelling, the headaches went away. But . . . I've still got my ulcer."

She took a part-time job cleaning the home of a Jewish couple who taught at the community college. "They are such neat people," she wrote in her journal. "I put a Book of Mormon under their tree at Christmas time. I have hoped and prayed they would use it."

Terri still believed that all truth was lodged in the four "sticks" of her religion: the Book of Mormon, the Bible, *The Pearl of Great Price,* and the *Doctrine and Covenants.* In the hours just before dawn, the Holy Spirit sometimes visited her in her room. She took note of the phenomenon in her journal:

> *The first time was last summer when Loyd's sister Diane was here. The Lord told me to help get Casey a blessing and he would be able to see. Satan really interferred. The second time was not too long ago, and he spoke two words to me*—food storage. *Then it happened just the other day, and he said one word*— Contrite. *I had to look it up in the dictionary. It means repentant. These experiences have really helped me.*

Instead of doubting her qualifications, she began to relish her responsibilities in the Relief Society. "I have such a strong desire to tell others who don't know the truth all about why we live on Earth, where we came from, what we are to do while we are here and where we will go when we leave here," she wrote. "Sometimes I feel like I want to stand on the roof and shout, 'Listen, people, the truth about life is on the earth again. Won't you please listen to the gospel?' "

Wanda Hammond couldn't shake her melancholia. There was always some new torment, some reminder. In 1987 she received a Christmas card bearing a picture of the Christ child and a hand-printed message: "Even tho a person is beautiful on the outside, that doesn't mean anything, cuz they're ugly on the inside. I hope you have a nice Christmas realizing that Doc is in prison because of the lies you told on the witness stand."

It made Wanda cry, but so did soap operas and phone calls from her children and almost anything else these days. At the Rose City Food Farm, owner Tom Cornwall finally had to let her go; he told her she could make the doughnut run to Powell each day, but she felt he was just being kind and refused his offer. Not long afterward, the market went under. Along with everyone else in town, Wanda now had to shop at the Big Horn IGA. It made her uncomfortable to patronize a merchant who treated her like a pariah but sent food baskets up the hill to Mrs. Story.

No one would ever convince her that she hadn't committed the sin of adultery. Counselors at the Behavioral Clinic stressed her innocence and Story's guilt, but to her it was just chatter. Another man's organ had soiled her. To Wanda, it was a wrong that could never be righted.

Diana Harrison received a Christmas card like Wanda's, but with an extra line of printing across the face: "To the ugliest woman in Lovell."

The former receptionist swore she would always love "Doctor," but she'd also begun to face certain realities. "I can see how he spent years manipulating me. He treated me like somebody special, lent me money to buy a car, told me how smart and pretty I was. It's all so obvious now. He knew that if he ever got in trouble, he'd need some LDS women to speak up for him. That's where Arden and I came in. We were his chief fools.

"He hated us Mormons from the beginning. When he dies, they ought to put on his tombstone, 'John Huntington Story. Loved God, hated people.' "

Ironically, Diana and her husband lost their chance at the Celestial Kingdom and the other divine rewards of their lifelong faith. In 1988 they were excommunicated for polygamy.

Terrill Tharp won easy reelection to the job that was all he'd ever asked of life. Sometimes it seemed he spent part of every day trying to answer the same question: What took the rape doctor's victims so long to stand up and be counted?

"Folks in these parts," he would explain, "are uncomfortable with change. They figure they can handle their own problems themselves. That's because they had no other choice back when the next ranch was twenty miles up a dirt road. A situation like that creates a feeling of insularity. 'What I do is my business, and I can handle it myself.' They'd rather be victimized than yell for help. They think it's a mark of weakness to run to cops or lawyers or social agencies. And Mormons are brought up to take their problems to the bishops, just like they did back in Joseph Smith's day. If the bishops don't do anything, that's the end of it.

"There's also the universal human reluctance to challenge authority figures. 'Who's gonna believe *me*?' Each victim was her own little island, and nobody knew there were other victims till Arden McArthur started keeping score. People have a misimpression about small towns.

They think that everybody knows everybody's business. That's only superficially true. They only know what they can see. They don't always see the deeper things."

The prosecutor heard from Story and his backers more frequently than he wished. "I get letters on his office stationery: 'John H. Story, M.D.' He's threatened to sue me and turn me in to the bar association. He's losing some of that smirky cool exterior now. He's mad as hell. Isn't that your typical rapist?"

Police Chief David Wilcock resigned, returned briefly to help clear a murder case, then took a security job west of the Cascade Mountains near Seattle, where his FM radio brought in classical music on two stations. He bought a bike and pedaled off a hundred pounds.

Despite her speeding ticket, Judi Cashel was promoted to lieutenant and placed in command of the Casper P.D.'s traffic division. She also taught sex crime investigation at the Wyoming Law Enforcement Academy.

The red-haired cop maintained her attitude of compassionate understanding, even toward the most rabid of Story's backers. "For all the hateful things they did," she reflected, "they thought they were protecting a wonderful, innocent man. He was an important figure to them, fatherly, almost saintly. He made them into victims, too."

Meg and Dan Anderson decided to tough it out in Lovell, their childhood "paradise on earth," and never wavered despite one test after another. Like so many other stores on Main Street, both Kids Are Special and the family's dry cleaners went under, and Meg stayed home with her husband and their four children.

The sisters' $3-million civil suit was settled for $3,000, barely enough to cover costs. Meg explained, "Our lawyers couldn't find Story's money. And with no money, there was no suit. So we had to settle."

One day Bob Asay knocked on the front door of the Andersons' small frame bungalow at 152 E. Eighth and asked if Meg intended to testify against him in his wife's threatened divorce action. Both Meg and Dan strongly recommended that the Asays settle any differences out of court. "I don't think you'd like what I might say under oath," Meg warned.

She stopped wearing makeup, and when she went downtown she wore loose, floppy clothes. She said she felt safer that way. Her commitment to her church remained absolute. She never missed a service or a meeting, and sometimes drove her children to the temple in Idaho Falls to perform the ordinance of baptism for the dead. "We do it for everybody that's ever lived," she explained. "If John Story dies tomorrow, his ordinance work will be done to get him into the Celestial Kingdom." She hesitated, then added, "But not by me."

After six years on the Lovell P.D., her husband Dan nursed hopes of making chief, but when he was passed over for the job, he redoubled his efforts toward a degree in psychology. In the first few months after the sentencing, Story supporters filed one petty complaint after another against him. Jan Hillman claimed that he'd been abusive to her customers while on a call to her bar. Her mother LaVera questioned his use of city-purchased fuel. Dan knew what was eating them, and he tried to forgive.

There was more than enough real crime to occupy him and the other Lovell policemen. Crack demoralized the little town and ruined lives. A "black Ninja" took to prowling at night in his pajamas. Dan had reason to believe that child abuse and incest were worse than ever, but sex offenses were still almost impossible to prosecute. The Story case, he knew, had been the rarest of exceptions.

Minda and Scott Brinkerhoff returned to Lovell, but not before a stern lecture to their two boys and two girls. "Lovell's a nice place to live," Minda said at her usual rapid pace, "but that doesn't mean it's completely safe. There are certain people you are to *absolutely* stay away from." She read off a short list. Number one was Bob Asay.

As always, she took on several jobs, including midnight-to-eight stints clerking at the new motel across Main Street from her house. In a Christmas newsletter, she told old friends:

My father used to say that work never killed anyone. I do not fully agree with that statement. My father was a work-aholic and we know where he is. But he was very happy working like he did. He felt good about Dean, and that is what work can do for all of us.

For the middle child, labor took her mind off the Story case and the childhood sexual abuse and the physical problems that seemed to be worsening as she approached thirty. Scott worked just as hard on an out-of-town computing job and flew home when he could. The Brinkerhoffs intended to buy a farm and bring up their children among cows and hogs and beets. It was not only their plan, Minda explained, but God's.

"We are not sure what the future brings to our little family," she wrote in her newsletter, "but we do know that we are loved. My Father in Heaven loves us dearly and is watching over us always."

5

Arden McArthur

That is the land of lost content,
I see it shining plain,
The happy highways where I went
And cannot come again.
                    —A. E. Housman

AFTER two years of fleeing from her memories, Arden settled in with friends in the LDS town of Orem, Utah, long enough to fall in love for the second time in her fifty-three years. Blaine Brailsford was a retired steelworker, a widower and devout Mormon, tall and slim, white-haired, gentle of voice and manner. He courted her in the old-fashioned way, with flowers and moonlit walks and long conversations on the sofa.

"But gol, Mom," Minda said when she heard their plans by telephone, "you and Dad were sealed in the temple. What's gonna happen, uh . . . later?"

Arden told her not to bother her head. "Blaine and I'll only be marrying for time," she told her daughter. "Not for time and all eternity."

Just before the wedding, Arden listened as Meg described a disturbing dream: "We were all sitting in our front room—me and Minda and the kids and grandkids, and you and Blaine side by side. Dad walked in with that big smile of his and took your hand. 'C'mon, girlie,' he said. 'Let's go.' You and Dad walked away together, and the rest of us just sat there laughing."

"Meggie," Arden said, "that's just the way it'll be. I'll get up and go with your dad, and Blaine'll pick up his wife, and we'll each go on our journeys."

After the wedding, "Papa Blaine" and Arden visited Lovell occasionally, but she preferred that her children drive to Orem to visit her. "I love the folks in Lovell," she explained. "I walk downtown and see so many friends. But sooner or later there's a sour note. One day I dropped into the IGA, flitting from person to person, having a good time vizting, and the mayor's wife sees me and runs for the other aisle. It made me feel too bad."

On one of her trips back home, she was consulted by Uncle Bob Asay, now sixtyish and worried that his wife might try to gain custody of their little daughter. He wanted a preview of what Arden would say if she were called to testify against him. "Why, I'd tell the truth, Bob," Arden said. "What would you expect?"

As she looked at her old family friend, she still considered him more sick than evil. She might have been able to forgive him if he'd ever 'fessed up and sought treatment. But he never had, as far as she knew. And now he had the nerve to sit across from her and claim that he'd always loved her daughters.

"Don't give me that, Bob," Arden said. "You didn't love 'em."

He finally admitted what he'd done. "Oh, Ard," he said tearfully, "how do I make amends?"

"Bob, you know the process of repentance."

He looked down. "It's so . . . humiliating."

Arden said, "We have to be humiliated before we can be humbled."

When he left, she told Minda, "I'm afraid Bob hasn't learned a thing about truth. All he's ever wanted was immediate gratification. The Holy Ghost isn't with him in any way. He can't progress." His continuing prominence as a Mormon was another reason she tried to stay away from Lovell.

It also demoralized her to look across the highway from Minda's house and see the Super 8 Motel and the Big Horn Restaurant and a truck-parking lot, all carved from lost McArthur farmland. "Your dad helped grub that ground out," she reminded her children.

Nothing was harder on her than a stroll down Main Street. So many landmarks were now empty shells: the Busy Corner Pharmacy, Montgomery Ward's, the Rose City Food Farm, gas stations, the women's shop, the car wash, six or eight small shops. The fine old Horseshoe Bend Motel barely bothered to keep up appearances; its sign read BEST

ROO S IN TO N. The Beverly Motel, once a family hospital owned by the brothers-in-law Horsley and Croft, had been up for sale for months. The handsome proprietress, Eloise Benson, had become disenchanted with Lovell after Dr. Story made unseemly remarks about her breasts and twice approached her in public to suggest that she come in for an exam.

Arden always hurried across the street when she came to the Hyart Theater, so she wouldn't have to read the yellowing signs in the window next door—"Kids Are Special. Childrens to adults T-shirts transfers. Fashion finish. Food for fabrics." Story's backers had hauled their dry cleaning thirty miles south to Greybull or twenty miles west to Powell rather than patronize the McArthurs. Arden still owned the business, but the $100,000 investment was as valueless on the open market as a played-out drift of bentonite.

"Lovell's gone," said the handsome woman sadly. "The new hospital's full of empty beds. The rescue helicopters land someplace else. Folks just won't go to a place like that. Why, they've still got staff people up there that call us all liars!

"That's what's finishing Lovell off—the gutter stuff, the name-calling, the nastiness. It stifles spirituality. What's life without spirituality? The unjust and the just get caught up together. I got a call from my son Mel in Venezuela the other day. He said, 'You know, Mother, all us missionaries can feel what some of the Saints are doing back in Lovell— and they're not doing right.' "

Arden had always tried to avoid simplistic devil theories, but she couldn't help drawing certain conclusions about the men Dr. Henry Eskens had tagged "those dirty little doctors from Lovell."

"What I resent about Dr. Story," she explained, "is that he manipulated the whole town, every danged one of us. But he didn't set the tone—our 'Rose Doctor' did that. Bill Horsley was angry when he was put out of the hospital for perversion. He sure got his revenge. He put his curse on the whole community.

"Story knew what was going on behind the rosebushes when he first came here—everybody knew. Lovell must've looked like the perfect place to him. So one sick doctor begat another. The two of 'em sure changed a nice little town."

Whenever she walked west on Main from the old family house where Minda now lived, Arden passed a small park festooned with roses under tall pines. The Lovell Women's club had installed a plaque in 1970, the year before Horsley died. The message read:

The beauty of these gardens is our enduring tribute to Dr. W. W. Horsley, the Rose Doctor, whose enthusiasm, dedication and service to our community made Lovell The Rose Town of Wyoming.

THE END

Author's Note

"*Doc*" is a true story, based on trial testimony, police reports, public documents, tape recordings, and the cross-checked memories of the people most intimately involved. It is neither a fictionalization, in which scenes are re-created from the author's imagination, nor a so-called "nonfiction novel," in which (to judge by various examples of the genre) time sequences are juggled and facts are altered to achieve a novelistic effect.

Nearly one hundred people were interviewed, many of them for days (and nights) on end. No author ever received more enthusiastic cooperation on both sides of an issue, or met advocates who were more honestly convinced of the righteousness of their position. On my first field trip to Lovell, eight of the rape victims assembled in a homey old parlor to grill me about my attitude and intentions. Over the next two years, these and other victims responded to the most personal questions with candor, sensitivity and insight. Through psychotherapy, they had cast off childhood mind-sets and reached the clear realization that the crime of rape casts neither guilt nor shame on its victims.

Unfortunately, not everyone in the Cowboy State (or elsewhere) has attained the same level of enlightened awareness. Because the subject of sexual abuse remains sensitive and misunderstood, I arbitrarily assigned pseudonyms to certain characters to spare them harassment or embarrassment. They include Margaret Anselm, Carol Beach, Julia Bradbury, Bettina Diaz, Mae Fischer, Juana Garcia, Rhea Jaffe, Alma Kent, Susan Moldowney, Irene Park, Dottie Parry and Molly Pratt.

I acknowledge an abiding indebtedness to Wayne Aarestad, Meg and Dan Anderson, Eloise and Dave Benson, Dr. Russell Blomdahl, Arden McArthur Brailsford, Dorothy and Gerald Brinkerhoff, Minda Brinkerhoff, Val Brinkerhoff, the Reverend Kenneth Buttermore, Judi Cashel, Charlotte Crispin, Aletha Durtsche, Hayla Farwell, Marie Fink, Wanda Hammond, Diana and Bill Harrison, Jan Hillman, Ronald Lewis, Pamela Mayer, Emma Lu Meeks, Beverly and Larry Moody, Rex and Cheryl Nebel, Annella and Nelson St. Thomas, Duane Shillinger, Inez Story, Dr. John Story, Marilyn Story, William Jerod Story, Cal Taggart, Terrill Tharp, Loyd and Terri Timmons, Catherine Warren, Ina Welling, Judy and David Wilcock, and other interviewees who asked to remain nameless.

And a special thanks to Tom Hill of Sacramento, California, a psychologist and criminal justice consultant, who alerted me to the goings-on in Wyoming and provided invaluable guidance along the way.

Jack Olsen
Bainbridge Island, Washington
February 20, 1989

JACK OLSEN is the author of twenty-four books published in eleven countries and nine languages, including the highly acclaimed *Give a Boy a Gun* and the bestselling *"Son."* A former bureau chief for *Time*, Mr. Olsen has won the National Headliners Award, citations for excellence from Indiana and Columbia universities, and the Special Edgar Award of the Mystery Writers of America. The *Detroit Free Press* has called him "the master" of true crime. He lives on Bainbridge Island, Washington.

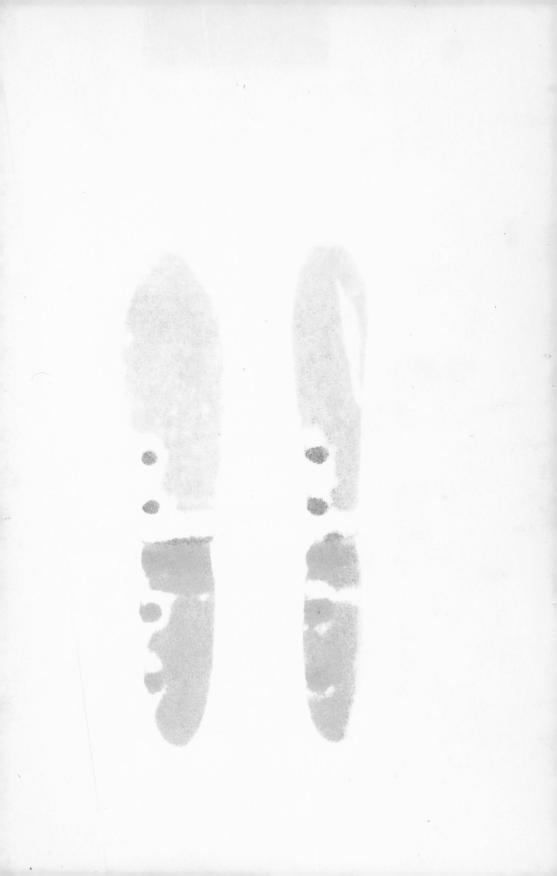

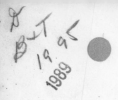

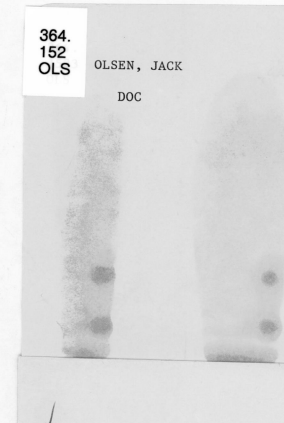